CASE REVIEW
Obstetric and Gynecologic Ultrasound

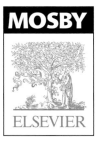

ELSEVIER

Karen L. Reuter, MD, FACR
Professor of Radiology,
Tufts University School of Medicine
Radiologist, Lahey Clinic Medical Center
Burlington, Massachusetts

T. Kemi Babagbemi, MD
Instructor, Harvard Medical School
Radiologist, Brigham & Women's Hospital
Boston, Massachusetts

CASE REVIEW

Obstetric and Gynecologic Ultrasound

SECOND EDITION

CASE REVIEW SERIES

1600 John F. Kennedy Blvd.
Suite 1800
Philadelphia, PA 19103-2899

OBSTETRIC AND GYNECOLOGIC ULTRASOUND   ISBN-13: 978-0-323-03976-5
Copyright © 2007, 2001 by Mosby, Inc., an affiliate of Elsevier Inc.   ISBN-10: 0-323-03976-6

NOTICE

Knowledge and best practice in this field are constantly changing. As new research and experience broaden our knowledge, changes in practice, treatment and drug therapy may become necessary or appropriate. Readers are advised to check the most current information provided (i) on procedures featured or (ii) by the manufacturer of each product to be administered, to verify the recommended dose or formula, the method and duration of administration, and contraindications. It is the responsibility of the practitioner, relying on their own experience and knowledge of the patient, to make diagnoses, to determine dosages and the best treatment for each individual patient, and to take all appropriate safety precautions. To the fullest extent of the law, neither the Publisher nor the Editors assume any liability for any injury and/or damage to persons or property arising out or related to any use of the material contained in this book.

Library of Congress Cataloging-in-Publication Data

Reuter, Karen L.
  Obstetric and gynecologic ultrasound / Karen L. Reuter, T. Kemi Babagbemi.—2nd ed.
    p. cm -- (Case review series)
  Rev. ed. of: Obstetric and gynecologic ultrasound / Pamela T. Johnson, Alfred B. Kurtz. c2001.
  Includes bibliographical references and index.
  ISBN-13: 978-0-323-03976-5   ISBN 10: 0-323-03976-6
  1. Generative organs, Female—Ultrasonic imaging. 2. Fetus—Diseases—Diagnosis. I. Babagbemi, T. Kemi. II. Johnson, Pamela T. (Pamela Teecc) Obstetric and gynecologic ultrasound. III. Title. IV. Series.
  RG107.5.U4J647 2007
  618'.047543—dc22

                                                              2006044958

ISBN-13: 978-0-323-03976-5
ISBN 10: 0-323-03976-6

Acquisitions Editor: Meghan McAteer
Developmental Editor: Ryan Creed
Project Manager: Bryan Hayward

Working together to grow
libraries in developing countries

www.elsevier.com | www.bookaid.org | www.sabre.org

ELSEVIER   BOOK AID International   Sabre Foundation

Printed in China

Last digit is the print number: 9   8   7   6   5   4   3

To the radiology residents and all those who
participate in the obstetrical and gynecological
care of women

I have been very gratified by the popularity and positive feedback that the authors of the Case Review Series have received upon the publication of the first editions of their volumes. Reviews in journals and word of mouth have been uniformly favorable. The authors have done an outstanding job in filling the niche of an affordable, easy-reading, case-based learning tool that supplements the material in THE REQUISITES series.

It was recognized that while some students learn best in a noninteractive study-book mode, others needed the anxiety or excitement of being quizzed, i.e., being put on the hot seat. The format that was selected for the Case Review Series—showing a limited number of images needed to construct a differential diagnosis and asking a few clinical and imaging questions—was designed to simulate the Boards experience (The only difference is that the Case Review books give you the correct answer and immediate feedback.) Cases are scaled from relatively easy to very hard to test the limit of the reader's knowledge. In addition, a brief authors' commentary, a link back to THE REQUISITES volume, and an up-to-date reference in the literature are provided.

Because of the success of the series, we have begun to roll out the second editions of the volumes. The expectation is that the second editions will bring the material to the state-of-the-art, introduce new modalities and new techniques, and provide new and even more graphic examples of pathology.

Drs. Reuter and Babagbemi have taken on the task of refreshing the *Obstetric and Gynecologic Ultrasound Case Review*, previously authored by Drs. Johnson and Kurtz. They have breathed new life into the edition and have used new cases that teach the fundamental principles of this high risk area of the body. Radiologists are on the hot seat when it comes to OB ultrasound and our tools have really progressed to the point of acquiring such fine anatomy that we may even be able to tell the color of a fetus' eyes in the not too distant future (just joking!). I commend them for their attention to detail and hard work.

I welcome the *Obstetric and Gynecologic Ultrasound Case Review* by Drs. Reuter and Babagbemi to the second edition series, which includes *Genitourinary Imaging* second edition by Drs. Zagoria, Mayo-Smith, and Fielding and *Head and Neck Imaging* second edition by David M. Yousem and Ana Carolina B. S. da Motta.

First edition volumes include *Cardiac Imaging Case Review* by Gautham Reddy and Robert Steiner; *Breast Imaging Case Review* by Emily Conant and Peggy Brennecke; *Vascular and Interventional Imaging Case Review* by Suresh Vedantham and Jennifer Gould; *Pediatric Imaging Case Review* by Rob Ward and Hans Blickman; *Nuclear Medicine Case Review* by Harvey A. Zeissman and Patrice Rehm; *General and Vascular Ultrasound Case Review* by William D. Middleton; *Musculoskeletal Case Review* by Joseph Yu; *Obstetric and Gynecologic Ultrasound Case Review* by Pamela Johnson and Al Kurtz; *Spine Imaging* by Brian Bowen; *Thoracic Imaging* by Phil Boiselle and Theresa McLoud; *Genitourinary Imaging* by Ron Zagoria, William Mayo-Smith, and Glenn Tung; *Gastrointestinal Imaging* by Peter Feczko and Robert Halpert; *Brain Imaging* by Laurie Loevner; and *Head and Neck Imaging* by David M. Yousem.

David M. Yousem, MD, MBA

This updated case review series focuses on ultrasound in obstetrics and gynecology, with a few pertinent comparisons drawing on the role of 3D ultrasound, body computed tomography and magnetic resonance imaging.

Our goals in making this case review more current were twofold. The first was to replace images whenever possible with higher resolution ones from more recently available equipment. We generally did not change the case material selected or the specific teaching points emphasized by the original authors, Drs. Johnson and Kurtz. Test questions related to the cases were modified as necessary. The second goal was to update the literature and cross-references to the new edition of THE REQUISITES on ultrasound.

Karen L. Reuter, MD, FACR
T. Kemi Babagbemi, MD

We thank all of those who contributed or assisted in obtaining cases, beginning of course with profound thanks to Drs. Pamela T. Johnson and Alfred B. Kurtz who wrote the original *Obstetric and Gynecologic Ultrasound: Case Review.* Much appreciation to Dr. Carol Benson and Dr. Sara Durfee who provided many of the obstetrical images and to Dr. Beryl Benacerraf, Dr. Mary Frates, Dr. Faye Laing, Dr. Don DiSalvo, Dr. George Bega, Dr. Beverly Coleman, Mr. Dennis Woods, Dr. Alda Cossi, and Dr. Cheryl Sadow, who contributed additional select images. Much gratitude also goes to the Brigham and Women's Hospital sonographers, specifically Linda Marquette, Jaclyn Sangco, Kris Ann Botka, Allison Forest, Denie Bernier, Regina Viner, Youssef Mina, Julie Mombourquette, Cherise Petersen, and Christine McDonald (Siemens) for their invaluable effort in acquiring top quality images.

— *K. L. R.*
— *T. K. B.*

A special thank you to my husband, Dr. John Krolikowski, for his loving encouragement and much appreciated technical expertise.　　　　— *K. L. R.*

A special thank you to Sal and Leo for their support, patience, and above all, love.　　　　— *T. K. B.*

Opening Round   1

Fair Game   117

Challenge   209

Index of Cases   261

Index of Terms   263

Opening Round

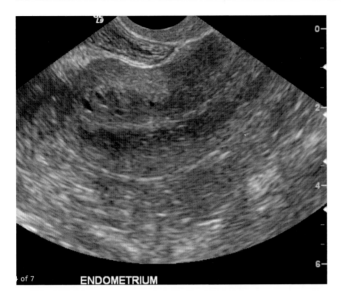

ENDOMETRIUM

1. A 61-year-old woman on long-term treatment with tamoxifen for breast cancer presents with a transvaginal sagittal image of the uterus (endometrial thickness of 18 mm). Is this considered normal?

2. What is the effect of tamoxifen on the uterus?

3. What spectrum of endometrial abnormalities does tamoxifen induce?

4. What is the cutoff measurement for abnormal endometrial thickness in a woman taking tamoxifen?

CASE 1

Tamoxifen

1. No this is not considered normal; it is diffuse endometrial thickening, which may be benign.

2. Estrogenic.

3. Endometrial hyperplasia, endometrial and endocervical polyps, subendometrial cysts, and endometrial cancer.

4. The cutoff measurement is 8 mm or greater.

References

Cohen I: Endometrial pathologies associated with postmenopausal tamoxifen treatment. *Gynecol Oncol* 96: 561, 2005.

Cohen I, Bernheim J, Azaria R, et al: Malignant endometrial polyps in postmenopausal breast cancer tamoxifen-treated patients. *Gynecol Oncol* 75:136–141, 1999.

DeKroon CD, Louwe LA, Trimbos JB, Jansen FW: The clinical value of 3-dimensional saline infusion sonography in addition to 2-dimensional saline infusion sonography in women with abnormal uterine bleeding. *J Ultrasound Med* 23:1433–1440, 2004.

Hann LE, Kim CM, Gonen M, et al: Sonohysterography compared with endometrial biopsy for evaluation of the endometrium in tamoxifen-treated women. *J Ultrasound Med* 22:1173–1179, 2003.

Hulka CA, Hall DA: Endometrial abnormalities associated with tamoxifen therapy for breast cancer: Sonographic and pathologic correlation. *AJR* 160:809–812, 1993.

Ramondetta LM, Sherwood JB, Dunton CJ, Palazzo JP: Endometrial cancer in polyps associated with tamoxifen use. *Am J Obstet Gynecol* 180:340–341, 1999.

Cross-Reference

Ultrasound: THE REQUISITES, 2nd ed, pp 542, 544, 546.

Comment

Tamoxifen is a widely used medication for patients with breast cancer because of its antiestrogenic effect on breast tissue. However, the medication can have an estrogenic effect on the endometrium. Accordingly, these patients are predisposed to develop a number of different endometrial abnormalities, including polyps of the endometrium and endocervix, subendometrial cysts, endometrial hyperplasia, and cancer (endometrial, malignant mixed mesodermal tumors, and sarcoma). The risk of developing one of these pathologic conditions relates to the duration of tamoxifen therapy; the most common abnormality is an endometrial polyp.

An endometrial thickness of 8 mm or greater warrants follow-up. Sonohysterography is an excellent modality to better delineate the endometrial contents. This imaging procedure is the most likely to reveal polyps, the most frequent abnormality in tamoxifen-treated women. Furthermore, tamoxifen-related polyps tend to be larger and have an increased rate of malignant changes compared to endometrial polyps in the general population. A hyperechoic endometrium with small cystic spaces is the classic finding with tamoxifen therapy (see figure). Many of these cystic spaces represent endometrial polyps; however, cystic hyperplasia may also have this appearance. Sonohysterograms, 2D or 3D, are often helpful to elucidate the cause of endometrial stripe thickening.

One study demonstrated that most women on tamoxifen *do not* have symptoms such as bleeding. Nonetheless, almost half of these women had abnormal endometrial thicknesses on ultrasound (defined as >8 mm). Although the risk may be increased as much as sixfold, fewer than 1% of the women taking tamoxifen therapy develop endometrial cancer. Most of *these* women have been receiving the treatment for more than 5 years, and most present with postmenopausal bleeding.

Notes

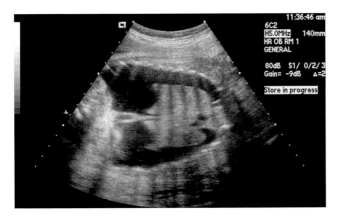

1. In this third-trimester fetus, what is the important finding on this coronal image of the fetal chest?

2. What are the potential complications of this finding?

3. Explain the spectrum of outcomes.

4. What is the treatment if this condition persists or recurs?

Pleural Effusions

1. Bilateral pleural effusions.

2. Inhibition of pulmonary development, hydrops, and polyhydramnios.

3. Variable, from normal development to fetal death.

4. Thoracocentesis and thoracoamniotic shunt if effusions are large and recurrent.

References

Achiron R, Weissman A, Lipitz S, et al: Fetal pleural effusion: The risk of fetal trisomy. *Gynecol Obstet Invest* 39:153–156, 1995.

Ahmad FK, Sherman SJ, Hagglund KH, et al: Isolated unilateral fetal pleural effusion: The role of sonographic surveillance and in utero therapy. *Fetal Diagn Ther* 11:383–389, 1996.

Hashimoto K, Shimizu T, Fukuda M, et al: Pregnancy outcome of embryonic/fetal pleural effusion in the first trimester. *J Ultrasound Med* 22:501–505, 2003.

Cross-Reference

Ultrasound: THE REQUISITES, 2nd ed, pp 249–250.

Comment

Fetal pleural effusion can present in the first, second, or third trimester of pregnancy. Ultrasound demonstrates fluid surrounding the lungs, which can have a "batwing" appearance when bilateral, as shown in this case. There are a number of possible causes, including chylothorax, chromosomal anomalies, cardiac malformations, infection, pulmonary lymphangiectasia, pulmonary mass, and hydrops fetalis in conjunction with accumulation of fluid (such as in the peritoneal cavity) and thickening of the skin.

Karyotyping is advised, irrespective of whether additional malformations are present to suggest a chromosomal anomaly. Isolated pleural effusion has been associated with trisomy 21 and Turner's syndrome and has been detected as early as the first trimester. The incidence of such a chromosomal anomaly is as high as 6%. A fetal pleural effusion in early pregnancy is associated with a poor outcome, such as spontaneous abortion or chromosomal anomaly.

The course of fetal pleural effusion is variable. Almost 10% of small effusions resolve spontaneously. If thoracocentesis is performed before delivery, some pleural effusions will not reaccumulate, and one lung can expand when the newborn attempts to breathe. However, small effusions can grow rapidly, with the risk of secondary polyhydramnios, nonimmune hydrops, and underdevelopment of the compressed lung. Thus, careful follow-up ultrasound studies, as frequently as twice a week, have been recommended. If a large volume of fluid reaccumulates, a thoracoamniotic shunt can be placed to improve the outcome.

Notes

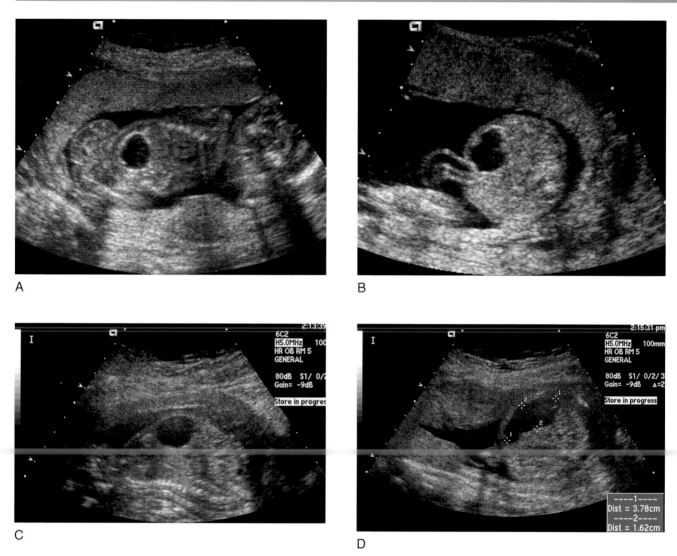

A

B

C

D

1. What is the location of the cystic abnormalities shown in these images of the fetal abdomen in these two third-trimester fetuses (Figs. A and B of one fetus and C and D of a second fetus), both in the anterior abdomen?

2. Name the type of fetal abdominal mass that can have both cystic and solid components.

3. Which cystic mass may have internal echoes?

4. Which associated anomalies may be seen with enteric duplication cysts?

Cystic Abdominal Mass

1. Intra-abdominal (not retroperitoneal).

2. Teratomas, either ovarian or retroperitoneal.

3. Meconium pseudocyst.

4. Spinal or gastrointestinal malformations.

References

Bryant AE, Laufer MR: Fetal ovarian cysts: Incidence, diagnosis and management. *J Reprod Med* 49:329–337, 2004.

Foster MA, Nyberg DA, Mahoney BS, et al: Meconium peritonitis: Prenatal sonographic findings and their clinical significance. *Radiology* 165:661–665, 1987.

Richards DS, Langham MR, Anderson CD: The prenatal sonographic appearance of enteric duplication cysts. *Ultrasound Obstet Gynecol* 7:17–20, 1996.

Cross-Reference

Ultrasound: THE REQUISITES, 2nd ed, pp 447, 464.

Comment

The differential diagnostic list for a cystic abdominal or pelvic mass in a fetus is long. Identification of associated findings may aid in determining the precise etiology. In these two cases, the cystic masses do not extend back to the spine and are not related to the kidneys so that renal and retroperitoneal masses do not need to be considered.

Ovarian cysts are among the most common cystic abdominal masses in females. With improved neonatal imaging, greater numbers of ovarian cysts are being diagnosed. The risks of acute and long-term complications must be weighed against the possibility of cyst regression. Cyst size is important. Simple cysts (Figs. A–D) and teratomas can arise from the ovary. Obstruction of the vagina or uterus may appear as a cystic mass in the pelvic midline.

A simple cyst may represent a mesenteric or omental cyst; additionally, enteric duplication cysts are located in the mesentery. Enteric duplication cysts are directly contiguous with the bowel and may communicate with the bowel lumen. Approximately 30% of fetuses with enteric duplication cysts have associated anomalies. Spinal or gastrointestinal malformations may be present with foregut or hindgut duplications, respectively.

A meconium pseudocyst forms from walled-off complicated ascites secondary to meconium peritonitis. The cyst typically contains internal echoes. Dilatation of the small bowel, peritoneal calcifications, and polyhydramnios can be seen. The obstructed bowel loop in bowel atresia can also present as an abdominal cystic mass, usually with hyperperistalsis.

Genitourinary cysts can arise from several sites. Renal causes such as multicystic dysplastic kidney have been eliminated in this case. However, posterior urethral valve (PUV) obstruction can result in urinoma formation. An obstructed bladder in PUV or other types of bladder outlet obstruction appears as large cystic pelvic-abdominal masses. The existence of a urachal cyst is an additional possibility.

Notes

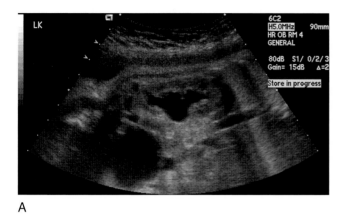

A

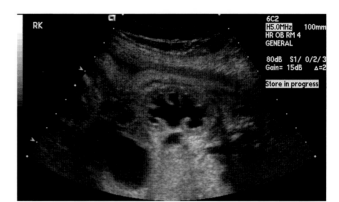

B

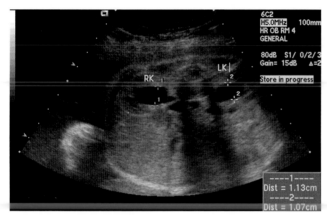

C

1. In this early third-trimester fetus, what do the coronal images (Figs. A and B) and transverse image (Fig. C) show in a fetal kidney?

2. What is the most common cause of hydronephrosis in the neonate?

3. What is the incidence of contralateral renal abnormalities with hydronephrosis?

4. Are extrarenal anomalies associated with this entity?

Ureteropelvic Junction Obstruction

1. Hydronephrosis.

2. Ureteropelvic junction (UPJ) obstruction.

3. 20%.

4. Yes.

Reference

Anderson N, Clautice-Engle T, Allan R, et al: Detection of obstructive uropathy in the fetus: predictive value of sonographic measurements of renal pelvic diameter at various gestational ages. *AJR* 164:719–723, 1995.

Bosman G, Reuss A, Nijman M, Wladimiroff JW: Prenatal diagnosis, management and outcome of fetal uretero-pelvic junction obstruction. *Ultrasound Med Biol* 17: 117–120, 1991.

Mandell J, Blyth BR, Peters CA, et al: Structural geni-tourinary defects detected in utero: *Radiology* 178: 193–196, 1991.

Cross-Reference

Ultrasound: THE REQUISITES, 2nd ed, p 465.

Comment

Ureteropelvic junction (UPJ) obstruction is the most common cause of hydronephrosis in the neonate. UPJ obstruction is considered to be an intrinsic functional obstruction of outflow from the renal pelvis owing to abnormal development. Infrequently, an obstructing vessel or other anatomic cause is implicated.

On prenatal ultrasound, dilatation of the renal pelvis is seen. The degree of dilatation has been classified using ultrasound, depending on the pelvic diameter (<1 cm, 1 to 1.5 cm, >1 cm) and the presence and degree of caliectasis (none, moderate, or marked). Kidneys with significant postnatal obstruction may have no dilatation of the renal pelvis before 23 weeks' gestation. During pregnancy renal pelvic diameter increases at a greater rate in kidneys later shown to be obstructed. Once dilata-tion has been detected, postnatal follow-up is essential to determine the degree of residual renal function in the obstructed kidney and also to evaluate the contralateral kidney. If residual renal function is adequate, pyeloplasty is the preferred treatment.

Contralateral renal anomalies can occur in 20% of cases of UPJ obstruction, including multicystic dysplastic kidney and renal agenesis. If the UPJ obstruction is severe in these cases, oligohydramnios will develop. Interestingly, unilateral UPJ obstruction may initially man-ifest with polyhydramnios. As opposed to a lower geni-tourinary tract obstruction, which has a 40% incidence of associated extrarenal anomalies, a UPJ obstruction has a lower incidence of gastrointestinal complications (esophageal and anal atresia, Hirschsprung's disease), neural tube defects, and cardiovascular anomalies (12%).

Notes

1. What is the major finding in this second-trimester fetal head scan (axial), and what is the incidence of detection of this finding by ultrasound?

2. Can this be a normal finding? Is it associated with any karyotypic abnormalities?

3. What factors are important when deciding whether amniocentesis is required?

4. Do any characteristics of these cysts (e.g., size and bilaterality) correlate with the presence of a karyotypic abnormality?

Choroid Plexus Cysts

1. Choroid plexus cyst. The incidence is 0.2% to 2.5%.

2. Yes, this is often a normal finding. It is associated with trisomies 18 and 21.

3. Serum triple screen results, maternal age, and the presence of additional ultrasound findings.

4. No.

References

Doubilet PM, Copel JA, Benson CB, et al: Choroid plexus cyst and echogenic intracardiac focus in women at low risk for chromosomal anomalies *J Ultrasound Med* 23:883–885, 2004.

Filly RA, Benacerraf RB, Nyberg DA, Hobbins JC: Choroid plexus cyst and echogenic intracardiac focus in women at low risk for chromosomal anomalies. *J Ultrasound Med* 23:447–449, 2004.

Gratton RJ, Hogge WA, Aston CE: Choroid plexus cysts and trisomy 18: Risk modification based on maternal age and multiple-marker screening. *Am J Obstet Gynecol* 175:1493–1497, 1996.

Reinsch RC: Choroid plexus cysts' association with trisomy: Prospective review of 16,059 patients. *Am J Obstet Gynecol* 176:1381–1383, 1997.

Turner SR, Samei ME, Hertzberg BS, et al: Sonography of fetal choroid plexus cysts. *J Ultrasound Med* 22:1219–1227, 2003.

Cross-Reference

Ultrasound: THE REQUISITES, 2nd ed, pp 395–397.

Comment

Choroid plexus cysts are detected in 0.2% to 2.5% of pregnant women with prenatal ultrasonography and are often normal variants. Improvement in ultrasound technology has led to an increased ability to visualize these cysts; unfortunately, their management is controversial.

Choroid plexus cysts occur in fetuses with trisomy 18, but not in all cases. Furthermore, they also occur in 1% to 2% of pregnant women. Detection of a choroid plexus cyst requires a careful search for other findings of trisomy 18, including a strawberry-shaped skull, micrognathia, overlapping fingers, and clubfoot. Some studies report an increased incidence of trisomy 21 in such fetuses. When another anomaly is detected on ultrasound, karyotypic evaluation is recommended.

The controversy arises when isolated choroid plexus cysts are detected. Reports in the literature vary. One recent publication recommends that when a choroid plexus cyst or an echogenic intracardiac focus is the only detected abnormality, the sonographic report should emphasize that either of these findings alone does not change the mother from a low- to a high-risk status. Advanced maternal age (quoted as greater than or equal to 37 years) or an abnormal serum triple screen may dictate amniocentesis. However, the size of the cysts, their site (unilateral versus bilateral), the gestational age at detection, the gestational age at resolution, and the fetal sex cannot be used to predict the presence or absence of a karyotypic abnormality. Although most cysts resolve by 22 to 26 weeks of gestation, resolution does not reduce the likelihood of karyotypic abnormality.

Notes

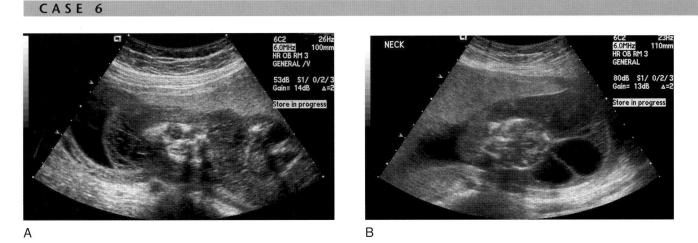

A   B

1. What is the chromosomal anomaly most likely to be present in this second-trimester fetus? Figure A is a coronal image of the facial region and upper body, and Figure B is an axial image of the posterior neck.

2. What cardiovascular anomaly is associated with this condition?

3. Does the triple screen aid in the detection of this chromosomal anomaly?

4. Is this chromosomal anomaly associated with advanced maternal age?

Turner's Syndrome

1. Turner's syndrome.

2. Coarctation of the aorta.

3. Yes, but only 30% of cases are detected.

4. No.

References

Bronshtein M, Zimmer EZ, Blazer S: A characteristic cluster of fetal sonographic markers that are predictive of fetal Turner syndrome in early pregnancy. *Am J Obstet Gynecol* 188:1016–1020, 2003.

Saenger P: Turner's syndrome. *N Engl J Med* 335: 1749–1754, 1996.

Shimizu T, Hashimoto K, Shimizu M, et al: Bilateral pleural effusion in the first trimester: A predictor of chromosomal anomaly and embryonic death? *Am J Obstet Gynecol* 177:470–471, 1997.

Wenstrom KD, Williamson RA, Grant SS: Detection of fetal Turner syndrome with multiple marker screening. *Am J Obstet Gynecol* 170:570–573, 1994.

Cross-Reference

Ultrasound: THE REQUISITES, 2nd ed, pp 394, 407, 409, 420–421.

Comment

Turner's syndrome is the most common anomaly of sex chromosomes in females with a karyotype of 45,X0. The X chromosome is of maternal origin in two thirds of the cases and of paternal origin in one third. Ninety-nine percent of all 45,X karyotype fetuses abort spontaneously. The chromosomal anomaly is *not* associated with advanced maternal age. The triple screen test may be abnormal. In most series, it is estimated that only 30% of cases are detected.

Although many cases are discovered by amniocentesis or chorionic villus sampling, ultrasound findings can be helpful in detecting Turner's syndrome. Nuchal abnormalities range from nuchal thickening to full-blown cystic hygromas, with dilatation of the lymphatics arising from the posterior jugular sac. This case demonstrates a more diffuse lymphangiectasia (see Figs. A and B). Cardiovascular malformations include coarctation of the aorta (<20%), often with a bicuspid aortic valve. Horseshoe kidney and other renal malformations are also associated with this abnormality. The fetuses often have mild intrauterine growth retardation. In one study, all fetal Turner's syndrome cases had huge septated cystic hygromas, severe subcutaneous edema, and hydrops in early pregnancy. A few cases of Turner's syndrome presenting in utero with transient pleural effusion have been described in the literature.

Almost 70% of fetuses with Turner's syndrome are lost from 16 weeks' gestation to term. Development of diffuse hydropic changes in the setting of a cystic hygroma is uniformly fatal. Survivors are monitored carefully for the multiple associated anomalies, which include hypothyroidism, otitis media, scoliosis, inflammatory bowel disease, mesenteric vascular anomalies, glucose intolerance, and hypertension. Estrogen is supplemented in these children, beginning in the early teenage years. With assisted fertility, 50% to 60% of women with Turner's syndrome can become pregnant.

Notes

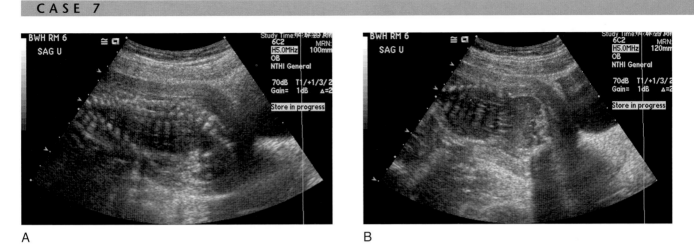

A

B

1. In this third-trimester fetus, what is the most likely diagnosis for the lack of amniotic fluid, and what is the most likely cause of death in the newborn? Figure A is a sagittal image of the fetal body; Figure B is an image of the fetal body in the plane of the cervix.

2. What factors predict the outcome in cases of spontaneous rupture of the membranes (SROM)?

3. What musculoskeletal complications result from this diagnosis?

4. What is the potentially serious short-term complication of membrane rupture?

Oligohydramnios (Secondary to Spontaneous Rupture of the Membranes)

1. Severe oligohydramnios secondary to SROM; pulmonary hypoplasia.

2. Severity of fluid loss, gestational age at the time of rupture, and the length of exposure to oligohydramnios.

3. Limb deformities, including hip dysplasia and clubfoot.

4. Infection (chorioamnionitis)

References

Cunningham FG, MacDonald PC, Gant NF, et al: Placental disorders: Disease and abnormalities of the fetal membranes. In Cunningham FG, Williams JW (eds): *Williams Obstetrics*, 20th ed. Stamford, CT, Appleton & Lange, 1997, pp 664–665.

Kilbride HW, Yeast J, Thibeault DW: Obstetrics: Defining limits of survival: Lethal pulmonary hypoplasia after midtrimester premature rupture of membranes. *Am J Obstet Gynecol* 175:675–681, 1996.

Ott WJ: Reevaluation of the relationship between amniotic fluid volume and perinatal outcome: *Am J Obstet Gynecol* 192:1803–1809, 2005.

Cross-Reference

Ultrasound: THE REQUISITES, 2nd ed, pp 458, 460.

Comment

This case of SROM shows that the degree of oligohydramnios can be severe (see Figs. A and B). The kidneys can frequently be seen and the urinary bladder can be identified. In cases of SROM in which the amniotic fluid index is less than 1 cm, the duration of this severe exposure to oligohydramnios and the gestational age at the time of membrane rupture are predictors of fetal outcome. Fetal mortality is higher than 90% if membranes rupture before 25 weeks and the exposure to severe oligohydramnios continues for more than 14 days. The mother is watched carefully for signs of infection (chorioamnionitis). However, a recent very large series found oligohydramnios to be a weak predictor of poor perinatal outcome as opposed to polyhydramnios.

Twenty percent of cases of membrane rupture result in lethal pulmonary hypoplasia. In those fetuses that survive severe oligohydramnios due to membrane rupture, limb deformities can occur. In fact, 80% of fetuses born after more than 2 weeks' exposure to severe oligohydramnios had such deformities, including clubfoot and congenital hip dysplasia.

In any case of newly diagnosed oligohydramnios with *intact* membranes, umbilical artery Doppler ultrasound should be performed to exclude placental insufficiency. The systolic to diastolic ratio (S/D) is measured and compared with the normal range defined for each gestational age. In normal patients, the diastolic flow increases with increasing gestational age. In cases of intrauterine growth restriction, decreasing diastolic flow results in an *increase* in the S/D ratio. When the ratio is above the 90th percentile, careful follow-up examinations are conducted to detect the absence or reversal of diastolic flow, which can prompt induction of delivery.

In gestations that extend beyond the expected due date, amniotic fluid can normally decrease. This may result occasionally in umbilical cord compression and fetal heart deceleration. Monitoring includes frequent amniotic fluid index measurements and subjective quantitative measurements of fluid volume, maternal assessment of fetal movement, and fetal nonstress cardiac testing.

Notes

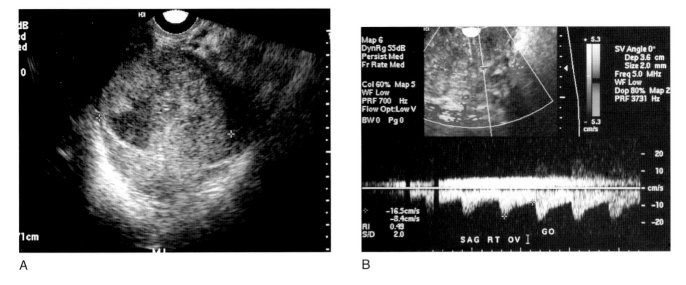

A

B

1. In this 55-year-old postmenopausal woman with a palpable right-sided pelvic mass, what is the most likely diagnosis and what are the differential diagnostic possibilities based on the ultrasound images of the right adnexa? (Figs. A and B)

2. Does this spectral waveform from the soft tissue component raise concern regarding a malignancy (Fig. B)?

3. Does the impedance (i.e., resistive index [RI] and pulsatility index [PI]) aid in making the correct diagnosis?

4. Which benign ovarian masses may demonstrate high diastolic flow?

Ovarian Cancer (Cystadenocarcinoma)

1. Ovarian cancer (cystadenocarcinoma). The differential diagnoses are cystadenoma, tubo-ovarian abscess, endometrioma, corpus luteum cyst, and dermoid.

2. Yes; although it occurs in some benign lesions, an arterial waveform with elevated diastolic flow may be seen in malignant ovarian lesions.

3. It can be helpful, but it is nonspecific.

4. Hormone-secreting or inflammatory lesions such as tubo-ovarian abscesses, endometriomas, and dermoids.

References

Alcazar JL, Galan MJ, Ceamanos C, Garcia-Manero M: Transvaginal gray scale and color Doppler sonography in primary ovarian cancer and metastatic tumors to the ovary. *J Ultrasound Med* 22:243–247, 2003.

Alcazar JL, Galal MJ, Garcia-Manero M, Guerriero S: Three-dimensional sonographic morphologic assessment in complex adnexal masses. *J Ultrasound Med* 22:249–254, 2003.

Alfuhaid TR, Rosen BP, Wilson S: Low-malignant potential tumor of the ovary: sonographic features with clinicopathologic correlation in 41 patients. *Ultrasound Q* 19:13–26, 2003.

Brown DL, Zou KH, Tempany CM, et al: Primary versus secondary ovarian malignancy: imaging findings of adnexal masses in the Radiology Diagnostic Oncology Study. *Radiology* 219:213–218, 2001.

Kinkel K, Lu Y, Mehdizade A, et al: Indeterminate ovarian mass at US: incremental value of second imaging test for characterization-meta-analysis and Bayesian analysis. *Radiology* 236:85–94, 2005.

Rieber A, Nussle K, Stohr I, Grab D: Preoperative diagnosis of ovarian tumors with MR imaging: comparison with transvaginal sonography, positron emission tomography, and histologic findings. *AJR* 177:123–129, 2001.

Cross-Reference

Ultrasound: THE REQUISITES, 2nd ed, pp 579–583.

Comment

Ultrasound is usually the first imaging modality for detection and characterization of ovarian cysts. Most simple cysts are benign follicles (usually <25 mm in long axis) that come and go with each menstrual cycle. Follow-up after one to two menstrual cycles is reasonable for any premenopausal woman with a simple or complex cyst, which could be a follicle or a hemorrhagic follicle, to see if resolution occurs.

Ovarian cancer demonstrates a number of the ultrasound criteria for a malignant mass. The presence of a solid component or solid papillary mural projections, particularly if they are *nonhyperechoic*, is worrisome. A hyperechoic solid component is seen more typically in a dermoid. If a fluid component is present, it is more commonly anechoic or hypoechoic. Septations may or may not occur in a malignant mass, but if present, they are usually 3 mm or thicker. The wall is often not discernible but can be thin or thick if seen. A malignant cyst is accompanied by ascites in 30% of cases, which suggests spread to the pelvis (stage 2) or abdomen (stage 3 or 4). Multilocularity favors the diagnosis of a primary ovarian neoplasm rather than a secondary one. A purely solid tumor indicates a higher probability of metastatic carcinoma rather than primary ovarian carcinoma.

The distinction of a benign from a malignant ovarian mass by Doppler ultrasound has been shown to be nonpredictive. Doppler ultrasound has been applied on the principle that low impedance flow should indicate a malignancy. When arterial signals are detected, the systolic and diastolic components can be evaluated. Measurements include RI [(peak systolic velocity − end-diastolic velocity) ÷ peak systolic velocity] and PI [(peak systolic velocity − end-diastolic velocity) ÷ mean velocity]. The standard cutoff level for malignancy is an RI less than 0.4 or a PI less than 1.0. It is not uncommon for a malignant lesion to have a borderline or low ratio that is suggestive of a malignancy. Conversely, arterial flow with systolic flow but little or no diastolic flow is a high-resistance signal that is seen almost exclusively in benign lesions.

However, considerable overlap has been shown between benign and malignant masses when the spectral waveform shows an arterial waveform with a high diastolic component (low impedance). In the example shown, the RI is borderline and the mass was pathologically malignant. Benign masses that are endocrine-secreting or inflammatory may have this flow pattern, particularly tubo-ovarian abscesses, endometriomas, and ovarian dermoids. A recent large study showed that in women with an indeterminate mass at gray scale ultrasound, the use of magnetic resonance imaging contributed to a change in probability of malignancy in both pre- and postmenopausal women more than did the use of computed tomography or combined gray-scale and Doppler ultrasound results.

Notes

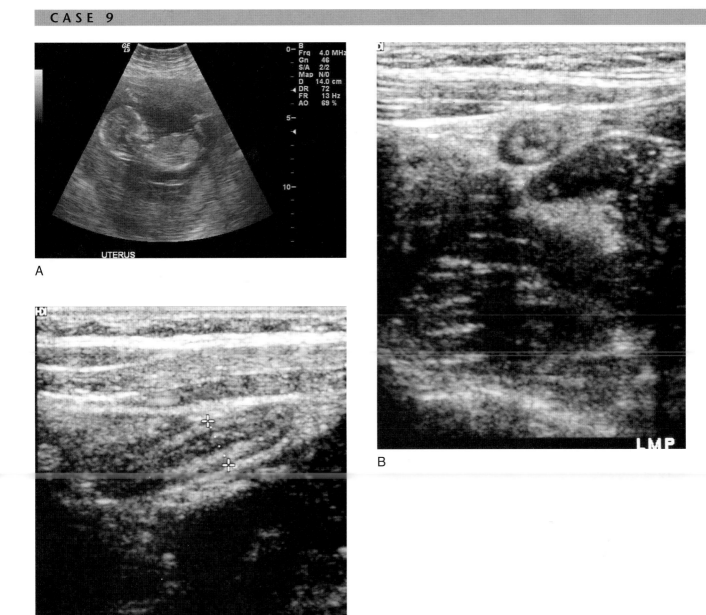

A

B

C

1. What is the most likely diagnosis in this transabdominal (Figs. A–C) late first-trimester ultrasound examination of a 25-year-old woman ? Figure A is an image of the gestational sac in the uterus containing the fetus. Figure B is an axial image to the right of the upper uterine body showing an adjacent structure measuring 10 mm in diameter. Figure C is a sagittal image of the same structure in Figure B.

2. Do leukocytosis and right lower quadrant pain indicate appendicitis?

3. Does appendicitis have a higher mortality rate in pregnancy?

4. What are the complications of appendicitis in pregnancy?

Appendicitis

1. Appendicitis.

2. No; leukocytosis can occur as part of a normal pregnancy.

3. Yes, particularly in the third trimester.

4. Preterm delivery, spontaneous abortion, maternal-fetal sepsis, and neonatal neurologic injury.

References

Abu-Yousef MM: Ulltrasonography of the right lower quadrant. *Ultrasound Q* 17:211–225, 2001.

Cobben LP, Groot I, Haans L, et al: MRI for clinically suspected appendicitis during pregnancy. *AJR* 184: 671–675, 2004.

Eyvazzadeh AD, Pedrosa I, Rofsky NM, et al: MRI of right-sided abdominal pain in pregnancy. *AJR* 183:907–914, 2004.

Kessler N, Cyteval C, Gallix B, et al: Appendicitis: evaluation of sensitivity, specificity, and predictive values of US, Doppler US and laboratory findings. *Radiology* 230:472–478, 2004.

Mourad J, Elliott JP, Erickson L, Lisboa L: Appendicitis in pregnancy: new information that contradicts long-held clinical beliefs. *Am J Obstet Gynecol* 185:259–260, 2001.

McGahan JP: What is the role of ultrasound in evaluating patients with right lower quadrant pain? *Appl Rad* 33:30–38, 2004.

Tracey M, Fletcher HS: Appendicitis in pregnancy. *Am Surg* 66:555–559, 2000.

Cross-Reference

Ultrasound: THE REQUISITES, 2nd ed, pp 224–225.

Comment

Appendicitis occurs in 1 in 1500 pregnant women. It can develop in the first, second, or third trimester. Unfortunately, the symptoms of appendicitis are identical to those that occur in a normal pregnancy. Leukocytosis and nausea are common. The enlarging uterus can cause severe right lower quadrant pain due to round ligament strain. The clinical differential diagnosis of right lower quadrant pain in pregnancy includes appendicitis, renal calculus, pyelonephritis, placental abruption, degeneration of myoma, ovarian cyst, and torsion. Right lower quadrant pain has been found to be the most common presenting symptom of appendicitis in pregnancy regardless of gestational age. Fever and leukocytosis are not clear indicators of appendicitis in pregnancy.

Ultrasound has been used to make the diagnosis, thereby avoiding the ionizing radiation of computed tomography. Early in pregnancy, the inflamed appendix may be visualized as a noncompressible tubular structure measuring 6 mm or more, as shown in this case (see Figs. B and C), with a diameter of 10 mm. Doppler ultrasound has been found to be a sensitive indicator of inflammation and increased diastolic flow with a low resistive index. Pain often occurs directly over this area. In the setting of perforation, a collection of peritoneal fluid may be detected. As the uterus enlarges, the appendix can move superiorly and toward the flanks.

Magnetic resonance imaging is a safe modality to evaluate pregnant patients clinically suspected of having acute appendicitis. Unnecessary operations can be avoided when a normal appendix is imaged. In one series, 50% of pregnant women who underwent surgery had appendicitis. If the diagnosis is missed, peritonitis results. In the third trimester, peritonitis has a poor prognosis, and maternal mortality is approximately 5%. Other complications include preterm labor, spontaneous abortion, and even fetal neurologic injury if maternal-fetal sepsis results.

Notes

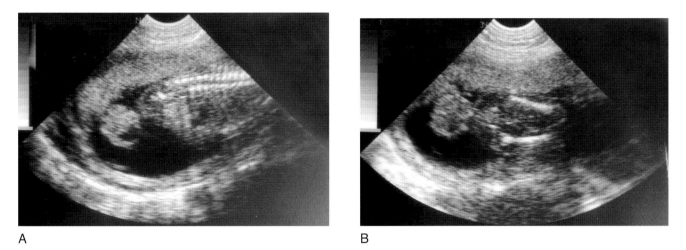

A   B

1. What is the abnormality shown on these sagittal (Fig. A) and axial (Fig. B) images of the lower spine in this third-trimester fetus?

2. What factor increases the risk of malignancy?

3. What associated findings may be seen on prenatal ultrasound?

4. What are the hyperechoic foci that may be seen in this type of mass?

Sacrococcygeal Teratoma

1. Sacrococcygeal teratoma.

2. Diagnosis after 2 to 4 months of *neonatal* age.

3. Bladder displacement, hydronephrosis, and polyhydramnios.

4. Calcifications due to dystrophic calcification or small bone fragments.

References

Hedrick HL, Flake AW, Crombleholme TM, et al: Sacrococcygeal teratoma: prenatal assessment, fetal intervention, and outcome. *J Pediatr Surg* 39:430–438, 2004.

Sheth S, Nussbaum SR, Sanders RC, et al: Prenatal diagnosis of sacrococcygeal teratoma: Sonographic-pathologic correlation. *Radiology* 169:131–136, 1988.

Westerburg B, Feldstein VA, Sandberg PL, et al: Sonographic prognostic factors in fetuses with sacrococcygeal teratoma. *J Pediatr Surg* 35:322–325, 2000.

Woodward PJ, Sohaey R, Kennedy A, Koeller KK: A comprehensive review of fetal tumors with pathologic correlation. *RadioGraphics* 25:215–242, 2005.

Cross-Reference

Ultrasound: THE REQUISITES, 2nd ed, pp 408–410.

Comment

Sacrococcygeal teratoma is the most common congenital tumor in the newborn and is more common in females. Seventy percent to 80% of all teratomas are located in this region. Interestingly, the tumor has been associated with twins and often affects only one of the two. Women often have a large-for-dates uterus owing to the frequently accompanying polyhydramnios, or to the neoplasm itself. The diagnosis is important, because most pregnancies result in premature deliveries. More important, if the mass is not diagnosed, vaginal delivery may lead to dystocia and intratumoral hemorrhage owing to a traumatic delivery. Amnio-reduction, cyst aspiration, and surgical debulking can be life-saving.

The mass may be one of four subtypes: (1) exterior with a minimal presacral component, (2) exterior with a significant presacral component, (3) both exterior and presacral, and (4) predominantly presacral. The latter has the worst prognosis and may not be detected at birth. The risk of malignancy increases with age after delivery (particularly after 2 to 4 months of age).

On ultrasound, a mass that is usually cystic and solid is seen in the region of the fetal sacrum. Calcifications are often present, owing to fragments of bone or dystrophic calcification. A review of several cases demonstrated three ultrasonographic patterns: (1) predominantly solid with small anechoic areas (as shown here), (2) a unilocular cystic mass, or (3) a mixed solid and cystic mass. Although the presacral component may be visualized on ultrasound, the internal component can go undetected, even when it is large. There is little or no distortion of the sacral spine (see Fig. A), but the tumor may spread into the spinal canal. Associated findings are important; if they include bladder displacement and hydronephrosis, severe renal dysfunction with oligohydramnios may result. Furthermore, because these tumors may be very vascular (often appreciated with Doppler ultrasound), the following can develop: high-output problems for the fetus, massive polyhydramnios necessitating therapeutic amniocentesis, placentomegaly, and hydrops. Fetuses with mainly solid vascular tumors have a higher risk of hydrops.

Most of the sacrococcygeal teratomas diagnosed in utero are benign. The presence of yolk sac tumor components may result in an elevated α-fetoprotein level, particularly in the rare malignant tumor. Cesarean section is often necessary to prevent traumatic delivery with an intratumor hemorrhage. The mortality rate for fetuses with sacrococcygeal teratomas is close to 50%. Surgical excision is the treatment; the coccyx must be excised in order to prevent a recurrence.

Notes

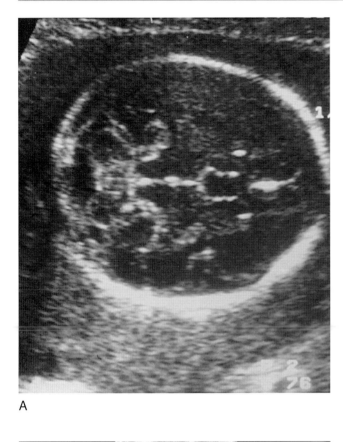

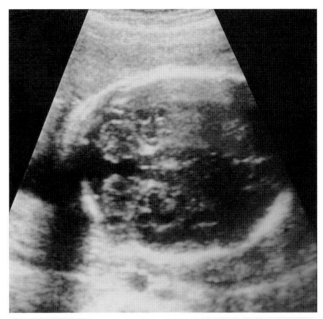

B

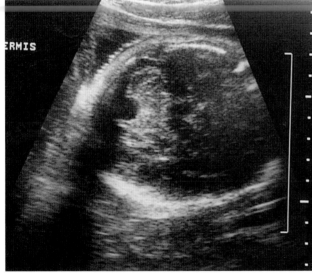

C

1. Three middle second-trimester fetal brains with axial scans of the posterior fossae. Which scans are abnormal, and what diagnoses do they indicate?

2. Does the presence of ventriculomegaly with this disorder have any prognostic significance?

3. Which portion of the cerebellar vermis fuses last?

4. When is the cerebellar vermis completely fused?

CASE 11

Dandy-Walker Malformation

1. A is normal; B is complete absence of cerebellum vermis; and C has partial absence of the cerebellar vermis in Dandy-Walker malformation.

2. Yes, there is an inverse relationship between the presence of ventriculomegaly and chromosomal anomalies.

3. Fusion begins superiorly and continues inferiorly.

4. Embryologically the cerebellar vermis may fuse by the end of the 15th week. Using ultrasound, an open vermis may be seen in normal patients before 18 weeks.

References

Baumeister LA, Hertzberg BS, McNally PJ, et al: Fetal fourth ventricle: US appearance and frequency of depiction. *Radiology* 192:333–336, 1994.

Bromley B, Nadel AS, Paulker S, et al: Closure of the cerebellar vermis: Evaluation with second trimester US. *Radiology* 193:761–763, 1994.

Chang MC, Russell SA, Callen PW, et al: Sonographic detection of inferior vermian agenesis in Dandy-Walker malformations: prognostic implications. *Radiology* 192:765–770, 1994.

Ecker JL, Shipp TD, Bromley B, Benacerraf B: The sonographic diagnosis of Dandy-Walker and Dandy-Walker variant: associated findings and outcomes. *Prenat Diagn* 20:328–332, 2000.

Frates MC, Kumar AJ, Benson CB, et al: Fetal anomalies: comparison of MR imaging and US for diagnosis. *Radiology* 232:398–404, 2004.

Cross-Reference

Ultrasound: THE REQUISITES, 2nd ed, pp 391–393, 398.

Comment

Dandy-Walker malformation consists of variable degrees of cerebellar vermian agenesis (see Figs. B and C), dilatation of the fourth ventricle, and enlargement of the posterior fossa. The cisterna magna communicates with the fourth ventricle. Ventriculomegaly may be present and was reported in 24% to 71% of cases. Nyberg described an inverse relationship between the presence of chromosomal anomalies and ventriculomegaly.

The cerebellar vermis is open early in gestation and closes in most normal patients by 18 weeks of age. Accordingly, an open cerebellar vermis on prenatal ultrasound *cannot* be considered abnormal until 18 weeks' gestation. Ultrasound criteria for a normal posterior fossa include a cisterna magna from 2 to 10 mm and a bilobed cerebellum. The normal fourth ventricle can be seen 70% of the time in the mid-second trimester and measures 3.5 × 3.9 mm on average. The posterior fossa should be imaged in an axial plane; semicoronal imaging toward the cervical spine often yields spurious enlargement of the cisterna magna. Magnetic resonance imaging has been used as an adjunct to prenatal ultrasound, especially in fetal anomalies of the central nervous system.

Because approximately 75% of afflicted fetuses with Dandy-Walker malformation have concomitant anomalies, the mortality rate has been reported to be as high as 70%. Chromosomal anomalies are present in almost one third of cases, including trisomy 13, trisomy 18, and trisomy 21. Additional central nervous system abnormalities include agenesis of the corpus callosum, aqueductal stenosis, microcephaly, and encephalocele. Cardiac, genitourinary, and facial malformations as well as polydactyly are common. An isolated Dandy-Walker variant has the highest chance of leading to a normal neonate.

Notes

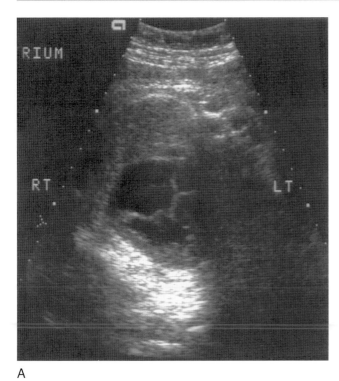

RIUM

RT   LT

A

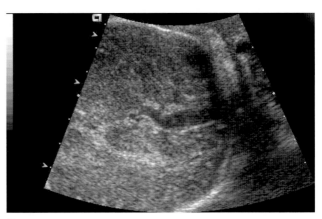

B

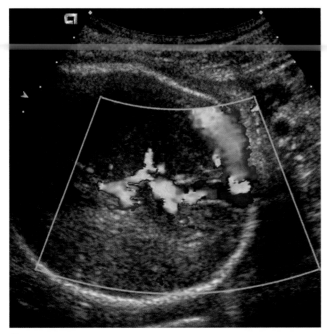

C

1. How does Figure A of the fetal heart relate to Figures B and C of the fetal head?

2. What are the central nervous system (CNS) complications of this condition?

3. Are other cardiovascular malformations associated with this cerebral abnormality?

4. When does this malformation present in utero?

Central Nervous System Arteriovenous Malformation

1. Cardiomegaly resulting from high-output heart failure due to an intracranial arteriovenous malformation (AVM).

2. Cerebral anoxia, porencephaly, and hydrocephalus.

3. Yes, coarctation of the aorta and transposition of the great vessels.

4. Usually after 30 weeks.

Reference

Comstock CH, Kirk JS: Arteriovenous malformations: Locations and evolution in the fetal brain. *J Ultrasound Med* 10:361–365, 1991.

Gailloud P, O'riordan DP, Burger I, et al: Diagnosis and management of vein of Galen aneurysmal malformations. *J Perinatol* 25:542–551, 2005.

Gerards FA, Engels MAJ, Barkhof F, et al: Prenatal diagnosis of aneurysms of the vein of Galen (vena magna cerebri) with conventional sonography, three-dimensional sonography, and magnetic resonance imaging. *J Ultrasound Med* 22:1363–1368, 2003.

Cross-Reference

Ultrasound: THE REQUISITES, 2nd ed, p 398.

Comment

Intracranial fetal AVMs almost always involve the vein of Galen, as shown in this case. Their occurrence is rare. Although traditionally called an "aneurysm," this malformation represents a direct arteriovenous anastomosis or arteriovenous fistula. The anterior and posterior circulations supply the malformation, stealing blood from the cerebral vasculature; the vein of Galen drains the malformation and dilates. Multiple arteriovenous shunts drain into a dilated median prosencephalic vein, an embryonic vessel normally absent in an adult. The outcome is usually poor, particularly if high-output heart failure develops, as shown by cardiomegaly in Figure A; the heart is greater than one half of the diameter of the chest. Associated cardiovascular malformations include coarctation of the aorta and transposition of the great vessels.

On prenatal ultrasound, these malformations do not become apparent until the third trimester, usually after 30 weeks. A cystic structure is identified posterior to the foramen of Monro (superior to the third ventricle), just superior and posterior to the thalamus. The structure is generally larger than 2.5 cm in its shortest diameter and fills on color Doppler imaging (see Fig. C). Arterial or high venous flow is detected with spectral Doppler, depending on the site of examination. Dilated intracerebral vessels may be detected around the AVM. The head circumference is normal. Hydrocephalus, usually seen in the neonate with a vein of Galen AVM, is not always present prenatally.

Because of the high flow through the AVM or possibly owing to pressure necrosis, cerebral anoxia may lead to microinfarcts and periventricular leukomalacia. The fetal heart or right ventricle is usually enlarged. Hydrops fetalis results from high-output heart failure and can cause pulmonary hypoplasia from pleural effusions. The prognosis relates to the presence of heart failure rather than to the size of the lesion. Ultrasound and magnetic resonance imaging help in determining the best possible care after birth.

Notes

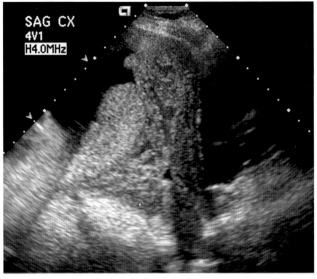

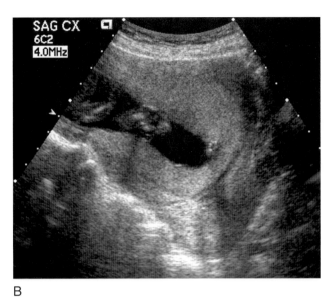

A

B

1. In this late second-trimester pregnancy, Figures A and B are transabdominal images of the lower uterine segment (LUS). Which is more diagnostic and why?

2. What are the best imaging techniques to evaluate for the presence of placenta previa?

3. Can the diagnosis of placenta previa be made from a transabdominal scan?

4. Name three complications of placenta previa.

C A S E 1 3

Placenta Previa

1. Figure B; the urinary bladder is empty.

2. Translabial and transvaginal ultrasound with an empty or minimally filled bladder.

3. Yes, if the bladder is empty or minimally distended.

4. Hemorrhage, placental invasion (accreta), and intrauterine growth restriction.

References

Hertzberg BS, Bowie JD, Carroll BA, et al: Diagnosis of placenta previa during the third trimester: Role of transperineal sonography. *AJR* 159:83–87, 1992.

Mabie WC: Placenta previa. *Clin Perinatol* 19:425–435, 1992.

Predanic M, Perni SC, Baergen RN, et al: A sonographic assessment of different patterns of placenta previa "migration" in the third trimester of pregnancy. *J Ultrasound Med* 24:773–780, 2005.

Wu S, Kocherginsky M, Hibbard JU: Abnormal placentation: twenty-year analysis *Am J Obstet Gynecol* 192:1458–1461, 2005.

Cross-Reference

Ultrasound: THE REQUISITES, 2nd ed, pp 488, 498–504.

Comment

Implantation of the placenta over the cervix (Fig. A) is described as placenta previa. Placenta previa can be complete (the internal os is covered by placenta), partial (partial coverage of the os), or marginal (the placental edge is at the margin of the os). A low-lying placenta (within 2 cm of the internal os) does not reach the internal os but may be clinically important because it can be incorporated into the dilated cervix at the time of delivery, leading to hemorrhage.

Complications can occur in addition to hemorrhage. An anterior placenta may invade the uterine wall (placenta accreta), particularly in patients with a previa and a history of cesarean section and advanced maternal age. Fetal complications include intrauterine growth restriction and subsequent development of cerebral palsy. Even the low-lying placenta may increase the incidence of small for gestational age fetuses.

Many cases can be diagnosed with transabdominal ultrasound. The bladder must be empty to make an accurate diagnosis. A distended bladder or uterine contraction can cause a false-positive result by compressing the LUS and making a low-lying placenta appear like a placenta previa. Translabial and transvaginal imaging after bladder emptying are often necessary to adequately visualize the LUS, particularly in the third trimester. The transvaginal probe should be inserted only partially in order to avoid direct contact with the cervix.

Most cases diagnosed early in pregnancy resolve, probably because of placental remodeling owing to poor blood supply of the LUS. Follow-up imaging is required in the third trimester (~30 weeks). A cesarean section is performed for a persistent placenta previa. A final placental distance of less than 2.0 cm from the internal os and a deceleration pattern of placental migration have been significantly associated with the need for a cesarean section delivery.

Notes

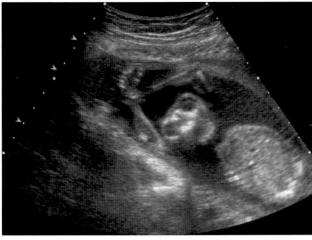

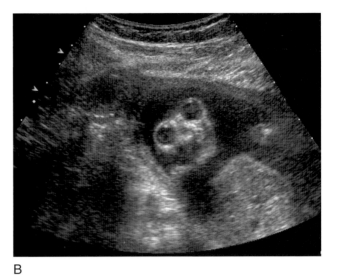

A   B

1. What is the diagnosis in these two images of an early second-trimester pregnancy?

   Figures A and B are coronal images of the head and upper body in the same fetus.

2. When can this disorder be reliably detected by ultrasound?

3. When does the neural tube close?

4. Which dietary deficiency is associated with this disorder?

Anencephaly

1. Anencephaly.

2. May be seen as early as 8 weeks but is seen reliably by the second trimester.

3. Twenty-four days of fetal life; 38 menstrual days.

4. Folic acid.

Reference

Goldstein RB, Filly RA: Prenatal diagnosis of anencephaly: Spectrum of sonographic appearances and distinction from the amniotic band syndrome. *AJR* 151:547–550, 1988.

Cross-Reference

Ultrasound: THE REQUISITES, 2nd ed, pp 374–376.

Comment

With an overall frequency of 1 in 1000, anencephaly is one of the most common neural tube defects. The incidence varies in different parts of the world. The cerebral cortex and skull are absent; orbits, brainstem, and skull base are present. In some cases, "angiomatous stroma" or vascular, dysmorphic tissue may cover the brainstem. As in other central nervous system anomalies, polyhydramnios is also often present, particularly later in the gestation period. Anencephaly is incompatible with life.

A deficiency of maternal folic acid has been shown to increase the risk of neural tube defects. It is recommended that women begin folic acid supplementation before becoming pregnant to decrease the risk of anencephaly and other neural tube defects.

Ultrasound demonstrates the absence of a calvarium and brain above the orbits (see Figs. A and B), cephalad to the brainstem. Although this may be detected as early as 8 weeks, it is diagnosed more reliably in the early second trimester.

Routine screening of maternal serum α-fetoprotein (AFP) is performed between 15 and 20 weeks as part of the serum triple screen (AFP, estriol, and human chorionic gonadotropin). The serum AFP is usually elevated in anencephaly, using either 2.0 or 2.5 multiples of the median (MOM) as the cutoff for detection. It is important that the pregnancy is dated accurately, as the levels vary with gestational age. The serum AFP level will also be abnormal in multiple gestations and obese women. The differential diagnosis for an elevated maternal AFP in pregnancy includes other open defects, such as gastroschisis, as well as fetal-maternal hemorrhage, maternal hepatitis, or maternal hepatocellular carcinoma.

Notes

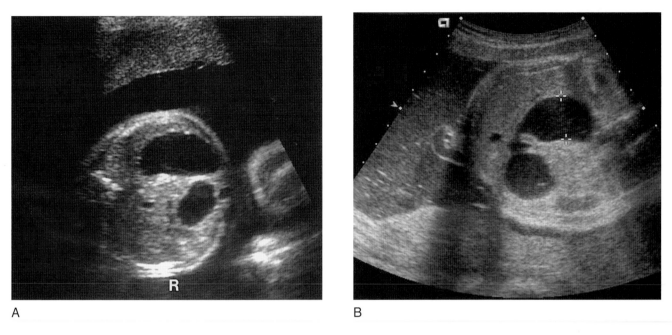

A   B

1. What are the two cystic structures shown on this axial image of the upper abdomen in this 24-week-old fetus (Fig. A; R = right side of the fetus)? Figure B shows the structures joining.

2. What is the most common cause of this finding?

3. What chromosomal anomaly is associated with this finding?

4. What prenatal complications are associated with it?

CASE 15

Duodenal Atresia

1. Stomach (larger) and duodenal bulb (smaller).

2. Duodenal atresia.

3. Down's syndrome.

4. Polyhydramnios (30% of cases) and premature birth (45% of cases).

Reference

Grosfeld JL, Rescorla RJ: Duodenal atresia and stenosis: Reassessment of treatment and outcome based on antenatal diagnosis, pathologic variance and long-term follow-up. *World J Surg* 17:301–309, 1993.

Traubici J: The double bubble sign: *Radiology* 220:463–464, 2001.

Cross-Reference

Ultrasound: THE REQUISITES, 2nd ed, pp 436–437.

Comment

Pathologically, a duodenal obstruction can be intrinsic or extrinsic. Causes of an extrinsic obstruction include annular pancreas, preduodenal portal vein, Ladd's bands, and malrotation. Duodenal obstruction is most commonly caused by duodenal atresia or stenosis, which is classically associated with Down's syndrome (trisomy 21). However, only 30% of the fetuses with duodenal atresia or stenosis have trisomy 21. Intrinsic stenosis/atresia is further categorized as mucosal atresia (type I), fibrous cord (type II), or complete separation of the duodenum (type III), usually near the ampulla of Vater. Concomitant biliary duct anomalies occur most commonly in the type III subset.

Prenatal ultrasound of a duodenal obstruction demonstrates a "double bubble," corresponding to a dilated stomach and duodenal bulb, as shown here. Polyhydramnios develops in 30% of cases (see Fig. A), and 45% are born premature. Both the "double bubble" appearance and polyhydramnios are often not detected until after 24 weeks. This is surprising, because the duodenal obstruction is typically complete by that time. It may be related to the examiner's failure to appreciate the second bubble, if small, as a distended duodenum and the slow accumulation of amniotic fluid, which may not appreciably increase until later in the pregnancy. All congenital causes of duodenal obstruction require surgery.

At least 50% of all fetuses with atresia or stenosis may have an additional anomaly, most commonly a complex cardiac malformation. The cardiac defects cause most of the deaths in these children; thus, although prenatal detection may lead to earlier gastrointestinal surgery, the outcome may still be poor. Other anomalies include esophageal atresia, imperforate anus, renal malformations, and biliary atresia. Once duodenal atresia is detected, a careful search should be conducted for other anomalies with prenatal ultrasound, including a fetal echocardiogram.

Notes

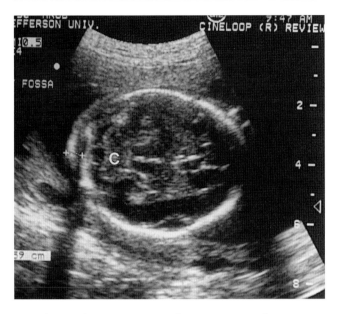

1. What is being measured posterior to the occiput in this 18-week-old fetus (+ signs)? It measures slightly less than 6 mm. Is this normal?

2. What are the proposed etiologies of thickening in this region?

3. What is the significance of thickening in this region that resolves later in the gestation?

4. In fetuses with such abnormal thickness and normal karyotype, is there any other significance?

CASE 16

Nuchal Skin Measurement: Second Trimester

1. Nuchal thickness. Yes.

2. Lymphatic obstruction and cardiac disease.

3. It still carries an increased risk of chromosomal anomaly.

4. Yes, cardiac malformations, various syndromes, and other complications are associated with these findings.

References

Cho JY, Kim KW, Lee YH, Toi A: Measurement of nuchal skin fold thickness in the second trimester: influence of imaging angle and fetal presentation. *Ultrasound Obstet Gynecol* 25:253–257, 2005.

Landwehr JB, Johnson MP, Hume RF, et al: Abnormal nuchal findings on screening ultrasonography: Aneuploidy stratification on the basis of ultrasonographic anomaly and gestational age at detection. *Am J Obstet Gynecol* 175:995–999, 1996.

McAuliffe FM, Hornberger LK, Winsor S, et al: Fetal cardiac defects and increased nuchal translucency thickness: a prospective study. *Am J Obstet Gynecol* 191:1486–1490, 2004.

Reynderes CS, Pauker SP, Benacerraf BR: First trimester isolated fetal nuchal lucency: Significance and outcome. *J Ultrasound Med* 16:101–105, 1997.

Vergani P, Locatelli A, Piccoli, MG, et al: Best second trimester sonographic markers for the detection of trisomy 21. *J Ultrasound Med* 18:469–473, 1999.

Cross-Reference

Ultrasound: THE REQUISITES, 2nd ed, pp 394–395, 473.

Comment

Nuchal thickening is a marker for chromosomal anomalies. In the second trimester (16 to 22 weeks), the nuchal thickness should be no greater than 6 mm. This 6 mm cutoff point is one independent predictor of trisomy 21. This measurement is performed in the axial plane at the level of the thalami. The transducer is *slightly* tilted so that the frontal region is more cephalad, and the posterior fossa is imaged. The region from the surface of the skin to the surface of the occipital skull is measured.

The etiology of nuchal thickening is controversial. Some believe that it is caused by edema owing to cardiovascular abnormalities. In fact, increased nuchal translucency in the first trimester has been shown to be more prevalent in fetuses with major cardiac defects. Lymphatic obstruction is another proposed etiology.

Nuchal thickening and cystic hygromas can resolve as the gestation evolves, although this does not decrease the risk of a karyotype abnormality or change the prognosis.

Nuchal thickening and translucencies can be seen in embryos/fetuses with no chromosomal anomalies. However, those with normal karyotypes have a higher risk of other malformations and syndromes, including Noonan's syndrome, Joubert's syndrome, and multiple pterygium syndrome. In addition, there is an increased risk of spontaneous miscarriage and premature delivery.

Notes

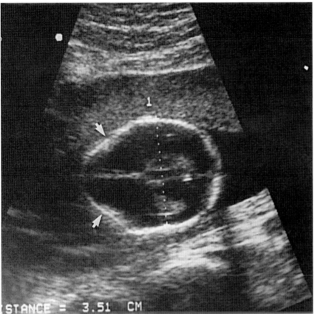
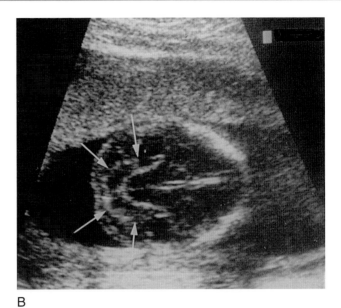

STANCE = 3.51 CM

A

B

1. Which is the most likely cause of the fetal head anomalies in these two second-trimester fetuses? Figures A and B are axial images.

2. Which of the head anomalies in this disorder are more common before 24 weeks' gestation? After 24 weeks?

3. When does the distal spine ossify in normal fetuses?

4. Name two associated musculoskeletal findings.

Myelomeningocele

1. Open spina bifida (meningocele and myelomeningocele).

2. Before 24 weeks: lemon head sign and banana-shaped cerebellum. After 24 weeks: ventriculomegaly and obliterated cisterna magna.

3. After 22 weeks.

4. Clubfoot and scoliosis/kyphosis.

References

Aaronson OS, Hernanz-Schulman M, Bruner JP, Reed GW: Myelomeningococele: prenatal evaluation-comparison between transabdominal US and MR imaging. *Radiology* 227:839–843, 2003.

Babcook CJ, Drake CM, Goldstein RB: Spinal level of fetal myelomeningocele: Does it influence ventricular size? *AJR* 169:207–210, 1997.

Babcook CJ, Goldstein RB, Barth RA, et al: Prevalence of ventriculomegaly in association with myelomeningocele: Correlation with gestational age and severity of posterior fossa deformity. *Radiology* 190:703–707, 1994.

Budorick NE, Pretorius DH, Nelson TR: Sonography of the fetal spine: Technique, imaging findings and clinical implications. *AJR* 164:421–428, 1995.

Thomas MT: The lemon sign. *Radiology* 228:206–207, 2003.

Sepulveda W, Corral E, Ayala C, et al: Chromosomal abnormalities in fetuses with open neural tube defects: prenatal identification with ultrasound. *Ultrasound Obstet Gynecol* 23:352–356, 2004.

Cross-Reference

Ultrasound: THE REQUISITES, 2nd ed, pp 402–406, 410.

Comment

Meningocele and myelomeningocele comprise the spectrum of open spina bifida; the latter contains nerve fibers in addition to meninges and cerebrospinal fluid. These spinal abnormalities can occur anywhere, but they are much more common in the lumbosacral region. (although these are most often not identified on US [see Fig. C]). Almost all are associated with a posterior fossa deformity (Chiari II-hindbrain malformation). A significant number of fetuses are chromosomally abnormal.

Four cranial abnormalities are associated with open spina bifida. As a result of the posterior fossa deformity (see Fig. B), the cerebellum becomes banana-shaped (usually seen before 24 weeks), and the cisterna magna is effaced (more common after 24 weeks). Before 24 weeks, the cranium may have a lemon shape (see Fig. A) (concave or inwardly scalloped frontal bones).

The lemon sign suggests the possibility of spina bifida. Ventriculomegaly is present in 70% to 80% of fetuses and 90% of infants with this disorder and becomes more prevalent after 24 weeks' gestation. It probably results from an obstruction of cerebrospinal flow by the posterior fossa deformity, as the presence of ventriculomegaly correlates with the severity of the posterior fossa defect. However, unlike infants in whom the degree of postoperative ventricular dilatation correlates with the level of the neural tube defect, the level in the fetus does not correlate with ventricular size.

There is increasing use of prenatal magnetic resonance (MR) imaging. However, it has been shown that little difference exists between prenatal MR imaging and ultrasound in determining the level of the lesion in a fetus with a myelomeningocele.

Notes

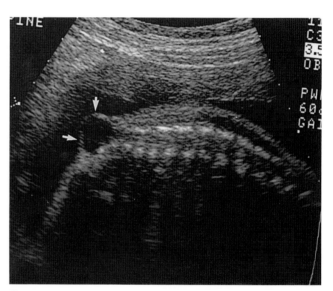

C

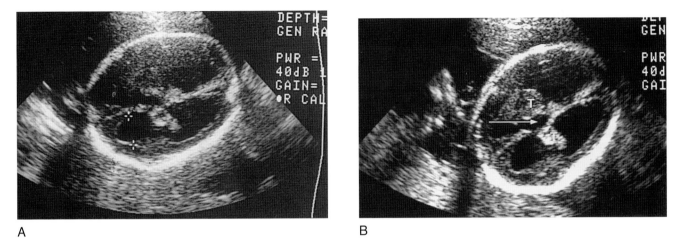

A   B

1. In this second-trimester fetus, what is the most likely etiology for its hydrocephalus (Fig. A, + signs measuring one of the dilated lateral ventricles)?

2. What percentage of causes of fetal hydrocephalus does this comprise?

3. Are other anomalies associated with these findings, and are they significant?

4. Is the outcome generally good?

Aqueductal Stenosis

1. Aqueductal stenosis.

2. 20%.

3. Yes; yes. Other anomalies are Chiari II malformation, Dandy-Walker complex, and agenesis of the corpus callosum.

4. No, mortality is 40%. Only 10% of these children are physically and neuropsychologically normal.

Reference

D'Addario V: The role of ultrasonography in recognizing the cause of fetal cerebral ventriculomegaly. *J Perinat Med* 32:5–12, 2004.

Levitsky DB, Mack LA, Nyberg DA, et al: Fetal aqueductal stenosis diagnosed sonographically: How grave is the prognosis? *AJR* 164:725–730, 1995.

Cross-Reference

Ultrasound: THE REQUISITES, 2nd ed, p 383.

Comment

Aqueductal stenosis is the cause of 20% of the cases of in utero hydrocephalus. It can be congenital, either X-linked or a part of an autosomal recessive disorder. Additionally, in utero infection and hemorrhage can result in aqueductal stenosis. This is a diagnosis of exclusion, once other causes of hydrocephalus have been investigated and ruled out.

The ultrasound findings, as shown by this case, are enlargement of the lateral and third ventricles (Fig. B: arrow = third ventricle; T = thalami). The third ventricle can usually be identified in the third trimester and sometimes in the second trimester. It is normally less than or equal to 2 mm in diameter and is situated between the thalami. In aqueductal stenosis, the dilatation is usually marked, ranging from 3 to 25 mm (mean=10 mm). Measurement of the atria of the lateral ventricles ranges from 15 to 70 mm. Thinning of the frontoparietal cortex may correlate with the degree of developmental impairment.

Associated anomalies can occur in 30% of cases, warranting a careful search with prenatal ultrasound. These anomalies include tracheoesophageal fistula, cleft palate, cardiac malformations (ventricular septal defect, atrial septal defect, transposition of the great vessels), renal agenesis, vertebral abnormalities, and polydactyly. In addition, adduction of the thumb, positioned on the palmar surface, is a characteristic hand configuration associated with aqueductal stenosis. Macrocephaly may dictate the requirement for cesarean section delivery.

Shunting is usually performed postnatally. The mortality rate is nevertheless high at 40%, owing to the associated anomalies; deaths occur in utero, in the neonatal period, and later. Most of the surviving children have degrees of developmental impairment, which relate to the central nervous system malformations.

Notes

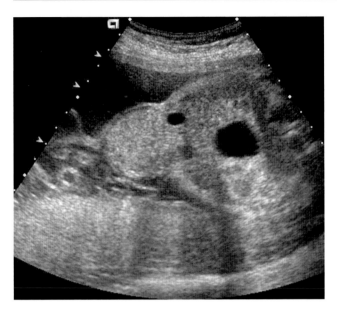

1. In this second-trimester fetus, what is the most likely diagnosis and what are the differential diagnoses of the abnormality projecting anteriorly from the abdomen?

2. Which entity has associated chromosomal anomalies?

3. How does the cord insertion aid in distinguishing the etiology?

4. At what gestational age can this abnormality be reliably diagnosed?

Omphalocele

1. Omphalocele. The differential diagnoses are gastroschisis and limb-body wall complex.

2. Omphalocele.

3. In small omphaloceles, usually containing only bowel, the cord inserts centrally. In large omphaloceles and in the limb-body wall complex, the cord insertion is displaced to the side of the defect. In gastroschisis, the normal cord insertion is identified away from the defect.

4. Because of normal midgut herniation in the first trimester, the diagnosis of omphalocele must await the second trimester.

Reference

Blazer S, Zimmer EZ, Gover A, Bronshtein M: Fetal omphalocele detected early in pregnancy: associated anomalies and outcomes: *Radiology* 232:191–195, 2004.

Emanuel PG, Garcia GI, Angtuaco TL: Prenatal detection of anterior abdominal wall defects with ultrasound. *Radiographics* 15:517–530, 1995.

Wilson RD, Johnson MP: Congenital abdominal wall defects: an update. *Fetal Diagn Ther* 19:385–398, 2004.

Cross-Reference

Ultrasound: THE REQUISITES, pp 443–444.

Comment

An omphalocele is a midline anterior abdominal wall defect that may contain varying amounts of abdominal contents. In those containing only bowel, the primitive body stalk or normal midgut herniation persists beyond 12 weeks. If the liver or other organs herniate into the omphalocele, the lateral body wall fails to migrate, thus precluding closure. A diagnosis with prenatal ultrasound is possible only after 12 weeks, when the normal herniation of the midgut has resolved.

In contradistinction to gastroschisis and the limb-body wall complex, the umbilical cord inserts into the apex of the defect in a small omphalocele. With larger omphaloceles, the cord insertion can be identified at the edge of the omphalocele. A covering membrane of peritoneum is present. In the larger defects, such as that shown in the figure, the hyperechoic areas can be either non–fluid-filled bowel or organs such as the liver. Cystic structures may be either fluid-filled bowel or ascites. Unlike most limb-body wall defects in which scoliosis is often associated with a spinal defect, the scoliosis in some cases of large omphaloceles (when present) represents an otherwise normal spine that "collapses" because of a lack of abdominal contents. Isolated omphaloceles diagnosed early in gestation usually have a good prognosis; small defects may actually disappear later in pregnancy.

Associated malformations are present in up to 90% of cases. Chromosomal anomalies are present in 30% to 40% of cases (most commonly trisomy 13 or 18), particularly those with small bowel involvement. Syndromes that include omphaloceles are Beckwith-Wiedemann syndrome, bladder exstrophy, and pentalogy of Cantrell. Central nervous system, cardiac, gastrointestinal, and genitourinary malformations may be also be associated. Malrotation and intestinal atresia, atrial septal defect, ventriculoseptal defect, tetralogy of Fallot, and ectopia cordis are among the specific anomalies reported. The presence of a concurrent malformation, particularly chromosomal or cardiac, increases mortality to almost 100%.

Notes

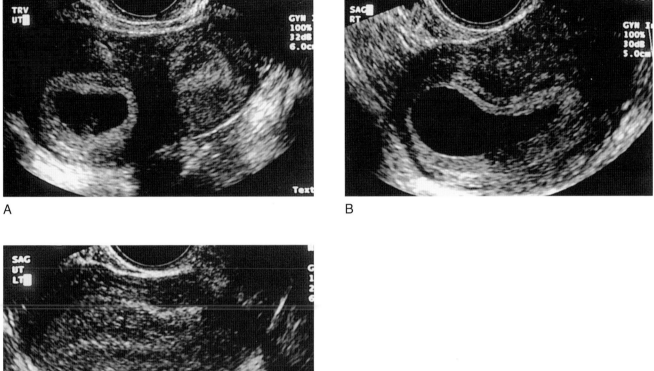

A

B

C

1. Figure A is an axial image of the uterus in the first trimester. Figure B is a sagittal image to the right and Figure C is a sagittal image to the left in the same uterus. What is the diagnosis?

2. Which uterine anomaly has the highest incidence of reproductive dysfunction?

3. Which uterine anomalies are most commonly associated with *early* pregnancy loss? With second- or third-trimester pregnancy loss?

4. Which uterine anomaly has an increased risk of cervical and vaginal neoplasia?

Congenital Uterine Anomalies and Pregnancy

1. Septate or bicornuate uterus with a pregnancy in the right horn.

2. Septate uterus.

3. Early loss: septate, diethylstilbestrol (DES)-related anomalies, and unicornuate uterus with a rudimentary horn. Later loss: bicornuate uterus.

4. DES-related anomalies of T-shaped uterus with a small uterine cavity and cervical constrictions.

Reference

O'Neill MJ, Yoder IC, Connolly SA, Mueller, PR: Imaging evaluation and classification of developmental anomalies of the female reproductive system with an emphasis on MR imaging. *AJR* 173: 407–416, 1999.

Monteagudo A, Strok I, Greenidge S, Timor-Tritsch IE: Quadruplet pregnancy: two sets of twins, each occupying a horn of a septate (complete) uterus. *J Ultrasound Med* 23:1107–1111, 2004.

Troiano RN, McCarthy S: Mullerian duct anomalies: imaging and clinical issues. *Radiology* 233:19–34, 2004.

Wagner BJ, Woodward PJ: Magnetic resonance evaluation of congenital uterine anomalies. *Semin Ultrasound CT MR* 15:4–17, 1994.

Cross-Reference

Ultrasound: THE REQUISITES, 2nd ed, pp 536–538.

Comment

A large study of fertile and infertile women showed that the most common müllerian duct anomaly is septate (55%) uteri. Bicornuate uteri comprised 10%, didelphic 11%, arcuate 7%, unicornuate 20%, and hypoplastic 5% to 10%. All have a higher incidence of renal anomalies, including unilateral agenesis and ptosis.

Uterine anomalies are present in a higher frequency in infertile women. Depending on the congenital anomaly, women may have difficulty with conception, early pregnancy loss, or later complications such as intrauterine growth restriction (IUGR). The septate uterus results in the highest incidence of reproductive difficulties (67%).

Problems with conception may occur with a septate uterus. This may be caused by implantation on the septum, which has an abnormal blood supply. Early pregnancy loss also occurs; other anomalies that have an increased incidence of early pregnancy loss include a unicornuate uterus with a rudimentary horn and DES-related anomalies.

This case shows a pregnancy in the right horn of a bicornuate uterus (see figures). Pregnancy loss occurs more frequently with a bicornuate uterus than with a uterine didelphys or a unicornuate uterus. Pregnancy loss can occur in the first 20 weeks or later in the second or third trimester. Three-dimensional sonography has been used to evaluate uterine malformations, especially when there have been inconsistent results from other imaging modalities and also to locate fetuses more precisely in the uterine horns.

Women whose mothers used DES during pregnancy can have a T-shaped uterus or uterine cavity constrictions that are not amenable to surgical correction. In addition, they have an increased risk of cervical and vaginal malignancies, mesonephric clear cell carcinoma of the cervix and vagina. There are no associated genitourinary anomalies in the DES-related uterine malformations.

Ultrasound and magnetic resonance imaging (MRI) are the best imaging modalities to diagnose a congenital uterine anomaly; the external uterine fundal contour is key. The signal intensity of the tissue separating the two endometrial cavities on MRI can be similar in both entities. In most septate uteri the inferior portion of the septum is uniformly T2 dark. The signal intensity of the upper portion of the septum is similar to that of the myometrium in many patients.

Notes

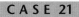

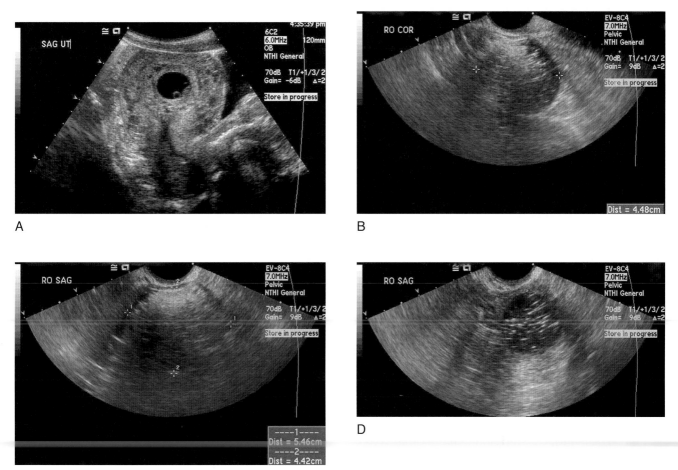

1. In this first-trimester ultrasound examination, where is the abnormality and what is the most likely diagnosis? Figure A is a transabdominal sagittal midline scan showing a living embryo within an intrauterine gestational sac. Figure B is a transvaginal coronal scan to the right of midline showing a mass. Figure C is a transvaginal sagittal image through the same structure (over 5 cm in length; see + signs), and Figure D is a sagittal image through another portion of the mass.

2. In a first-trimester pregnancy, what are the most likely differential diagnoses of a mass detected lateral to the uterus?

3. Do extrauterine masses need to be removed during pregnancy?

4. If it is necessary to perform surgery to remove an extrauterine mass, what would be the best time for this operation?

Normal First-Trimester Intrauterine Pregnancy with Extrauterine Mass, a Cystic Teratoma (Dermoid)

1. An extrauterine mass, probably a cystic teratoma (dermoid).

2. If the mass is cystic, a prominent corpus luteum cyst or nonfunctioning ovarian cyst. If complex, predominantly cystic, a hemorrhagic cyst, endometrioma, cystic teratoma, neoplasm, either benign or malignant, or rarely a concomitant ectopic pregnancy. If solid, a solid ovarian mass (benign or malignant), exophytic fibroid, ovarian torsion, or pelvic kidney.

3. If large, yes.

4. In the early to mid-second trimester, after the fourth month of pregnancy.

Reference

Choi RJ, Levine D, Finberg H: Luteoma of pregnancy: sonographic findings in two cases. *J Ultrasound Med* 19:877–881, 2000.

Di Salvo DN: Sonographic imaging of maternal complications of pregnancy. *J Ultrasound Med* 22:69–89, 2003.

Eastman NJ, Helman LM (eds): *Williams Obstetrics*, 13th ed. Stanford, CT, Appleton Century Crofts, 1966, pp 909–919.

Cross-Reference

Ultrasound: THE REQUISITES, 2nd ed, pp 568–584.

Comment

Extrauterine masses associated with pregnancy can be detected by both transabdominal and transvaginal ultrasound examinations. Their detection is commonly an incidental finding, although occasionally the physical examination may suggest the abnormality. These masses are usually ovarian in origin. When cystic, they may be a corpus luteum cyst or nonfunctioning ovarian cyst. If complex, they can be a hemorrhagic cyst, cystic teratoma, or neoplasm (cystadenomas and cystadenocarcinomas). Although endometriomas are often associated with infertility, they may be seen following pregnancy and can be extraovarian or, less commonly, ovarian. Solid masses are often exophytic fibroids, solid benign ovarian masses, ovarian carcinoma, or a pelvic kidney. Ovarian luteomas are rare non-neoplastic usually solid masses that regress spontaneously after delivery. Abscesses can vary in their appearance and typically are accompanied by significant symptoms. A hydrosalpinx appears tubular, especially on a transvaginal study. Ovarian torsion is more often solid and related to pain. Although usually associated with a lead mass, necrosis tends to produce an amorphous solid appearance.

This case shows a fairly typical appearance for one of the more common extrauterine masses (a cystic teratoma [dermoid]) detected during pregnancy (see Figs. B, C, and D). The mass is well circumscribed with hyperechoic areas and low-level or fine linear echoes.

Ovarian tumors may cause complications during pregnancy. These tumors are associated with the increased possibility of a spontaneous abortion; they may undergo torsion and they may pose obstacles to vaginal delivery. The second trimester is generally the time for exploration of worrisome adnexal masses, since the risk of spontaneous abortion is highest in the first trimester and in the third trimester the risk of preterm labor is highest. Even after spontaneous labor, the tumors may cause disturbances in the postpartum period. Although all types of ovarian tumors may complicate pregnancy and delivery, most of them are cystic. They occur once in every 81 pregnancies, but the ones that are of sufficient size to constitute a hazard to pregnancy are considered to have an incidence of only 1 in 328. Dermoids have been described comparatively frequently. The most frequent and serious complication of ovarian cystic masses is torsion, which frequently occurs after 9 weeks. The cysts may rupture and extrude their contents into the peritoneal cavity during spontaneous labor or as a result of operative interference. If the tumor blocks the pelvis, it can rupture the uterus or be forced into the vagina and occasionally even into the rectum.

Many ovarian tumors complicating pregnancy are asymptomatic and therefore unsuspected. Ultrasound can detect extrauterine tumors, particularly smaller ones that may not cause many of these complications. However, if these tumors are clinically considered to be large enough to cause problems (usually >4 to 5 cm), they should be removed. There is a pregnancy loss rate from surgery, and it is therefore thought that the early to mid-second trimester (after the fourth month of pregnancy) offers the most opportune time for removal of these masses. Although there is still a chance that the operation may lead to a spontaneous abortion, the danger is minimal compared with that of possible torsion or rupture of the cyst or interruption of later labor and delivery. If the diagnosis of an extrauterine mass is not made until later in the pregnancy, however, it is usually advisable to postpone surgery until term unless there is a high suspicion of cancer.

Notes

A

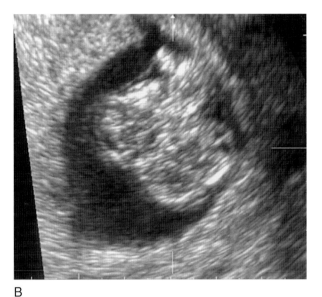

B

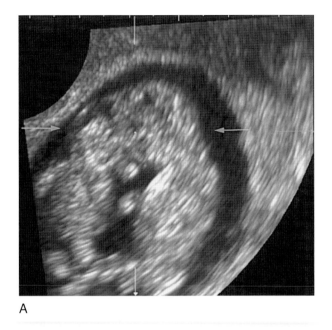

C

1. A woman presents because of uncertain menstrual dates in the late first trimester for evaluation of embryonic age. What are the findings on this transvaginal examination? (Figs. A and B are both three-dimensional [3-D] multiplanar reconstructed images. Fig. A is taken obliquely through the gestational sac, and Fig. B is taken through a plane of section at the arrows in Fig. A.)

2. In the first trimester, what are the ultrasound findings that allow the examiner to determine that a twin gestation is dichorionic-diamniotic (Di-Di)?

3. In the first trimester, the failure to identify an interposed membrane makes the diagnosis of what type of twinning most likely?

4. The detection of conjoined (Siamese) twins raises what possible problems in utero for the twins? For the pregnant woman?

Conjoined (Siamese) Twins in the First Trimester

1. Conjoined (Siamese) twins, joined at the heads.

2. Either two separate sacs, or if the sacs abut one another, a thick (>2 mm) interposed membrane.

3. A monochorionic-monoamniotic (Mono-Mono) twinning.

4. In utero, there are no problems for either the conjoined twins or the pregnant woman. At birth, cesarean section delivery is required.

Acknowledgment

Figures courtesy of Dr. George Bega.

References

Bromley B: Using the number of yolk sacs to determine amnionicity in early first trimester monochorionic twins: *J Ultrasound Med* 14:415–419, 1995.

Feldstein VA: Complications of monochorionic twins. *Radiol Clin North Am* 41:709–727, 2003.

Fong KW, Ants T, Salem S, et al: Detection of fetal structural abnormalities with US during early pregnancy. *RadioGraphics* 24:157–174, 2004.

Hertzberg BS, Kurtz AB, Choi HY, et al: Significance of membrane thickness in the sonographic evaluation of twin pregnancies. *AJR* 148:151–153, 1987.

Kurtz AB, Wapner RJ, Mata J, et al: Twin pregnancies: Accuracy of first trimester abdominal ultrasound in predicting chorionicity and amnionicity. *Radiology* 185:759–762, 1992.

Cross-Reference

Ultrasound: THE REQUISITES, 2nd ed, pp 516, 525–526.

Comment

Most twins (80%) are "fraternal," originating from two separate fertilized ova that develop within separate sacs (their own amniotic and chorionic sacs) and are therefore Di-Di twins. Their ultrasound detection, particularly in the first trimester, is often straightforward: either two separate sacs or a distinct separating intervening membrane (>2 mm) if the sacs impinge on each other. In the first trimester, it is estimated that the accuracy of detection of a Di-Di twinning by transabdominal imaging is approximately 100%; if uncertainty remains, twinning can be detected by a transvaginal study.

In the remaining 20% of twin pregnancies, a single fertilized ovum starts to develop and then splits into "identical" twins of the same gender. If this split occurs before the first day (20–30% of cases), the twins develop in completely separate Di-Di sacs similar to true "fraternal" twins.

In the remaining cases of "identical" twins, the fertilized ovum splits later and is enveloped by a single chorion (monochorionic). The twins then share the same environment, either partially (monochorionicdiamniotic [Mono-Di]) or completely (Mono-Mono).

Mono-Di twinning (70–75% of identical twins) occurs 1 to 7 days after fertilization. The ultrasound finding of a thin intervening diamniotic membrane is difficult to detect at any time in the pregnancy but is seen most consistently in the first trimester. This may require transvaginal imaging.

In the remaining 1% to 3% of cases of "identical" twins, with the split occurring between days 7 and 13, the twins completely share the same environment. This is a Mono-Mono pregnancy without an intervening membrane. A transvaginal study is needed in the first trimester. Despite the concern that a thin diamniotic membrane may not have been appreciated, the diagnosis of no interposed membrane is fairly accurate. Later in the pregnancy, the diagnosis of a Mono-Mono twinning is less certain. However the presence of one yolk sac early in the first trimester should prompt a follow-up ultrasonogram to assign a definitive amnionicity. Yolk sacs can be seen in the amnionic membrane before 8 weeks' gestation. All twin pregnancies are at risk for perinatal morbidity and mortality compared with singleton gestations, but the potential for problems is much greater when the twins share the same amnionic sac.

In rare instances, far fewer than 1%, the fertilized ovum separates after 12 to 13 days. The twins not only share the same sac (Mono-Mono twinning) but also cannot be completely separated, called a conjoined (Siamese) twinning. This most commonly occurs in the thoracic region (thoracopagus). When the thorax and abdominal regions fail to separate, this is called thoracoabdominopagus. Conjoined twins can be joined anywhere from the head (craniopagus) to the pelvis (ischiopagus).

Conjoined twins can share very little or a great deal of their internal structures. Regardless, their in utero development and the mother's welfare, aside from being Mono-Mono twinning with the additional complication of entangled umbilical cords, is unaffected. However, the mode of delivery must be by cesarean section because the overall size of the twins is too large for vaginal delivery.

The late first-trimester diagnosis of conjoined twins is possible, particularly with transvaginal imaging. To accurately make this diagnosis, not only is it necessary to show that the twins are inseparable (e.g., in Figure A, which suggests that the fetal heads are joined) but also to show that they share internal structures. This is further, but not definitively, shown in Figure B, which shows a scan through the fetal heads. To help further define this case of craniopagus, a 3-D surface imaging reconstruction was performed (Fig. C). All three images make this diagnosis highly likely; however, when doubt remains, it is suggested that the pregnancy be re-examined in the second trimester to confirm the diagnosis and determine the extent of shared internal anatomy.

In this case (see Figs. A–C), 3-D reformatting was important and should be considered whenever the fetal anatomy is difficult to image. The conjoined twins were in an unusual oblique presentation, and standard 2-D images failed to obtain good planes of section. At present, however, the 3-D reconstructed images are not of the same high resolution as 2-D images, although this situation has been gradually improving.

Notes

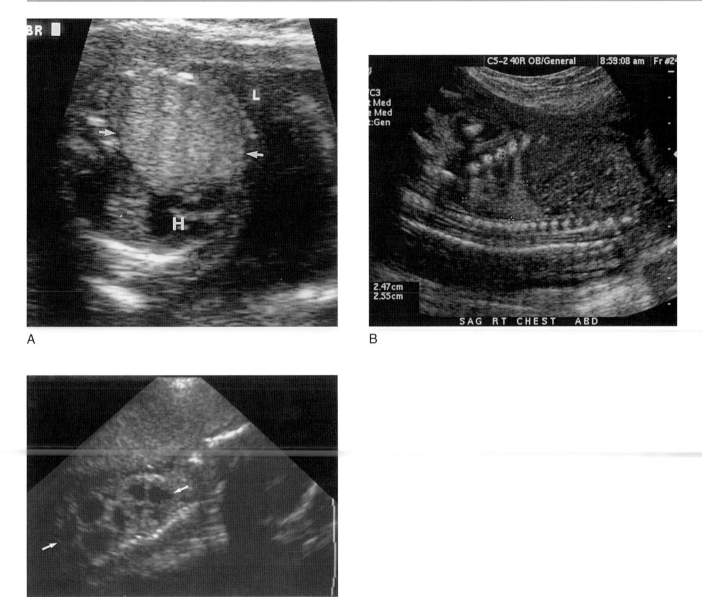

A

B

C

1. Three presentations of the same abnormality are shown in these images of the fetal chest (Fig. A, axial: arrows = an anomaly. H = heart; L = left side of fetus. Fig. B, sagittal: fetal head toward the reader's left; x = an anomaly. Fig. C, sagittal: fetal head toward the reader's right; arrows = an anomaly). What is the diagnosis in these second-trimester fetuses?

2. Which fetal lung masses may appear cystic on a prenatal ultrasound scan?

3. Which fetal lung masses may have associated anomalies?

4. What predicts the outcome of the neonate with a cystic adenomatoid malformation (CAM)?

Cystic Adenomatoid Malformation

1. CAM type III (see Figs. A and B) and type I (see Fig. C).

2. CAM type I or II, bronchogenic cyst, lobar emphysema, or diaphragmatic hernia containing bowel.

3. CAM type II, extralobar sequestration, and diaphragmatic hernia.

4. Associated anomalies and the amount of residual functioning lung.

Acknowledgment

Figure B courtesy of Beverly Coleman, M.D.

References

Ankermann T, Oppermann HC, Engler S, et al: Congenital masses of the lung, cystic adenomatoid malformation versus congenital lobar emphysema. *J Ultrasound Med* 23:1379–1384, 2004.

Johnson JA, Rumack CM, Johnson ML, et al: Cystic adenomatoid malformation: Antenatal demonstration. *AJR* 142:483–484, 1984.

King SJ, Pilling DW, Walkinshaw S: Fetal echogenic lung lesions: Prenatal ultrasound diagnosis and outcome. *Pediatr Radiol* 25:208–210, 1995.

Winters WD, Effmann EL: Congenital masses of the lung: Prenatal and postnatal imaging evaluation. *J Thorac Imaging* 16:196–206, 2001.

Cross-Reference

Ultrasound: THE REQUISITES, 2nd ed, pp 424–426.

Comment

Congenital CAM is a hamartomatous mass of pulmonary tissue in the lung. It can arise in any lobe of the lung. The classification depends on the size of the cysts. Type I has large cysts (>2 cm), and type II has small cysts. Type III consists of multiple tiny bronchiolar structures and appears as a solid mass. Concomitant renal and gastrointestinal anomalies are present with type II cysts.

On ultrasound, a mass that is cystic (see Fig. C), solid and hyperechoic (see Figs. A and B), or both, can be seen. Type II CAM can also appear solid on prenatal ultrasound scans if it consists of tiny cysts. In any of these types, the heart and mediastinum may shift (see Fig. A); the cardiac shift and caval compression can result in hydrops. Polyhydramnios is common, probably due to esophageal compression. Detection of a large mass is imperative, because the neonate with a large CAM often has severe respiratory distress necessitating immediate surgery. With large lesions, the outcome depends on the amount of residual functional lung and the presence of associated malformations.

The differential diagnosis of a chest mass depends on the ultrasound characteristics, and serial prenatal ultrasound studies are important.. A solid hyperechoic mass may represent a sequestration, type III CAM, a diaphragmatic hernia containing the liver, or a focal hyperechoic lung due to bronchial obstruction (atresia or mucous plug). A cystic mass could be a type I or II CAM, lobar emphysema, a bronchogenic cyst, or a bowel containing a diaphragmatic hernia.

Detection of any fetal mass warrants a careful search for associated anomalies, present infrequently with extralobar sequestration, and described in association with type II CAM. Close follow-up is required to detect the complication of hydrops if a large mass is present. Postnatal resection of CAM is recommended because of its malignant potential.

Notes

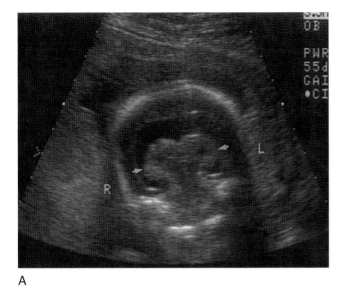

A

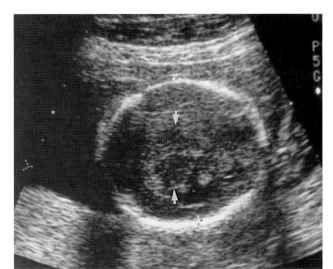

B

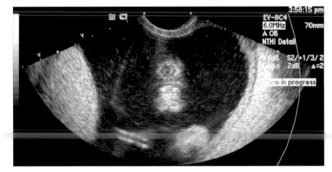

C

(Reprinted with permission from Doubilet P, Benson C: Atlas of Ultrasound and Obstetric Gynecology. Philadelphia, Lippincott Williams and Wilkins, 2003.)

1. What is the spectrum of abnormalities characteristic of the disorder demonstrated by these coronal (Fig. A) and axial (Fig. B) ultrasound images of the fetal brain and coronal image of the fetal face (Fig. C). Among this spectrum, which subtype is shown in this case?

2. Are chromosomal anomalies associated with this disorder?

3. What extracranial malformations have been described in association with this abnormality?

4. What is the prognosis?

Holoprosencephaly

1. Holoprosencephaly: alobar (most severe), semilobar, and lobar (least severe). Alobar subtype.

2. Yes, most commonly trisomy 13.

3. Omphalocele, polydactyly, renal dysplasia, and complex cardiac defects.

4. Dismal, for both alobar and semilobar holoprosencephaly. Variable for the lobar form.

Reference

Blaas HG, Eriksson AG, Salvesen KA, et al: Brains and faces in holoprosencephaly: pre- and postnatal description of 30 cases. *Ultrasound Obstet Gynecol* 20:304–305, 2002.

Fitz CR: Holoprosencephaly and septo-optic dysplasia. *Neuroimaging Clin North Am* 4:263–281, 1994.

Nyberg DA, Mack LA, Bronstein A, et al: Holoprosencephaly: Prenatal sonographic diagnosis. *AJR* 149:1050–1058, 1987.

Sepulveda W, Dezerega V, Be C: First-trimester sonographic diagnosis of holoprosencephaly: value of the "butterfly" sign. *J Ultrasound Med* 23:761–765, 2004.

Cross-Reference

Ultrasound: THE REQUISITES, 2nd ed, pp 383–387, 389.

Comment

Holoprosencephaly consists of a spectrum of midline brain and facial malformations caused by incomplete cleavage of the forebrain during early fetal development at about 6 weeks. The classification consists of alobar holoprosencephaly (most severe), semilobar (often difficult to distinguish from alobar on prenatal ultrasound), and lobar (least severe). Alobar holoprosencephaly includes a small head, fused thalamus (see Figs. A, B, and C), a monoventricle, and absence of the corpus callosum, falx cerebri, optic tracts, and olfactory bulbs. Incomplete fusion of the thalami and partial segmentation of the ventricle distinguish semilobar from alobar holoprosencephaly. The mildest form, lobar holoprosencephaly, consists of an absence of optic tracts and olfactory bulbs, similar to septo-optic dysplasia.

The appearance of the ventricular system varies with the severity of the disorder. In alobar holoprosencephaly, there is a monoventricle, with occipital, temporal, and frontal horns absent. Occipital horns may be present in semilobar holoprosencephaly. In the least severe lobar variant, the lateral ventricles are present, but frontal horns do not form. Failure to identify the "butterfly" sign of both choroid plexuses in the cross-section fetal brain image is a warning sign of holoprosencephaly in the first trimester.

Chromosomal anomalies and extracranial and facial malformations have all been associated. Approximately 55% of cases have chromosomal anomalies—most commonly trisomy 13. Facial anomalies are more common in the alobar form and include various orbital and nasal malformations (see Fig. C) ranging from fused orbits with supraorbital proboscis (cyclopia), hypotelorism with midline proboscis (ethmocephaly), hypotelorism, single nostril (cebocephaly) to a medial facial cleft. Extracranial abnormalities described include omphalocele, renal dysplasia, polydactyly, and complex cardiac anomalies.

Notes

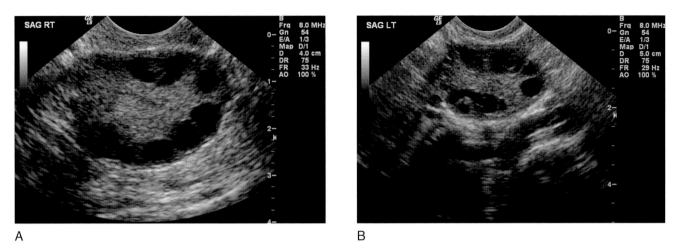

A

B

1. This 25-year-old woman presents with infertility. The ultrasound appearance and size of her ovaries (the volume of the right ovary is 18 mL, and that of the left ovary is 14 mL) suggest what diagnosis?

2. Is surgery necessary in this type of condition? If not, what is the alternative?

3. Is there an associated syndrome with these ultrasound findings of the ovaries?

4. What are the typical findings in this syndrome, and is the syndrome often present?

Polycystic Ovarian Disease

1. Polycystic ovarian disease (PCOD). Multiple small peripherally placed follicles.

2. No; fertility medication, particularly clomiphene citrate (Clomid), may cause successful ovulation and pregnancy.

3. Yes, Stein-Leventhal syndrome.

4. Hirsutism, infertility, and polycystic ovaries; no, the entire syndrome is not typically present.

References

Atiomo WU, Pearson S, Shaw S, Prentice A, et al: Ultrasound criteria in the diagnosis of polycystic ovary syndrome (PCOS). *Ultrasound Med Biol* 26:977–980, 2000.

Balen AH, Laven JS, Tan SL, Dewailly D: Ultrasound assessment of the polycystic ovary: international consensus definitions. *Hum Reprod Update* 9:505–514, 2003.

Dolz M, Osborne NG, Blanes J, et al: Polycystic ovarian syndrome: assessment with color Doppler angiography and three-dimensional ultrasonography. *J Ultrasound Med* 18:303–313, 1999.

Franks S: Polycystic ovary syndrome. Review article. *NEJM* 13:853–861, 1995.

Cross-Reference

Ultrasound: THE REQUISITES, 2nd ed, pp 566–567, 569.

Comment

PCOD has a spectrum of findings, both sonographic and clinically. Ultrasound findings do not always correlate with clinical and biochemical ones. Polycystic ovaries (PCOs) can be detected incidentally in normally fertile women who do not have additional problems. The most common ovarian feature is multiple small follicles between 5 and 8 mm in size, typically peripherally located (see Figs. A and B). The classic appearance of PCOD is that of rounded enlarged ovaries, commonly at least greater than 10 mL in volume (length × width × height ÷ 2). However, PCOs may be normal in size, ovoid instead of round, and not enlarged. Polycystic ovaries are more vascular than normal. A more recent international joint consensus meeting concluded that the definition of PCOs should have at least one of the following: either 12 or more follicles measuring 2 to 9 mm in diameter or increased ovarian volume >10 cm. A description of the stroma is not required for the diagnosis under these new criteria.

Although PCOD may be incidentally noted, without clinical or physical examination findings, it can also be associated with various clinical and laboratory findings.

The full-blown clinical syndrome is hirsutism, infertility, and oligomenorrhea, and it is then called Stein-Leventhal syndrome. In these cases, there are frequently abnormal serum antigens or an increased luteinizing hormone/follicle-stimulating hormone ratio.

The diagnosis of PCOD is, therefore, based primarily on the ultrasound examination. The clinical significance of PCOs is based on clinical symptoms and laboratory findings.

PCOs are known pathologically to have fibrous capsules. The capsules cannot be appreciated by ultrasound imaging, but their presence has been thought to be the cause of the infertility, since the follicles could not rupture and release their ova. As a result, past treatment was surgical wedge resection of the ovary to disrupt this capsule. With the advent of fertility medicines, however, in particular clomiphene citrate, the treatment has become hormonal. Gonadotropins are often used.

Notes

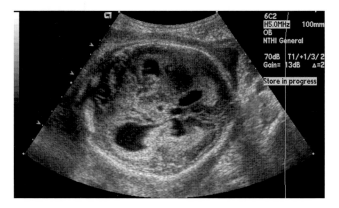

1. In this second-trimester fetal head, the atrium of the lateral ventricles measures 15 mm. What is the normal range of size for the atrium of the lateral ventricle?

2. List three causes of hydrocephalus.

3. Is there an association of hydrocephalus with other central nervous system (CNS) or systemic malformations?

4. Does postnatal ventricular shunting benefit noncommunicating or communicating hydrocephalus?

Hydrocephalus

1. Four to 8 mm (up to 10 mm).

2. Aqueductal stenosis, Arnold-Chiari malformation, mass (rare).

3. Yes; with CNS malformations, systemic malformations, and chromosomal anomalies.

4. Obstructive or noncommunicating hydrocephalus.

References

D'Addario V: The role of ultrasonography in recognizing the cause of fetal cerebral ventriculomegaly. *J Perinat Med* 32:5–12, 2004.

Davis GH: Fetal hydrocephalus. *Clin Perinatol* 30:531–539, 2003.

Durfee SM, Kim, FM, Benson CB: Postnatal outcome of fetuses with the prenatal diagnosis of asymmetric hydrocephalus. *J Ultrasound Med* 20:179–181, 2001.

Hertzberg BS, Kliewer MA, Bowie JD: Fetal cerebral ventriculomegaly: Misidentification of the true medial boundary of the ventricle at ultrasound. *Radiology* 205:813–816, 1997.

Hilpert PL, Hall BE, Kurtz AB: The atria of the fetal lateral ventricles: A sonographic study of normal atrial size and choroid plexus volume. *AJR* 164:731–734, 1995.

Cross-Reference

Ultrasound: THE REQUISITES, 2nd ed, pp 376, 379, 381–383, 404–406.

Comment

Fetal hydrocephalus can be diagnosed with prenatal ultrasound by detecting an enlarged atrium of the lateral ventricle. The upper limits of normal are 8 mm before 25 weeks' gestation and 10 mm later in the gestation period. The normal choroid plexus should fill 50% to 60% of the lateral ventricle. In the setting of hydrocephalus, choroid is surrounded by fluid within the dilated ventricle and appears to dangle, an important secondary sign.

Care must be taken to obtain an accurate measurement of the lateral ventricle. The atrium must be measured perpendicularly at the edge of the choroid plexus. False enlargement can be diagnosed if the interface with the subarachnoid space is misinterpreted as the lateral border of the ventricle; additionally, the medial boundary of the cerebral hemisphere must not be mistaken for the medial border of the lateral ventricle. Typically, the lateral ventricle farther from the transducer is better seen, whereas the closer ventricle is obscured by reverberation artifact from the overlying calvarium (see figure).

The etiology of hydrocephalus may be difficult to determine in utero. Its natural progression is not entirely understood. It is almost always associated with other intracranial and extracranial anomalies. Aqueductal stenosis presents with enlarged third and lateral ventricles but a small fourth ventricle. Arnold-Chiari malformation consists of a myelomeningocele, a small posterior fossa, and associated ventriculomegaly as well as a lemon-shaped skull early in the gestation. An obstructing mass is an uncommon cause of fetal hydrocephalus. Asymmetric hydrocephalus has fewer associated anomalies compared with symmetric hydrocephalus, and the asymmetric type has a better prognosis.

Notes

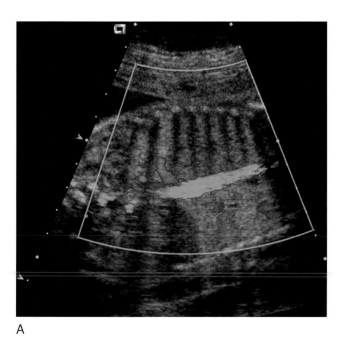

A

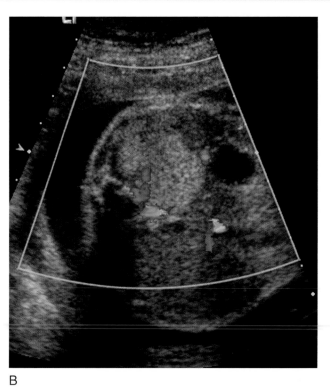

B

1. What is the most likely diagnosis of the thoracic mass shown in the coronal and axial color Doppler images of the fetal chest?

2. How does color Doppler imaging help in making the diagnosis?

3. Are there any anomalies associated with this entity?

4. Where are such masses typically located?

C A S E   2 7

Sequestration

1. The diagnosis is sequestration.

2. By means of identification of a systemic feeding artery.

3. Infrequently with the extralobar type of sequestration.

4. Typically in the lower lobe; on the left side more than the right side.

References

Bromley B, Parad R, Estroff JA, Benacerraf BR: Fetal lung masses: Prenatal course and outcome. *J Ultrasound Med* 14:927–936, 1995.

Felker RE, Tonkin IL: Imaging of pulmonary sequestration. *AJR* 154:241–249, 1990.

Hernanz-Schulman M, Stein SM, Neblett WW, et al: Pulmonary sequestration: Diagnosis with color Doppler sonography and new theory of associated hydrothorax. *Radiology* 180:817–821, 1991.

Dhingsa R, Coakley FV, Albanese CT, et al: Pictorial essay; prenatal sonography and MR imaging of pulmonary sequestration. *AJR* 180:433–437, 2003.

Cross-Reference

Ultrasound: THE REQUISITES, 2nd ed, p 426.

Comment

Pulmonary sequestration is defined as a portion of the lung that receives systemic rather than pulmonary arterial supply and is separated from the tracheobronchial tree. Intralobar sequestration is most common, contained within the normal pleura. Extralobar sequestration has its own pleura. Because intralobar sequestrations present in infants older than 2 months, many believe that sequestration is an acquired entity. Accordingly, most prenatally diagnosed sequestrations are extralobar. Extralobar sequestrations can be located between the lower lobe and the hemidiaphragm, within the diaphragm or lung, in the pleural or pericardial space, and even in the retroperitoneum. Most occur on the left side. Both intralobar and extralobar sequestrations have systemic arterial supply, usually from the aorta.

Prenatal ultrasound shows a supradiaphragmatic or infradiaphragmatic hyperechoic mass, usually on the left side. Mediastinal and cardiac shift will result if the sequestration is large. In some cases, as the fetus grows, the sequestration becomes relatively smaller. Blood flow may be evident on color Doppler imaging, and in some cases the systemic arterial supply may be visible from the aorta (see Fig. A). Polyhydramnios may be present. Rarely, tension hydrothorax and hydrops may occur and are believed to result from torsion of the sequestration.

Extralobar sequestration has an excellent prognosis and frequently regresses spontaneously.

Notes

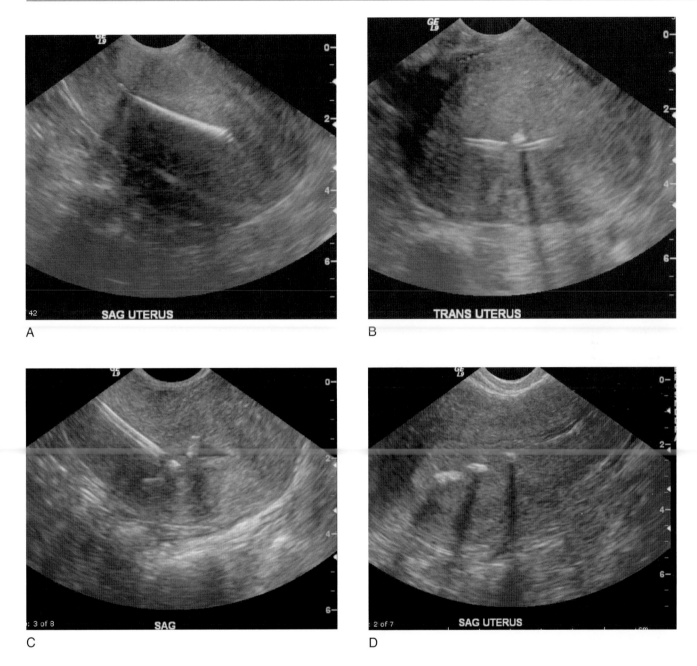

A   SAG UTERUS

B   TRANS UTERUS

C   SAG

D   SAG UTERUS

1. A 30-year-old woman with a previously inserted intrauterine contraceptive device (IUCD-T-shaped) presents for ultrasound of the uterus because of menorrhagia (Fig. C). What does the image show? Figures A and B are of a second asymptomatic patient with the same IUCD as patient in C, and Figures D and E are of a third asymptomatic patient with a different type of IUCD (Lippes loop). Figures F and G (coronal and sagittal transabdominal and sagittal transvaginal views) are of a fourth asymptomatic patient with a new type of IUCD that is often difficult to discern on ultrasound images; see arrow showing shadowing from the device.

2. What is the role of ultrasound in the evaluation of an IUCD?

3. On physical examination of the pelvis, if the string is not identified, what are the three diagnostic possibilities?

4. Are IUCDs currently used in the United States?

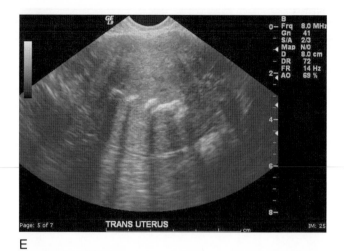

E

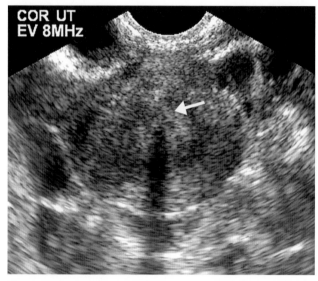

F

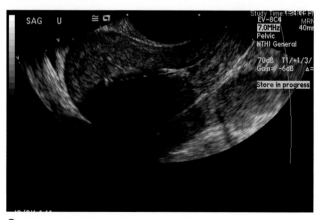

G

Intrauterine Contraceptive Device

1. The image shows that the IUCD is embedded in the uterine wall; it is improperly positioned.

2. To evaluate for the intrauterine presence and position of the IUCD.

3. The three diagnostic possibilities are that (a) the IUCD is in correct position, but the string has pulled back into the cervical or uterine canal; (b) The IUCD has been expelled along with the string; and (c) the IUCD has partially or completely perforated the uterine wall and the string has, therefore, been pulled up into the uterine canal or into or through the myometrium.

4. Yes.

Reference

Copeland LJ: *Textbook of Gynecology.* Philadelphia, WB Saunders, 1993, pp 164–169.

Grimes DA, Jones KP, Knutson CC, Wysocki S: New Developments in Intrauterine Contraception. Assoc. of Reproductive Health Professionals. *ARHP Clinical Proceedings,* Sept 2004, pp 1–20.

Cross-Reference

Ultrasound: THE REQUISITES, 2nd ed, pp 544–549.

Comment

IUCDs have been used since the early 1900s to prevent pregnancy. Since then, the devices have been steadily refined, and today many types are available. IUCDs are better suited for older women who have already been pregnant. Younger IUCD users experience higher pregnancy rates and more expulsions, and they have the devices removed more frequently for medical reasons. Contraindications to use of an IUCD include pregnancy, a history of pelvic inflammatory disease, undiagnosed vaginal bleeding, uterine anomalies, and large fibroid tumors. Primarily for these reasons, IUCD use has significantly decreased in the United States.

IUCDs have a number of different ultrasound appearances, depending on their shape and composition. They use thin plastic tubing, metal wrapping, or a combination of both. A Copper 7, for example, has a long arm of wrapped copper along the long axis of the uterus and a small arm of plastic in transaxial view in the upper body or fundus. The metal wrapping exhibits a "reverberation artifact," a series of parallel lines that get weaker and weaker from the IUCD posteriorly when the IUCD is parallel to the ultrasound beam. The plastic tubing appears as two parallel lines, an entrance and an exit echo.

Ultrasound is very accurate in detecting an IUCD when it is correctly positioned. When the uterus is normal and there is no distortion of the endometrial canal, the IUCD has a midline position. However, with an IUCD in place, the thickness of the endometrial complex is difficult to evaluate. When fibroids or a retroverted or retroflexed uterus (typically a globular-appearing uterus) is present, the determination of the exact position of the IUCD in relation to the endometrial complex may become difficult. Fibroids may change the position of the uterine cavity so that the IUCD may appear to be partially perforating the uterine wall.

One of the most common clinical uses of ultrasound in the evaluation of IUCDs is to determine whether the IUCD is still present within the uterus when the string is no longer present on pelvic examination. Because of the potential for expulsion and for perforation either into or through the uterine wall (Fig. C), failure to detect a string within the vagina often leads to an ultrasound examination. If the IUCD is well positioned within the uterus, then the retracted string is of no consequence. Conversely, the failure to detect an IUCD is often an accurate determination of expulsion. When clinical symptoms still make perforation likely, a negative uterine study does not entirely rule out perforation, and a plain anteroposterior radiograph of the pelvis may be used to detect the perforated radiopaque IUCD.

IUCDs have complications. In addition to unexpected pregnancies, infections are more common. Although typically bacterial, there may also be fungal infections including actinomycosis. Expulsion may also occur. If a pregnancy occurs after implantation of an IUCD, the role of ultrasound is to detect whether it is still present. The IUCD does not create a risk to the pregnancy, because it is in the endometrial cavity and is not within the chorionic sac. However, if on physical examination, the string is still projecting into the vagina, the cervical plug will not form and there is a potential for an ascending infection. The IUCD should then be removed, often under ultrasound guidance

A new IUCD has recently come into use in the United States. See Figs. F and G. This levonorgestrel intrauterine contraceptive device (LNG IUS) commonly known as Mirena is growing in popularity because it is so well tolerated even in primiparous women. The LNG IUS consists of a small T-shaped frame with a steroid reservoir which contains levonorgestrel. This hormone is a potent progestin found in many combination oral contraceptives. Unlike other IUCDs, the main frame of this levonorgestrel intrauterine contraceptive device is often poorly delineated on even the best quality ultrasound images. This IUCD is identified mostly by the shadowing it produces at specific points. It is important to be familiar with the different appearances of the IUCDs in order to accurately assess their appropriate positions.

Notes

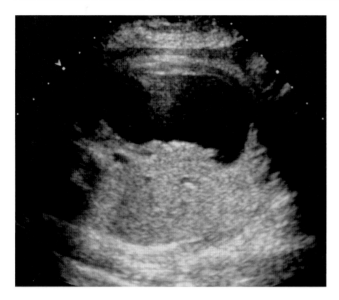

1. What is the cystic structure in the left upper quadrant in this second-trimester fetus (axial image of the upper abdomen)? Is it enlarged?

2. Name a potential cause of a distended stomach.

3. When is the stomach reliably visualized?

4. When does the fetus begin swallowing?

Enlarged Fetal Stomach

1. Stomach. Yes.

2. Duodenal atresia.

3. By 19 weeks.

4. At 11 gestational weeks.

References

Blaas HG, Eik-Nes SH, Kiserud T, Hellevik LR: Early development of the abdominal wall, stomach and heart from 7 to 12 weeks of gestation: A longitudinal ultrasound study. *Ultrasound Obstet Gynecol* 6:240–249, 1995.

Ozmen MN, Onderoglu L, Ciftci AO, et al: Prenatal diagnosis of gastric duplication cyst. *J Ultrasound Med* 16:219–222, 1997.

Zimmer EZ, Chao CR, Abramovich G, Timor-Tritsch IE: Fetal stomach measurements: Not reproducible by the same observer. *J Ultrasound Med* 11:663–665, 1992.

Cross-Reference

Ultrasound: THE REQUISITES, pp 431, 434–436.

Comment

Visualization of a normal fetal stomach is important in order to exclude esophageal disease, cardiovascular disease, and gastric and small bowel anomalies. The fetal stomach should be seen in normal patients by 19 weeks; one series using transvaginal ultrasound demonstrated gastric visualization in all normal cases by 11 weeks. The location and size of the stomach are specific criteria that are assessed in utero. An abnormal location with regard to the heart is an indicator of cardiovascular disease.

Reference charts are available describing the normal mean gastric size at any gestational age. Because the stomach is dynamic, measurements are difficult to reproduce reliably in normal patients. The fetus initiates swallowing movements at 11 weeks. As early as 14 weeks' gestational age, the stomach can be shown to fill and empty. A small or absent stomach can be seen with several abnormalities, including esophageal atresia, oligohydramnios, and central nervous system or neck malformations that prevent swallowing.

Enlargement of the fetal stomach (see figure) is a less well-known potential sign of abnormality. It has been described in cases of duodenal atresia. The differential diagnosis of a cystic mass in the region of the stomach includes the rare gastric duplication cyst. These cysts occur most commonly along the greater curvature and do not usually communicate with the stomach; thus they remain fixed in size.

Notes

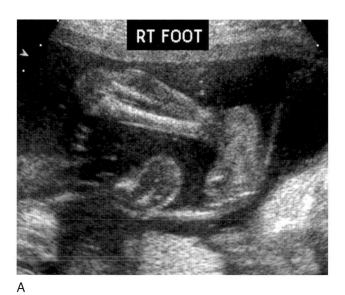

A

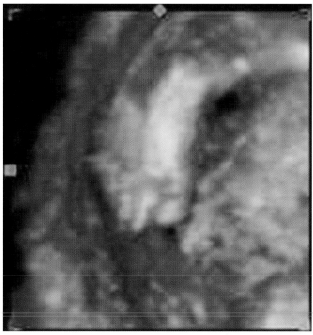

B

1. In this late second trimester fetus, what is the finding on this image of its right leg (Fig. A)? Figure B is a 3-D image of another patient with the same anomaly.

2. What percentage of cases are bilateral?

3. Are chromosomal anomalies associated with this finding?

4. Name two extrinsic causes of this entity.

Clubfoot

1. Clubfoot.

2. Slightly more than half.

3. Yes.

4. Oligohydramnios and amniotic band syndrome.

References

Benacerraf BR, Frigoletto TD: Prenatal ultrasound diagnosis of clubfoot. *Radiology* 155:211–213, 1985.

Hashimoto BE, Filly RA, Callen PW: Sonographic diagnosis of clubfoot in utero. *J Ultrasound Med* 5:81–83, 1986.

Shipp TD, Benacerraf BR: The significance of prenatally identified isolated clubfoot: Is amniocentesis indicated? *Am J Obstet Gynec*ol 178:600–602, 1998.

Mammen L, Benson C: Outcome of fetuses with clubfeet diagnosed by prenatal sonography. *J Ultrasound Med* 23:497–500.

Cross-Reference

Ultrasound: The REQUISITES, 2nd ed, pp 480–482.

Comment

Clubfoot is a common congenital anomaly that occurs bilaterally in slightly more than half of the cases. Many cases are familial, and the risk is as high as 25% for the fetus if the parent has a clubfoot. Although the most common cause is idiopathic, possible associated abnormalities warrant a careful search with prenatal ultrasound once clubfoot is detected.

Clubfoot is associated with chromosomal anomalies such as trisomy 13 and trisomy 18. Even if the prenatal sonogram fails to detect other malformations, the incidence of a karyotype abnormality is 6%. The rates for aneuploidy have been found to be similar for unilateral and bilateral clubfeet.

In addition to chromosomal anomalies, clubfoot deformity is associated with other malformations in 10% of cases. Cleft lip and palate, micrognathia, facial deformities, congenital heart disease, and hip dislocations are among the associated anomalies. Neurologic abnormalities associated with clubfoot include meningomyelocele and hydrocephalus. Numerous congenital syndromes and musculoskeletal disorders include clubfoot in their spectrum of anomalies: Gordon's syndrome (camptodactyly and cleft palate), distal arthrogryposis (fixated hands and feet), nail-patella syndrome, muscular dystrophies, and Pierre Robin syndrome (congenital heart disease). Other musculoskeletal anomalies besides clubbed feet, neural tube defects, and cardiovascular anomalies have been found to be more common in fetuses with bilateral clubbed feet compared with those with unilateral deformity. Extrinsic causes can also lead to clubfoot deformity, including oligohydramnios and amniotic band syndrome.

The ultrasound appearance relies on an unusual configuration between the foot and the lower leg (see Fig. A). Once seen, careful evaluation of the other extremities for bilaterality and clubhands should be undertaken. The more the limbs are affected, the greater is the possibility of the presence of a congenital syndrome or a musculoskeletal disorder.

Notes

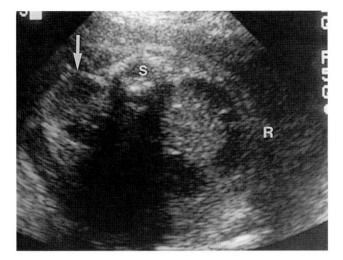

1. What does the arrow point to in this mid-abdominal axial image of a second-trimester fetus, and what is the abnormal finding? What are possible etiologies? (S = spine; R = toward the fetal right.)

2. What are the three criteria for prenatal ultrasound diagnosis if this anomaly is bilateral?

3. How early can the diagnosis be made?

4. How can color Doppler imaging be useful in the diagnosis?

Renal Agenesis

1. The arrow points to the normal left kidney. The right kidney is not in its usually paraspinal location. Possible etiologies are unilateral renal agenesis, ectopically placed kidney such as a pelvic kidney, or crossed fused ectopia.

2. If the finding is bilateral, in addition to the absence of the kidneys, the urinary bladder is not visualized, and oligohydramnios is present.

3. Early second trimester (12 to 13 weeks).

4. It can identify the abdominal aorta by its flow, even when severe oligohydramnios is present, and can confirm the absence of renal arterial flow to the suspected side where the kidney is absent.

References

Mackenzie FM, Kingston GO, Oppenheimer L: The early prenatal diagnosis of bilateral renal agenesis using transvaginal sonography and color Doppler ultrasonography. *J Ultrasound Med* 13:49–51, 1994.

Sherer DM, Thompson HO, Armstrong B, Woods JR: Prenatal sonographic diagnosis of fetal renal agenesis. *J Clin Ultrasound* 18:648–652, 1990.

Cross-Reference

Ultrasound: THE REQUISITES, 2nd ed, pp 104, 451, 458–459, 461.

Comment

The fetal kidneys can be seen as early as 12 to 14 weeks. By 12 weeks, the urinary bladder can be seen in approximately half of cases. Renal agenesis can be unilateral (see figure), or bilateral; the latter case is fatal (Potter's syndrome). Autopsy studies report the incidence of unilateral agenesis to be 1 in 400 and bilateral agenesis to be 1 in 2653. Bilateral renal agenesis is an autosomal recessive condition.

Routine prenatal sonography requires the identification of both fetal kidneys. On an axial image of the fetal mid-abdomen, both kidneys should be detected on the same image. If one is not visualized, as in this case (see figure), the abnormal renal region should be evaluated. Occasionally, bowel with peristalsis can be seen. The adrenal glands, however, are much more prominent in utero and are up to one third of the size of the kidneys. To the casual observer, when unilateral (or bilateral) renal agenesis occurs, the adrenal glands, which are discoid and of the same echogenicity as the kidneys, can fill the renal beds and mimic the kidneys.

If it can be established that one kidney is not in its normal position, an ectopic location should be sought. In particular, the fetal pelvis should be examined for a pelvic kidney. The normal side should be further examined for a possible cross-fused ectopia. If unilateral agenesis is confirmed, the contralateral kidney should also be carefully inspected to exclude other genitourinary anomalies such as an associated multicystic dysplastic kidney. Additional associated anomalies include congenital uterine anomalies in females and seminal vesicle cysts and cryptorchidism in males.

In unilateral renal agenesis, the amniotic fluid remains normal. Bilateral renal agenesis leads to marked oligohydramnios, which results in pulmonary hypoplasia in utero. This condition is incompatible with life. The urinary bladder is not visualized (or appears to be very small), and the stomach may be secondarily small or absent due to oligohydramnios. The ultrasound examination becomes technically difficult in the setting of severe oligohydramnios. Doppler ultrasound has proved helpful in confirming the absence of renal artery flow bilaterally.

Notes

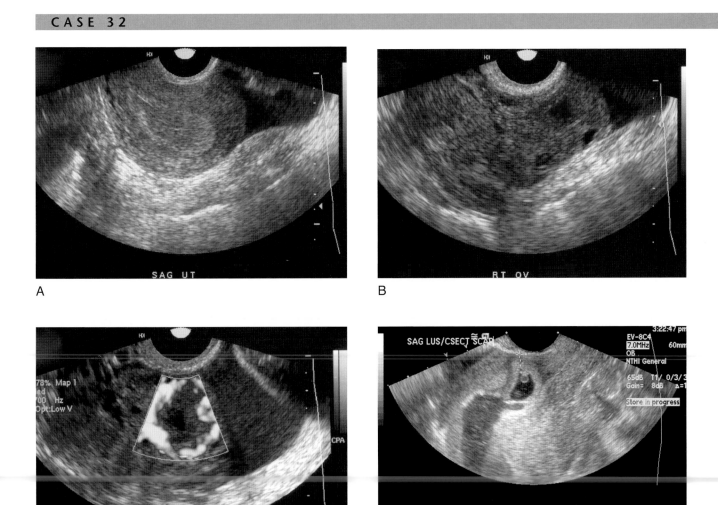

A

B

C

D

1. What accounts for the ultrasound finding in this first-trimester examination? Figure A is a transvaginal image of the uterus; Figure B is a transvaginal image of the right adnexa; and Figure C is a Doppler image of the right adnexa. Figure D is a transvaginal image showing a similar diagnosis in a patient with a prior cesarean section.

2. What is the intradecidual sign?

3. What is the double decidual reaction?

4. What is the significance of decidual cysts?

5. What is the finding in Figure D?

Ectopic Pregnancy

1. Right ectopic pregnancy with an intrauterine pseudogestational sac.

2. The early intrauterine sac is situated adjacent to or abutting the uterine cavity and is embedded in the decidua.

3. Two concentric hyperechoic rings that surround the early intrauterine gestational sac.

4. The decidual cysts indicate decidual breakdown.

5. Ectopic pregnancy in a cesarean section scar.

References

Ackerman TE, Levi CS, Lyons EA, et al: Decidual cyst: Endovaginal sonographic sign of ectopic pregnancy. *Radiology* 189:727–731, 1993.

Botash RJ, Spirt BA: Ectopic pregnancy: review and update. *Appl Radiol* 29:7–12, 2000.

Chiang G, Levine D, Swire M, McNamara A, et al: The intradecidual sign: Is it reliable for diagnosis of early intrauterine pregnancy? *AJR* 183:725–731, 2004.

Dialani V, Levine D: Ectopic pregnancy: a review. *Ultrasound Q* 20:105–117, 2004.

Farquhar CM: Ectopic pregnancy. *Lancet* 366:583–591, 2005.

Maymon R, Halperin R, Mendlovic S, Schneider D, et al: Ectopic pregnancies in cesarean section scars: the 8 year experience of one medical center. *Hum Reprod* 19:278–284, 2004.

Parvey HR, Dubinsky TJ, Johnston DA, Maklad NF: The chorionic rim and low impedance intrauterine arterial flow in the detection of early intrauterine pregnancy. *AJR* 167:1479–1485, 1996.

Cross-Reference

Ultrasound: THE REQUISITES, 2nd ed, pp 357–370.

Comment

Detection of a true intrauterine gestational sac is paramount to the exclusion of an ectopic pregnancy, which usually occurs in the distal fallopian tube. An intraendometrial fluid collection, also known as "decidual cast," should not be misinterpreted as a gestational sac. This field collection is often called a pseudogestational sac (see Fig. A). These collections can be seen in the setting of an ectopic pregnancy and are caused by the hormonal influence of the ectopic pregnancy. Several characteristics of a true early intrauterine gestational sac have been shown to be helpful in distinguishing this from intraendometrial fluid when the intrauterine pregnancy (IUP) is visualized before the development of a yolk sac or fetal pole.

Before the double decidual sac becomes apparent, the location of the sac is an important criterion. The "intradecidual sign" refers to a sac located adjacent to or abutting the endometrial lining, embedded within the decidual reaction. The decidual cast or intraendometrial fluid, which is seen in cases of ectopic pregnancies, is located within the uterine cavity. This ultrasound finding of "intradecidual sign" has recently been shown to reliably exclude an ectopic pregnancy. Use of transvaginal ultrasonography and human chorionic gonadotropin (beta-hCG) has led to a reduction in the need for diagnostic laparoscopy.

The double decidual reaction refers to two concentric hyperechoic rings that surround the early intrauterine gestatational sac. Unfortunately, this sign may not be present with a normal intrauterine gestational sac. The chorionic rim, a hyperechoic rim bordering an intrauterine collection of fluid, has been shown to be a more sensitive indicator of an IUP, particularly if there is an associated high diastolic flow. Although color Doppler imaging can be used, care must be taken to avoid using pulsed Doppler on or near a normal early embryo.

Decidual cysts are 1- to 5-mm diameter simple cysts that are located in the decidual reaction and are remote from the endometrial canal. They may be found at the junction of the endometrium and myometrium. They do not have a hyperechoic trophoblastic ring and are believed to represent an early breakdown of the decidua.

Figure D shows a rare life-threatening ectopic pregnancy developing in a cesarean section scar. Women at risk for this development are those with a history of placental pathology, ectopic pregnancy, multiple cesarean sections, and cesarean breech delivery.

Notes

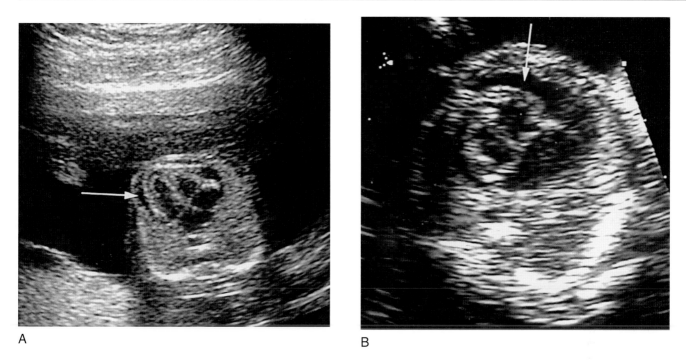

A

B

1. What is the finding (denoted by an arrow) on these images of the fetal chest?

2. What percentage of normal fetuses have minimal pericardial fluid in the second trimester?

3. What amount of pericardial fluid is considered to be normal in these fetuses?

4. What viruses may cause fetal pericardial fluid?

Pericardial Effusion

1. Pericardial effusions; Figure A's is small; Figure B's is moderate in size.

2. Greater than 70%.

3. Up to 2 mm.

4. Maternal parvovirus, cytomegalovirus (CMV), and human immunodeficiency virus (HIV).

Acknowledgment
Figures for Case 33 courtesy of Mr. Dennis Wood.

References
Di Salvo DN, Brown DL, Doubilet PM, et al: Clinical significance of isolated fetal pericardial effusion. *J Ultrasound Med* 13:291–293, 1994.

Dizon-Townson DS, Dildy GA, Clark SL: A prospective evaluation of fetal pericardial fluid in 506 second-trimester low-risk pregnancies. *Obstet Gynecol* 90:958–961, 1997.

Sharland G, Lockhart S: Isolated pericardial effusion: An indication for fetal karyotyping? *Ultrasound Obstet Gynecol* 6:29–32, 1995.

Slesnick TC, Ayres NA, Altman CA, Bezold LI, et al: Characteristics and outcomes of fetuses with pericardial effusions *Am J Cardiol* 96:599–601, 2005.

Cross-Reference
Ultrasound: THE REQUISITES, 2nd ed, pp 421–422.

Comment
A small amount of pericardial fluid is normal in the second trimester. A study of more than 500 low-risk pregnancies demonstrated that between 16 and 25 weeks of gestation, a small quantity of pericardial fluid (defined as 2 mm or less) is a normal finding detected in 71% of the cases.

Larger quantities of pericardial fluid can be associated with additional abnormalities. Structural cardiac anomalies and arrhythmias must be excluded with fetal echocardiography. Fetuses with hydrops can have pericardial effusions. Viral causes have been reported, most commonly parvovirus, CMV, and HIV. Intrauterine growth restriction has also been associated.

If the pericardial effusion is determined to be the only abnormality, the outcome is controversial. One study demonstrated that fetuses with isolated significant pericardial effusion had a higher incidence of chromosomal anomalies (31%), particularly Down's syndrome. However, a separate study demonstrated that 52 fetuses with pericardial effusions ranging from 2 to 7 mm in thickness had no significant differences in outcome compared with all neonates born during the same period.

According to a recent publication, most pericardial effusions resolve, and fetuses with isolated pericardial effusions have a good prognosis.

Notes

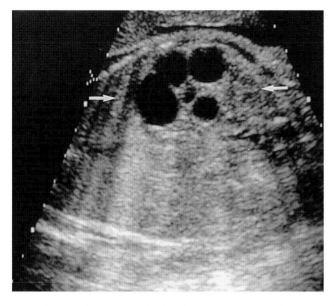

1. What is the most likely diagnosis and what are the differential diagnoses of the abnormality (arrows) adjacent to the spine on this sagittal view of the fetal abdomen?

2. Why is it important to evaluate the other kidney?

3. Is there any risk of malignant degeneration of a multicystic dysplastic kidney (MCDK) postnatally?

4. What is the typical outcome of an MCDK?

Multicystic Dysplastic Kidney

1. MCDK is the most likely diagnosis. Differential diagnoses are hydronephrosis, cystic mesoblastic nephroma, and a rare cystic Wilms' tumor.

2. Contralateral renal anomalies occur in 40%.

3. Yes.

4. The kidney usually regresses.

References

De Oliveira-Filho AG, Carvalho MH, Sbragia-Neto L, et al: Wilms' tumor in a prenatally diagnosed multicystic dysplastic kidney. *J Urol* 158:1926–1927, 1997.

Minevich E, Wacksman J, Phipps L, et al: The importance of accurate diagnosis and early close follow-up in patients with suspected multicystic dysplastic kidney. *J Urol* 158:1301–1304, 1997.

Van Eijk L, Cohen-Overbeek TE, den Hollander NS, et al: Unilateral multicystic dysplastic kidney: a combined pre-and postnatal assessment: *Ultrasound Obstet Gynecol* 19:180–183, 2002.

Cross-Reference

Ultrasound: THE REQUISITES, 2nd ed, pp 465–466.

Comment

Pathologically, a multicystic dysplastic kidney is replaced by noncommunicating cysts of varying sizes, composed of dilated collecting tubules. The etiology is believed to be either an obstruction during embryogenesis or primary dysplasia due to abnormalities of metanephric blastema and ureteral bud. In one recent large study, the dysplastic kidney was left-sided in 53% and right-sided in 47% of cases. Sixty-three percent of the affected fetuses were male and 37% were female. Fetal outcome is determined by the associated renal or nonrenal structural pathology or both and not by the size or location of the unilateral multicystic dysplastic kidney.

MCDK is often diagnosed with prenatal ultrasound; it can present as an abdominal mass in the neonate. The differential diagnosis of a multicystic renal mass in the fetus includes hydronephrosis (in which the cystic areas communicate), cystic mesoblastic nephroma (the most common neonatal genitourinary neoplasm), and cystic Wilms' tumor.

On prenatal ultrasound, the kidney is replaced by multiple simple cysts. In utero, growth of the dysplastic tissue can cause an MCDK to enlarge, warranting follow-up ultrasound examinations. Careful evaluation of the contralateral functioning kidney is essential, because additional congenital renal anomalies occur in up to 40% of cases. Contralateral MCDK (a lethal condition) comprises half of these, with ureteropelvic junction obstruction and renal agenesis accounting for the remaining 20%. Contralateral reflux is also common.

MCDK regresses with increasing age postnatally. Complications include hypertension, which is uncommon, and malignant degeneration, which is rare. Both Wilms' tumor and renal cell carcinoma have been described arising from an MCDK. Close follow-up is recommended. Although some physicians advocate surgical removal of the kidney, the current trend is toward conservative, nonsurgical management.

Notes

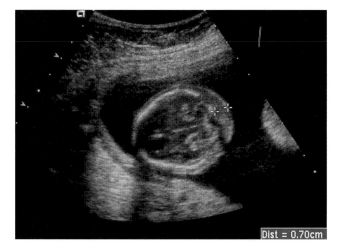

Dist = 0.70cm

1. What is the soft tissue abnormality (+ signs) posterior to the occiput in this 20-week-old fetus? What is the most commonly associated karyotype abnormality?

2. What constitutes nuchal thickening?

3. At what age do most women have a fetus with this disorder?

4. What serum screening test is used, and what is the sensitivity?

Trisomy 21 (Down syndrome)—Basic

1. Nuchal skin thickening. Trisomy 21 (Down syndrome).

2. Nuchal translucency greater than 3 mm in the first trimester or greater than 6 mm between 16 and 22 weeks.

3. Most cases occur in women younger than 35 years of age.

4. The triple screen measures maternal serum α-fetoprotein (AFP), estradiol, and β-human chorionic gonadotropin (hCG). Its sensitivity for Down syndrome is 60%.

References

Benacerraf BR: Use of sonographic markers to determine the risk of Down syndrome in second trimester fetuses. *Radiology* 201:619–620, 1996.

Nyberg DA, Souter VL, El-Bastawissi A, Young S: Isolated sonographic markers for detection of fetal Down syndrome in the second trimester of pregnancy. *J Ultrasound Med* 20:1053–1063, 2001.

Rotmensch S, Liberati M, Bronshtein M, et al: Prenatal sonographic findings in 187 fetuses with Down syndrome. *Prenat Diagn* 17:1001–1009, 1997.

Wong G, Levine D: Fetuses with trisomy 21 having conflicting findings on antenatal testing for fetal well-being. *J Ultrasound Med* 24:1541–1545, 2005.

Cross-Reference

Ultrasound: THE REQUISITES, 2nd ed, pp 394, 396, 400, 453, 475.

Comment

Down syndrome, or trisomy 21, is the most common chromosomal anomaly diagnosed in newborns. Although advanced maternal age is a known risk factor, most cases occur in women younger than 35 years of age. The maternal serum triple screen of AFP, estradiol, and β-HCG, which is obtained at 15 weeks, has a sensitivity of only 60% for detection of Down syndrome.

Ultrasound can detect a number of normal anatomic variants as well as malformations associated with Down syndrome. Sensitivity for prenatal detection is as high as 80% using these markers. Nuchal translucency (thickening) greater than 3 mm in the first trimester or greater than 6 mm between 16 and 22 weeks (see figure) carries an increased risk of aneuploidy, most commonly trisomy 21. Nuchal thickening was the most common sonographic marker of Down syndrome in some studies. A short humerus and femur, dilatation of the renal pelves, and hyperechogenic (echogenic) bowel may also be present, and a combination of these findings makes the diagnosis more certain.

Additional associated malformations, which can be detected prenatally, include cystic hygroma, duodenal atresia, and hydrocephalus as well as cardiac abnormalities (atrioventricular canal, ventricular septal defect, tetralogy of Fallot, and transposition of the great vessels).

Ultrasound scans *may* appear normal in the setting of Down syndrome. Conversely, any abnormal finding does not definitively make the diagnosis of Down syndrome.

Notes

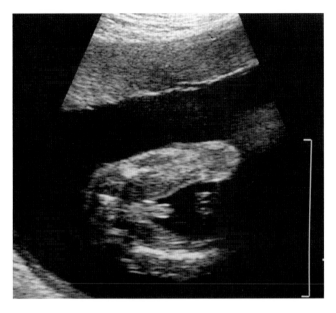

1. In addition to the gender of this fetus, what does this image reveal?

2. What are two common fetal organ systems that have anomalies associated with this condition?

3. What renal mass is associated with this condition?

4. Is there an increased incidence of chromosomal anomalies associated with this entity?

C A S E   3 6

Polyhydramnios

1. Polyhydramnios.

2. Gastrointestinal (GI) and central nervous system.

3. Mesoblastic nephroma.

4. Yes.

Reference

Barnhard Y, Bar-Hava I, Divon MY: Is polyhydramnios in an ultrasonographically normal fetus an indication for genetic evaluation? *Am J Obstet Gynecol* 173: 1523–1527, 1995.

Cross-Reference

Ultrasound: THE REQUISITES, 2nd ed, pp 375–376, 378, 435–437.

Comment

Polyhydramnios, shown in this image, may not present until after 24 weeks' gestation. The causes include maternal, fetal, and placental abnormalities. The quantity of fluid can be an indicator of the cause. Mild increases in amniotic fluid are often idiopathic. Larger volumes of fluid more commonly indicate the presence of an anomaly. The ability to make the diagnosis based on this one image emphasizes the importance of subjective evaluation of the fluid volume; in addition, the amniotic fluid index (AFI) can be calculated and compared with the range of normal for the specific gestational age.

Fetal anomalies are present in approximately 12% to 20% of cases. These relate to the inability of the fetus to swallow the amniotic fluid or an obstruction to the passage of amniotic fluid through the GI tract. Central nervous system malformations such as anencephaly, encephalocele, and Dandy-Walker malformation can cause decreased swallowing. Esophageal atresia and duodenal atresia result in a GI obstruction. Thoracic masses that obstruct the esophagus, such as a large congenital cystic adenomatoid malformation or diaphragmatic hernia, result in polyhydramnios. Fetal hydrops that develops from any underlying cause is another etiology.

Fetal masses can manifest with secondary polyhydramnios. These masses include head, neck, and sacrococcygeal teratoma. Several unusual associations include mesoblastic nephroma and a large fetal ovarian cyst.

Fetal chromosomal anomalies are present in 4% of cases. These should be suspected if specific associated fetal anomalies are documented or if the fetus develops intrauterine growth retardation.

Certain causes may not be apparent on prenatal sonography, including maternal diabetes mellitus or infection (the cause in this case) triggered by cytomegalovirus infection or toxoplasmosis.

Notes

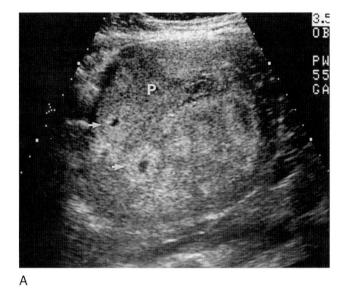

A

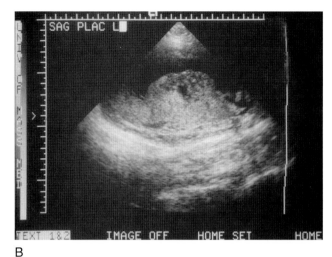

B

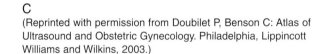

C

(Reprinted with permission from Doubilet P, Benson C: Atlas of Ultrasound and Obstetric Gynecology. Philadelphia, Lippincott Williams and Wilkins, 2003.)

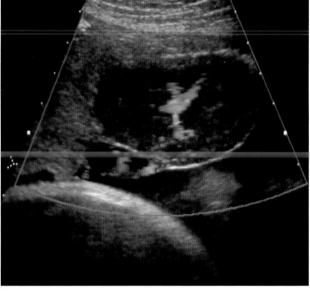

D

(Reprinted with permission from Doubilet P, Benson C: Atlas of Ultrasound and Obstetric Gynecology. Philadelphia, Lippincott Williams and Wilkins, 2003.)

1. What is the differential diagnosis of these lesions (arrows) within the placenta (P) (Fig. A)?

2. Which lesion occurs more commonly on the maternal side of the placenta?

3. Which laboratory abnormality is associated with several of these entities?

4. What is the typical ultrasound appearance of this pathologic condition?

Placental Infarct

1. Placental infarct, intervillous thrombus, fibrin deposition, and (less likely) hematoma.

2. Infarct.

3. Elevated α-fetoprotein (AFP).

4. Many are nonvisualized; hypoechoic or echogenic.

References

Harris RD, Simpson WA, Pet LR, et al: Placental hypoechoic/anechoic areas and infarction: Sonographic-pathologic correlation. *Radiology* 176: 75–90, 1990.

Levine AB, Frieden FJ, Stein JL, Pisnanont P: Prenatal sonographic diagnosis of placental infarction in association with elevated maternal serum alpha-fetoprotein. *J Ultrasound Med* 3:169–171, 1993.

Polat P, Suma S, Kantarcy M, Alper F, et al: Color Doppler US in the evaluation of uterine vascular abnormalities. *RadioGraphics* 22:47–53, 2002.

Sepulveda W, Alcalde JL, Schnapp C, Bravo M: Perinatal outcome after prenatal diagnosis of placental chorioangioma. *Obstet Gynecol* 102:1028–1033, 2003.

Cross-Reference

Ultrasound: THE REQUISITES, 2nd ed, pp 510–511.

Comment

Small placental infarcts, as shown in this case (see Fig. A), are not uncommon and occur in approximately 25% of pregnancies. Larger infarcts are associated with complications, including intrauterine growth retardation (IUGR) and increased perinatal mortality. These infarcts are more common in pregnancies complicated by pre-eclampsia or in women with essential hypertension. Placental infarcts are associated with an elevated maternal AFP.

The ultrasound appearance of a placental infarct has been described in several studies, and the descriptions vary. Harris and associates reported that placental infarcts are not visible with ultrasound unless they are complicated by hemorrhage. Other series have demonstrated that infarcts can be seen, can be hyperechoic acutely and become isoechoic with time, or present as hypoechoic lesions. Placental infarcts typically occur along the *maternal* plate of the placenta (see Fig. A).

The differential diagnosis of larger infarcts includes hemorrhage or hematoma, which decreases in size and changes in appearance with time. Three additional focal placental abnormalities include fibrin deposition, chorioangioma (Fig. B from one patient and Figs. C and D from another), and intervillous thrombosis. Fibrin deposition is more common on the *fetal* side of the placenta.

Chorioangiomas are benign vascular masses with arterial and venous flow (Fig. D), of mixed echogenicity with numerous cystic spaces (Fig. B) that usually present in the first half of the gestation period. A chorioangioma is the most common abnormality affecting the placenta. The most common complications from this entity are polyhydramnios and preterm labor. Later in gestation, an intervillous thrombosis may be detected as a hypoechoic region with slow, turbulent flow.

Notes

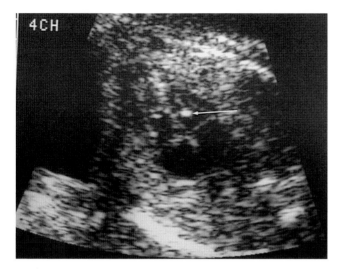

1. In this four-chamber image of the fetal heart, what is the finding denoted by an arrow in the left ventricle?

2. What is the incidence of this finding in fetuses with Down syndrome?

3. What is the hyperechoic focus pathologically?

4. Does the side of the heart (right versus left ventricle) where the calcification is seen have prognostic significance?

Papillary Muscle Calcification (Intraventricular Hyperechoic Focus)

1. Papillary muscle calcification.

2. Histologic studies show an incidence of 17%.

3. Calcification in a papillary muscle.

4. No, except if calcifications are bilateral.

References

Coco C, Jeanty P, Jeanty C: An isolated echogenic heart focus is not an indication for amniocentesis in 12,672 unselected patients. *J Ultrasound Med* 23:489–496, 2004.

Manning JE, Ragavendra N, Sayre J, et al: Significance of fetal intracardiac echogenic foci in relation to trisomy 21: A prospective sonographic study of high-risk pregnant women. *AJR* 170:1083–1084, 1998.

Wax JR, Cartin A, Pinette MG, Blackstone J: Are intracardiac echogenic foci markers of congenital heart disease in the fetus with chromosomal abnormalities? *J Ultrasound Med* 23:895–898, 2004.

Wax JR, Philput C: Fetal intracardiac echogenic foci: Does it matter which ventricle? *J Ultrasound Med* 17:141–144, 1998.

Cross-Reference

Ultrasound: THE REQUISITES, 2nd ed, p 417.

Comment

The intracardiac hyperechoic focus is a 1- to 2-mm punctate bright reflector as bright as bone within a papillary muscle and moving with the atrioventricular valves. It is found most commonly in the left ventricle but can arise in the right ventricle or can be biventricular. Biventricular calcification is more frequently associated with aneuploidy. Isolated right or left ventricular calcification is often an isolated finding without significance, but it may occasionally be associated with structural anomalies.

Pathologically, the focus represents papillary muscle microcalcification. Histologic studies have shown that this calcification is present in 15% to 17% of aneuploid fetuses versus 2% to 5% of normal fetuses. The significance of this finding is controversial when seen on an ultrasound examination. In a *high-risk* population, a statistically significant association has been shown with Down syndrome (trisomy 21). Because this finding is present in only 13% of fetuses with Down syndrome compared with 2% of normal fetuses, the positive predictive value is low. Many other studies have shown no increased incidence of Down syndrome in fetuses with an intracardiac hyperechoic focus. At present, the incidence of gross calcifications detected by ultrasound probably increases the risk of Down syndrome by no more than a factor of 2. The intracardiac echogenic focus is a poor screening marker for congenital heart disease in fetuses with congenital abnormalities, including trisomy 21.

Detection of this as an isolated finding in the general population necessitates at most an echocardiographic examination for structural anomalies. Amniocentesis need not be offered. In a high-risk population (e.g., advanced maternal age, abnormal triple screen), an additional careful evaluation for other systemic malformations is warranted.

Notes

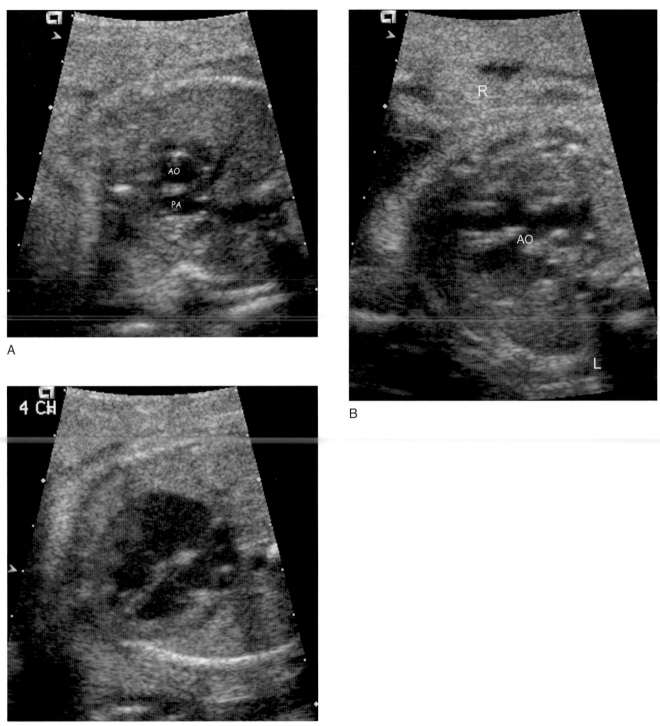

A

B

C

1. What abnormalities are demonstrated on these images of a third-trimester fetal heart (Figs. A and B)? (AO = aorta, PA=pulmonary artery, R=right; L=left)?

2. What is the most likely cause?

3. How do the ventricles appear on a four-chamber view (Fig. C) in tetralogy of Fallot?

4. What is the differential diagnosis of aortic enlargement with a small pulmonary artery?

Tetralogy of Fallot

1. Enlarged overriding aorta and an accompanying relatively smaller pulmonary artery.

2. Tetralogy of Fallot.

3. Most commonly normal.

4. Tetralogy of Fallot and a hypoplastic right side of the heart.

References

Benacerraf BR: Sonographic detection of fetal anomalies of the aortic and pulmonary arteries: Value of the four-chamber view vs. direct images. *AJR* 163:1483–1489, 1994.

Brown DL, DiSalvo DN, Frates MC, et al: Sonography of the fetal heart: Normal variants and pitfalls. *AJR* 60:1251–1255, 1993.

Kirk JS, Comstock CH, Lee W, et al: Sonographic screening to detect fetal cardiac anomalies: A 5-year experience with 111 abnormal cases. *Obstet Gynecol* 89:227–232, 1997.

Pinsky WW, Arciniegas E: Tetralogy of Fallot. *Pediatr Clin North Am* 37:179–192, 1990.

Sable CA: Ultrasound of congenital heart disease: A review of prenatal and postnatal echocardiography. *Semin Roentgenol* 39:215–233, 2004.

Cross-Reference

Ultrasound: THE REQUISITES, 2nd ed, pp 419–420.

Comment

Tetralogy of Fallot is one of the more common complex cardiac malformations of children born with cyanotic heart disease (10% of congenital heart disease patients) and includes a ventricular septal defect with overriding aorta, pulmonic stenosis, and right ventricular infundibular obstruction. There are variable degrees of pulmonary artery atresia. Tetralogy of Fallot can be seen in various syndromes, including Down syndrome. In addition, the branchial arch defects are associated with tetralogy of Fallot (DiGeorge's syndrome, velocardiofacial syndrome, and conotruncal anomaly face syndrome). Almost 40% of patients with tetralogy of Fallot have additional cardiac anomalies, particularly if it is associated with one of these syndromes. In addition, all patients have an increased incidence of noncardiac as well as chromosomal anomalies.

On prenatal sonogram, the four-chamber view is most commonly normal, with symmetric ventricular size. However, outflow views reveal a large overriding aorta and a VSD. It is important to recognize that one can create a "pseudo-overriding aorta" on the long axis view of the left ventricular outflow tract. If the aorta is truly overriding in the setting of tetralogy of Fallot, the vessel should be enlarged, and the abnormality will persist despite the orientation of scanning. The pseudo-overriding aorta may be due to volume averaging with the pulmonary artery or sinus of Valsalva.

Tetralogy of Fallot is the most common anomaly with a discrepancy in the size of the aorta and the pulmonary outflow tract. The differential diagnosis includes hypoplastic right side of the heart.

Notes

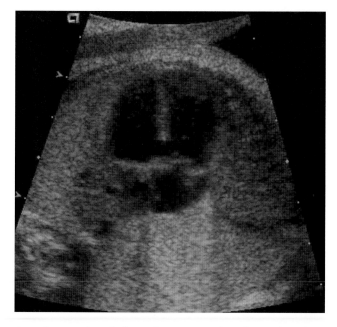

1. What is the defect shown on this four-chamber view of a middle second-trimester fetal heart?

2. What are the four types?

3. What fetal echocardiographic view best demonstrates this anomaly?

4. What is the effect on fetal cardiac hemodynamics?

Ventriculoseptal Defect

1. Ventriculoseptal defect (VSD).

2. Perimembranous (lower membranous septum defect), muscular septum defect, supracristal defect, and atrioventricular (AV) canal.

3. The four-chamber view.

4. Usually has no effect on *fetal* cardiac hemodynamics.

References

Haak MC, van Vugt JMG: Echocardiography in early pregnancy; review of the literature. *J Ultrasound Med* 22:271–280, 2003.

Nacht A, Kronzon I: Intracardiac shunts. *Crit Care Clin* 12:295–319, 1996.

Soto B, Bargeron LM, Diethelm E: Ventricular septal defect. *Semin Roentgenol* 10:200–213, 1985.

Cross-Reference

Ultrasound: THE REQUISITES, 2nd ed, pp 416–417, 419–420.

Comment

A VSD is the most common isolated congenital cardiac defect. In addition, it is present in conjunction with numerous other cardiac malformations, including tetralogy of Fallot, transposition of the great vessels, pulmonic atresia, and double-outlet right ventricle.

There are four types of VSDs, depending on their location. The most common type involves the lower membranous septum. The second type occurs in the muscular septum and can have multiple defects. Trisomy 21 is associated with the third type, an AV canal. In these cases, atrial and ventricular defects are present with anomalous AV valves. The last type is the supracristal defect, which is located directly below the aortic valve and is associated with aortic insufficiency.

Prenatal diagnosis of low membranous and muscular defects relies on adequate four-chamber views of the heart and outlet views. The diagnosis of a VSD can be made in the late first trimester with the use of high-frequency transvaginal probes. Whereas the four-chamber view detects approximately 50% of cases, the sensitivity is approximately 80% when outlet views are incorporated. Ultrasound can demonstrate an interruption in the ventricular septum (see the figure). It is essential to image the septum perpendicular to the beam of the ultrasound transducer to avoid a pseudo-defect caused by dropout of ultrasound signal. Color Doppler imaging can be used to depict the flow between the ventricles. Small defects can be missed, and high defects require special views to image the subaortic region. Once the defect is diagnosed, a careful search should be conducted for other cardiac anomalies (present in 40% of cases) using longitudinal and short axis views of the great vessels.

Notes

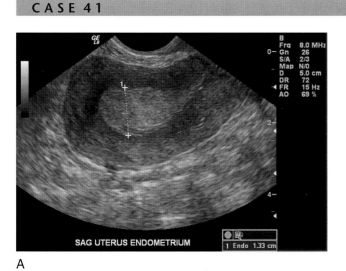

A

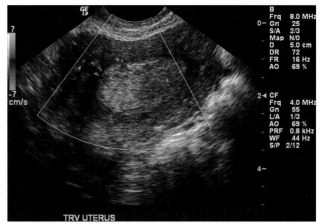

B

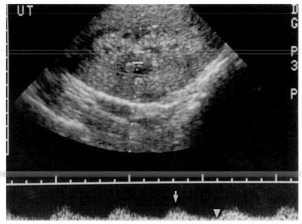

C

1. In this 67-year-old woman with vaginal bleeding, what is the primary finding, and what is the most likely diagnosis (Figs. A and B)? Figure B shows a transverse transvaginal color Doppler image.

2. Does spectral Doppler imaging (see another postmenopausal patient in Fig. C) confirm the diagnosis)? Figure C is a split image. The upper half shows a sagittal transvaginal study of the uterus with the Doppler cursor on the thickened endometrium. The lower half shows an arterial waveform; peak systole is noted by arrow and end-diastole is marked by an arrowhead.

3. What is an important question to ask the patient with a thickened endometrium?

4. Is endometrial hyperplasia considered to be premalignant?

Endometrial Cancer

1. Marked heterogeneous endometrial thickening. Endometrial cancer.

2. Yes. High diastolic flow suggests a malignancy.

3. For a premenopausal woman, "When was the last menstrual period?" For a postmenopausal woman, "Are you taking hormonal replacement supplements?"

4. Yes, the atypical subtype.

References

Gull B, Karlsson B, Milsom I, Granberg S: Can ultrasound replace dilation and curettage? A longitudinal evaluation of postmenopausal bleeding and transvaginal sonographic measurement of the endometrium as predictors of endometrial cancer. *Am J Obstet Gynecol* 188:401–408, 2003.

Kurjak A, Shalan J, Sosic A, et al: Endometrial carcinoma in postmenopausal women: Evaluation by transvaginal color Doppler ultrasonography. *Am J Obstet Gynecol* 169:1597–1602, 1993.

Smith-Blindman R, Weiss E, Feldstein V, et al: How thick is too thick? When endometrial thickness should prompt biopsy in postmenopausal women without vaginal bleeding. *Obstet Gynecol* 24:558–565, 2004.

Williams PL, Laifer-Narin SL, Ragavendra N: US of abnormal uterine bleeding. *RadioGraphics* 23:703–718, 2003.

Cross-Reference

Ultrasound: THE REQUISITES, 2nd ed, pp 540–544.

Comment

Endometrial cancer usually occurs in women over 50 years of age, most of whom have postmenopausal bleeding. These cases of endometrial cancer demonstrate that the neoplasm often causes greater degrees of endometrial thickening than benign etiologies (see Figures), although hyperplasia can cause a very thick endometrium. One series using transvaginal ultrasound demonstrated that the endometrium in endometrial cancer was almost always thicker than 10 mm (90% of cases) and usually thicker than 20 mm. The thickened endometrium is usually hyperechoic or heterogeneous and is rarely hypoechoic. Vascularity can be seen in or around the tumor in most cases; the arterial flow often demonstrates a low resistive index (<0.4) and elevated peak systolic velocity. Color Doppler sonography can confirm myometrial invasion by detecting an interruption of the zone of decreased echogenicity in the subendometrial region.

Thickening of the endometrium is the first indicator on ultrasound that an endometrial abnormality is present.

It has been shown in a recent publication that a threshold value of endometrial thickness for considering an endometrial biopsy in postmenopausal women *without* vaginal bleeding is 11 mm. In young women, the normal endometrium can measure up to 15 mm, depending on the phase of their menstrual cycle. Postmenopausal women should have a double-layer thickness of less than 5 mm. If they have this thin an endometrial lining and have vaginal bleeding, their incidence of endometrial cancer has been shown to be about .07% and 7.3% if it is thicker. However, postmenopausal women without vaginal bleeding and an endometrial stripe of less than or equal to 11 mm had a risk of endometrial cancer of about .002%, and 6.7% if the endometrial stripe was greater than 11 mm. Thus, the history of vaginal bleeding is key to the risk of endometrial cancer. In one recent publication postmenopausal bleeding incurred a 64-fold increase risk for endometrial cancer. Furthermore, studies over the last few years have shown that patients on tamoxifen therapy and women taking hormone supplements postmenopausally and not bleeding may be allowed a normal thickness up to 8–10 mm, depending on the patient population. Decision to biopsy in this group is at the discretion of the clinician.

Notes

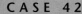

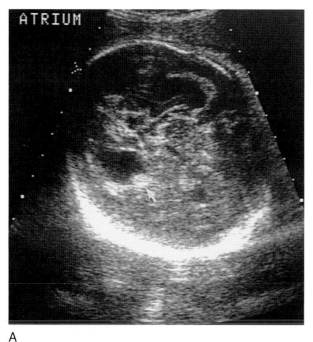

A

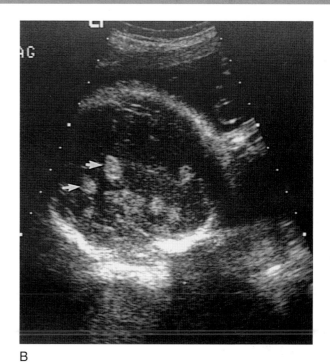

B

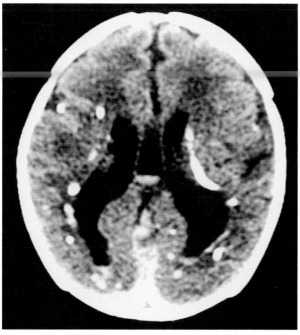

C

1. In this middle second-trimester ultrasound, the fetal head is small. In transaxial and oblique views, what are the most likely causes of the hyperechoic areas denoted by arrows, and what is the most likely diagnosis (Figs. A and B)?

2. What is the most common in utero infection in the United States?

3. What are the central nervous system (CNS) findings in the fetus with a TORCH (*t*oxoplasmosis, *o*ther infections, *r*ubella, *c*ytomegalovirus [CMV], *h*erpes/human immunodeficiency virus [HIV]) infection?

4. What is the prognosis for the fetus?

C A S E   4 2

In Utero Infection

1. Arrows = parenchymal calcifications.
   Cytomegalovirus (CMV).

2. CMV.

3. Microcephaly, periventricular calcifications, hydrocephalus, cerebellar aplasia, encephalomalacia, and porencephaly.

4. The prognosis is poor.

Reference

Drose JA, Dennis MA, Thickman D: Infection in utero: US findings in 19 cases. *Radiology* 178:369–374, 1991.

Cross-Reference

Ultrasound: THE REQUISITES, 2nd ed, pp 214–215.

Comment

In utero infection in the United States is most often caused by CMVs. Other common infections include varicella, syphilis, herpes simplex type 2, listeriosis, and toxoplasmosis as well as human immunodeficiency virus. Death can occur in utero or in the neonatal period, and those infants that survive may have developmental impairment or mental retardation.

The infection is often subclinical in the mother and is detected by the development of serum antibodies or by isolating the virus from urine or the cervix. Alternatively, amniocentesis or cordocentesis documents exposure of the fetus to the infection but does not predict the impact on fetal development.

Anomalies can occur in various organs. CNS malformations include hydrocephalus, microcephaly, cerebellar aplasia, encephalomalacia, or porencephaly. Ultrasound may demonstrate periventricular and parenchymal calcifications (see Figs. A and B). Much less commonly, the tubers of tuberous sclerosis may present in a microcephalic fetus as hyperechoic intracranial masses.

Cardiac anomalies include septal defects, cardiomegaly, and pulmonary stenosis. Hepatosplenomegaly, pleural effusion, ascites, and hydrops may be identified as well as intra-abdominal (including hepatic) calcifications. The amount of amniotic fluid can vary from oligohydramnios to polyhydramnios. Intrauterine growth retardation develops in some cases. The placenta was enlarged in 30% of one series. In some cases, the abnormalities may not be present on the first ultrasound but may develop later in the gestation period. In any prenatal sonogram in which unusual or atypical anomalies are detected, in utero infection should be considered.

Notes

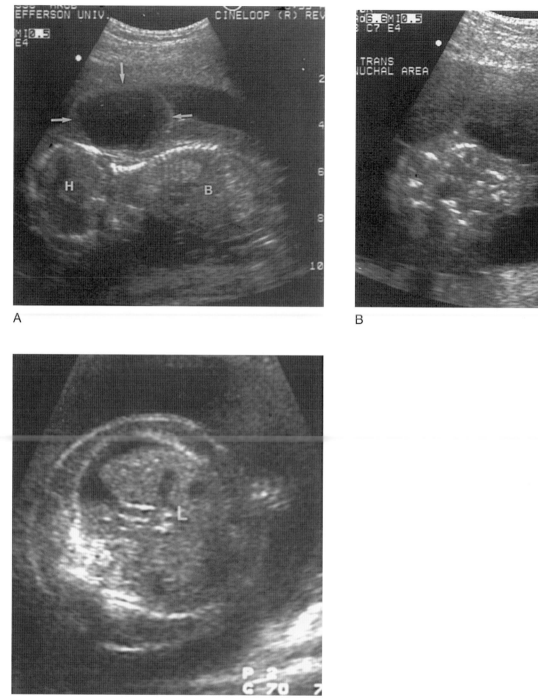

A

B

C

1. What is the abnormality located posterior to the fetal neck, and what is the most common chromosomal abnormality associated with it? (Fig. A is a sagittal view: H = head; B = body.) Figure B is an axial view of the neck. Is there an association with any other aneuploid states?

2. What percentage of pregnancies with this anomaly results in a healthy neonate with a normal karyotype?

3. What structure accounts for the midline septum (see Fig. B, curved arrow) in this cystic lesion?

4. What additional diffuse fetal findings may be associated with these findings?

Cystic Hygroma

1. Cystic hygroma. Turner's syndrome (XO). Yes, also with trisomy 21, 18, 13, and others.

2. Very few—only 9%.

3. Nuchal ligament or septation.

4. Nonimmune hydrops. (Fig. C, axial image of the abdomen [L = liver].)

Reference

Descamps P, Jourdain O, Paillet C, et al: Etiology, prognosis and management of nuchal cystic hygroma: 25 new cases and literature review. *Eur J Obstet Gynecol Reprod Biol* 71:3–10, 1997.

Machado LE, Osborne NG, Bonilla-Musoles F: Three-dimensional sonographic diagnosis of a large cystic neck lymphangioma. *J Ultrasound Med* 23:877–881, 2004.

Merbnagh JR, Mohide PT, Lappalainen RE, Fedoryshin JG: US assessment of the fetal head and neck: A state-of-the-art pictorial review. *RadioGraphics* 19:5229–5241, 1999.

Cross-Reference

Ultrasound: THE REQUISITES, 2nd ed, pp 406–410.

Comment

Cystic hygroma (see Figs. A and B) is a multiloculated septated cystic neck mass composed of dilated lymphatics, probably resulting from congenital blockage of the lymphatic drainage. The incidence is 1 per 6000 pregnancies. Ninety percent are unilateral. Three-dimensional sonography has confirmed the presumptive diagnosis of this cystic neck mass by giving more detailed visual information about the nature and extent of the abnormal structure. Cystic hygromas are most commonly associated with Turner's syndrome, but other chromosomal anomalies associated include trisomies 13, 18, and 21 as well as more rare mendelian chromosomal abnormalities. Only 9% of neonates born with this anomaly are healthy with normal chromosomes. Associated nonchromosomal abnormalities include Noonan's syndrome, multiple pterygium disease, Cowchock's syndrome, and Robert's syndrome as well as chondrodystrophies.

The α-fetoprotein (AFP) level varies, ranging from normal to very high. Lymphedema is present in slightly more than 50% of cases. Nonimmune hydrops is a complication that carries almost 100% mortality because of a diffuse lymphatic obstruction (see Fig. C); the risk correlates with the size of the hygroma. Oligohydramnios is commonly present.

Cystic hygroma may resolve in utero; nonetheless, karyotyping should be performed in all cases. In fetuses with a normal karyotype, parental karyotyping is advised to predict the risk of a recurrence. If parents have a normal karyotype, there is no increased risk in subsequent pregnancies. Cases that appear late (usually anterior or lateral in the neck) may have a different pathophysiology with a better prognosis.

The differential diagnosis of a posterior cystic neck mass includes an occipital encephalocele and a cervical myelomeningocele.

Notes

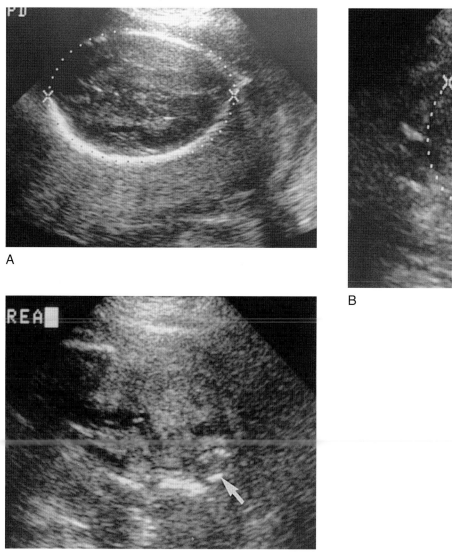

A

B

C

1. What are the findings identified in this second-trimester fetus (Figs. A to C), and what is the most likely diagnosis? Figure A is an axial image of the fetal head, Figure B is an axial image of the upper fetal abdomen, and Figure C is an axial image of the renal areas (arrow = spine.)

2. What quantitative measure is used to evaluate the severity of decreased amniotic fluid?

3. What clinical symptom(s) might the mother report in the setting of severe oligohydramnios?

4. What additional evaluation should be performed once this symptom is found?

Oligohydramnios (Secondary to Renal Agenesis)

1. Severe oligohydramnios and absence of the kidneys. The most likely diagnosis is bilateral renal agenesis.

2. An amniotic fluid index (AFI).

3. Decreased fetal movement, leaking amniotic fluid.

4. Umbilical artery Doppler imaging.

References

Cunningham FG, MacDonald PC, Gant NF, et al: *Williams Obstetrics*, 20th ed. Stamford, CT, Appleton & Lange, 1997, pp 664–665.

Sepulveda W, Stagiannis KD, Flack NJ, Fisk NM: Accuracy of prenatal diagnosis of renal agenesis with color flow imaging in severe second-trimester oligohydramnios. *Am J Obstet Gynecol* 173:1788–1792, 1995.

Chow JS, Benson CB, Lebowitz R: The clinical significance of an empty renal fossa on prenatal sonography. *J Ultrasound Med* 24:1049–1054, 2005.

Cross-Reference

Ultrasound: THE REQUISITES, 2nd ed, pp 458–463, 466.

Comment

Abnormalities in amniotic fluid volume reflect underlying fetal, maternal, and placental conditions. Oligohydramnios is defined as fluid volume less than the fifth percentile for a specific gestational age. The amniotic fluid volume varies with the gestational age and peaks in the second trimester. Although the diagnosis can be made by measuring the fluid (usually in the four uterine quadrants) as four perpendicular measurements added together, a subjective evaluation of the amount of fluid is usually just as accurate.

As this case of bilateral renal agenesis demonstrates, the abnormality in amniotic fluid volume may be immediately apparent (see Figs. A to C). Severe oligohydramnios should prompt a directed scan to identify the cause. The anatomy should be evaluated for the presence of both kidneys (see Fig. C) and fluid in the urinary bladder, both of which are absent in bilateral renal agenesis. The adrenal glands are large in utero and can resemble the kidneys; the urinary bladder will still not be present. A severe bilateral renal obstruction or any other bilateral renal anomaly that affects function (i.e., a multicystic dysplastic kidney with a contralateral ureteropelvic junction obstruction) would also lead to severe oligohydramnios.

If the fluid volume is very low, fetal anatomy can be difficult to assess. Color Doppler imaging has been shown to be useful in documenting the presence of renal arteries to exclude renal agenesis in these cases. In cases where there is the unilateral absence of a kidney ("empty renal fossa") the majority of cases are related to an ectopic location of the kidney or a congenital absence. Even though there is not a risk of oligohydramnios, an empty renal fossa is often associated with other congenital anomalies.

Alternative causes of oligohydramnios include growth restriction (intrauterine growth restriction or retardation), chromosomal anomalies, some congenital anomalies (e.g., cystic hygroma), and fetal demise. Hypertension, diabetes, and pre-eclampsia are among the maternal causes. Placental insufficiency, a cause of oligohydramnios later in the gestation period, warrants umbilical artery Doppler imaging whenever the fluid volume appears low. To exclude rupture of the membranes as the cause, the mother should be asked about fluid leakage. A physical examination must be conducted immediately by the obstetrician to exclude ruptured membranes, and the examination should be performed using a sterile speculum and the "fern test."

Notes

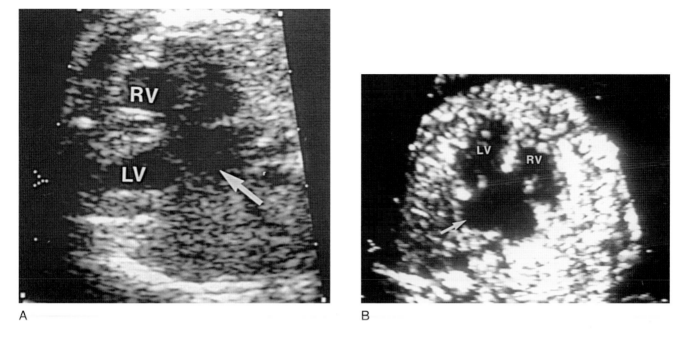

A

B

1. What is the anomaly shown in the four-chamber cardiac images of two second-trimester fetuses (Figs. A and B)? LV = left ventricle; RV = right ventricle; arrow = left atrium. What chromosomal anomaly is associated with this cardiac malformation?

2. What other cardiac malformations are associated with this cardiac malformation?

3. What subtype of this cardiac anomaly includes obstructive lesions of the right or left ventricle?

4. What percentage of cases have significant atrioventricular (AV) valve regurgitation?

CASE 45

Endocardial Cushion Defect

1. Endocardial cushion AV canal defects. Down syndrome (70%).

2. Tetralogy of Fallot (10%).

3. Unbalanced AV canal.

4. 20%.

Acknowledgment

Figures for Case 45 courtesy of Mr. Dennis Wood.

Reference

Pearl JM, Laks H: Intermediate and complete forms of atrioventricular canal. *Semin Thorac Cardiovasc Surg* 9:8–20, 1997.

Driscoll DJ: Left-to-right shunt lesions. *Pediatr Clin North Am* 46:355–368, 1999.

Cross-Reference

Ultrasound: THE REQUISITES, 2nd ed, p 416.

Comment

The AV canal, or endocardial cushion defect, is a cardiac malformation defined by a common AV valve with superior and inferior bridging leaflets that divide an otherwise continuous septal defect of atria and ventricles. An endocardial cushion defect is one of the right-to-left shunt lesions. Both of these cases demonstrate the AV septal defect. A classification system has been described by Rastelli (types A to C), depending on the morphology of the superior bridging valve leaflet.

Ten percent of patients with AV canal also have tetralogy of Fallot. A complete endocardial cushion defect is associated with Down syndrome in 70% of cases and is the most common congenital cardiac malformation in this syndrome. In non-Down syndrome cases, there is an increased incidence of an "unbalanced AV canal," where an obstructive lesion or hypoplasia of one of the ventricles is also present and dictates a different type of surgical repair.

A four-chamber view of the fetal heart easily identifies this abnormality by the mid-second trimester. Whereas ventricular and atrial septal defects by themselves could be small and missed, the combined defect forming an AV canal (see Figs. A and B) is accurately diagnosed. Accompanying arrhythmias may also be detected.

Treatment usually entails complete surgical repair in infancy. The older treatment of preliminary pulmonary banding is now reserved for infants who are not good surgical candidates, either because of sepsis, congestive heart failure, organ dysfunction, associated malformations, or small infants whose anatomy is difficult to correct surgically. The long-term outcome appears to be worse for those with Down syndrome and is attributed to the degree of pulmonary vascular disease in these patients.

Notes

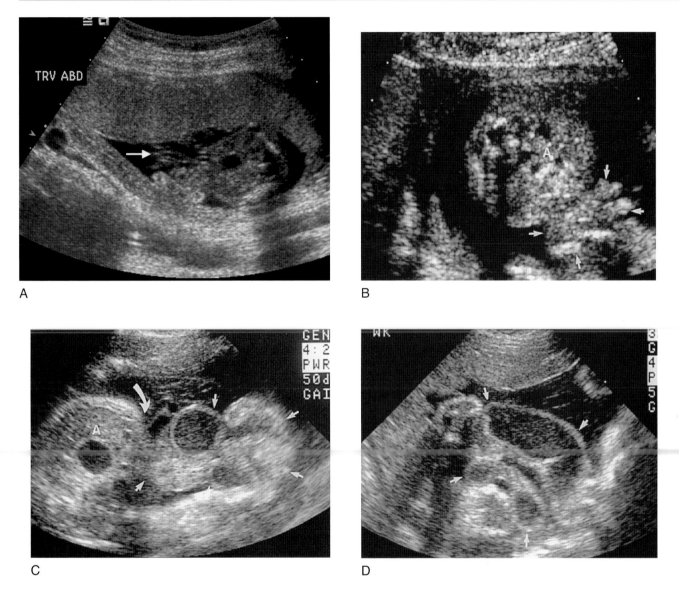

A

B

C

D

1. What type of anterior abdominal wall defect is shown in these two second-trimester fetuses? (Fetus 1, Figs. A and B; fetus 2, Figs. C and D; A = fetal abdomen.) What do the long straight and long curved arrows in Figures A and C represent?

2. How is gastroschisis distinguished from an omphalocele by prenatal ultrasound?

3. What prenatal ultrasound finding carries a higher incidence of postnatal bowel complications in gastroschisis?

4. Are there any associated anomalies?

Gastroschisis

1. Gastroschisis. Long straight and curved arrow = a normal umbilical cord insertion.

2. Paraumbilical location of the defect, and the lack of a covering peritoneal membrane.

3. Small bowel diameter greater than 11 mm.

4. Only secondary gastrointestinal abnormalities. This literature does not consistently report increased incidence of other anomalies.

References

Babcook CH, Hedrick MH, Goldstein RB, et al: Gastroschisis: Can sonography of the fetal bowel accurately predict postnatal outcome? *J Ultrasound Med* 13:701–706, 1994.

Bonilla-Musoles F, Machado LE, Bailao LA, et al: Abdominal wall defects: Two-versus three-dimensional ultrasonographic diagnosis. *J Ultrasound Med* 20: 379–389, 2001.

Durfee SM, Downard CD, Benson CBN, Wilson JM: Postnatal outcome of fetuses with the prenatal diagnosis of gastroschisis. *J Ultrasound Med* 21:269–274, 2002.

Emanuel PG, Garcia GI, Angtuaco TL: Prenatal detection of anterior abdominal wall defects with ultrasound. *Radiographics* 15:517–530, 1995.

Cross-Reference

Ultrasound: THE REQUISITES, 2nd ed, pp 443-446.

Comment

Gastroschisis is an isolated, eccentrically placed, anterior abdominal wall defect. It occurs in 1 to 6 per 10,000 live births and tends to occur in younger mothers, especially those less than 20 years old. As opposed to an omphalocele, the abdominal wall defect in gastroschisis is paraumbilical, usually on the right side in the lower quadrant (see Figs. A and C), but occasionally it is found in the left lower quadrant. This defect is typically <2 cm. The anterior abdominal wall defect is caused by ischemia secondary to early right umbilical artery failure or obstruction.

Bowel herniates through the defect with no overlying membrane, accounting for the absence of fetal ascites, and the much higher maternal serum AFP levels compared with those associated with an omphalocele.

Gastrointestinal abnormalities can result, including malrotation, bowel atresia, or stenosis. It is important to evaluate the caliber of the bowel, because dilatation indicates an increased incidence of postnatal bowel complications (fetus 2, see Figs. C and D). A study by Babcook and associates demonstrated that on prenatal ultrasound, a maximum small bowel diameter of greater than 11 mm was seen more frequently in fetuses that had complications such as obstruction or atresia, necrosis, or the need for postnatal bowel resection. Others have thought that the bowel caliber had to be greater (as large as 17 mm in diameter) before these complications could occur universally. Meconium peritonitis is suggested by dilatation and wall thickening of bowel within the abdomen (see Fig. C, a cystic structure adjacent to the letter A).

Most of the literature reports no increased incidence in other anomalies compared with normal patients. Accordingly, the prognosis is better than that with an omphalocele. The condition of the bowel at the time of delivery dictates the postnatal prognosis. Ischemic bowel, sepsis, and premature delivery are leading causes of death.

Notes

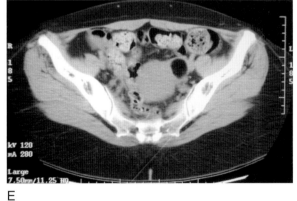

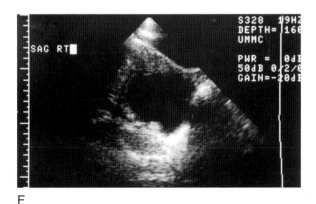

1. Four women, who are 20 to 35 years of age, present with ovarian masses on ultrasound: Figures A and B are transvaginal sagittal and coronal images of the right ovary in the same patient. Figures C and D are transvaginal sagittal and coronal images of the left ovary in another patient. Figure E is a computed tomographic (CT) scan of the left ovary in this second patient. Figure F is a transabdominal sagittal image of the right ovary in a third patient. Figures G and H are images of the left ovary on ultrasound and CT in the fourth patient. What is the most likely common diagnosis in these cases?

2. What are three complications associated with this mass?

3. What structure(s) account for the "bright lines and dots" often seen in these masses on sonography?

4. What endocrine syndrome is rarely associated and why?

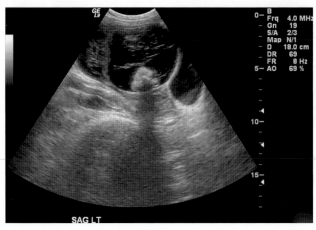

G

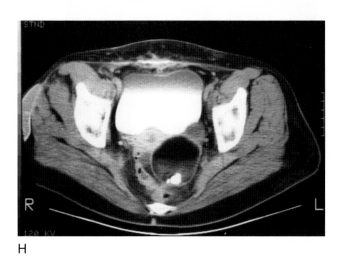

H

Dermoid

1. Dermoid (cystic teratoma).

2. Torsion, infection, and rare malignant degeneration.

3. Hair.

4. Thyrotoxicosis; the presence of struma ovarii in the tumor.

References

Mlikotic A, McPhaul L, Hansen GC, Sinow RM: Significance of the solid component in predicting malignancy in ovarian cystic teratomas. *J Ultrasound Med* 20:859–866, 2001.

Outwater EK, Siegelman ES, Hunt JL: Ovarian teratomas: Tumor types and imaging characteristics. *Radiographics* 21:475–490, 2001.

Patel MD, Feldstein VA, Lipson SD, et al: Cystic teratomas of the ovary: Diagnostic value of sonography. *AJR* 171:1061–1065, 1998.

Ueno T: Spectrum of germ cell tumors from head to toe. *Radiographics* 24:387–404, 2004.

Zalel Y, Caspi B, Tepper R: Doppler flow characteristics of dermoid cysts: Unique appearance of struma ovarii. *J Ultrasound Med* 16:355–358, 1997.

Cross-Reference

Ultrasound: THE REQUISITES, 2nd ed, pp 567–570, 572–573.

Comment

Mature cystic teratomas, also known as dermoid cysts, are the most common ovarian tumors, comprising up to 10% to 15% of all ovarian neoplasms. Most teratomas are benign. They are often incidental findings on cross-sectional imaging and are bilateral in 10% of cases. These masses, especially if large, can cause ovarian torsion. Other complications include infection, and rare malignant degeneration; the latter typically affects patients over 40 years of age, is usually less malignant than other ovarian neoplasms, and constitutes 1% to 2% of mature teratomas. Once a mature cystic teratoma is discovered, management is usually by surgical excision to prevent the known complications. If the dermoid is small, it may be removed without loss of the entire ovary.

The ultrasound appearance depends on which components are present (see Figs. A to H). Dermoids are composed of mature epithelial elements: skin, hair, desquamated epithelium, and teeth. Macroscopically, they contain variable amounts of sebum, hair, and teeth. Fat and calcifications are hallmarks of teratomas. The dermoid plug, or Rokitansky protuberance, consists of sebaceous material (Fig. F) as well as calcifications or teeth (see Figs. G and H), hair, and other soft tissue; this dermoid plug (Fig. F shows hyperechoic nodule) is present in most teratomas and varies in size. It is seen on ultrasound as a hyperechoic nodule or mass with shadowing, often within a more simple-appearing cyst. The cyst is filled with homogeneous sebaceous fluid, which accounts for the lack of internal echoes. Several characteristic ultrasound findings have been described for dermoids. Diffuse or regional bright echoes may be seen (see Figs. A, B, C, D). As in Figures C and D, the echogenicity is brightest at the top, with absorption of sound internally, called the "tip of the iceberg" sign. The presence of hair accounts for hyperechoic lines and dots (see images B and C from Case 21). A fluid-fluid level can also be present. In CT scans fat attenuation within a cyst is diagnostic (Figs. E and H). In magnetic resonance imaging the sebaceous component is identified with fat-saturation techniques.

In up to 20% of cases, thyroid tissue is present microscopically. When thyroid tissue constitutes a large portion of the lesion, it is called struma ovarii. In these cases, women may present with thyrotoxicosis or thyroid enlargement. On ultrasound, if the mass is endocrine secreting, a solid component will be seen in the dermoid with low impedance arterial flow detected by Doppler ultrasound imaging.

Notes

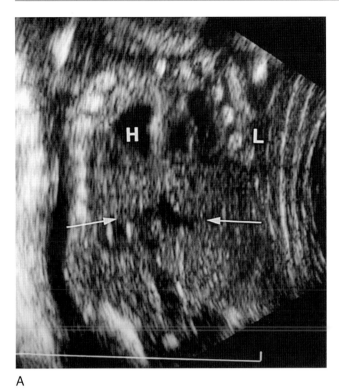

A

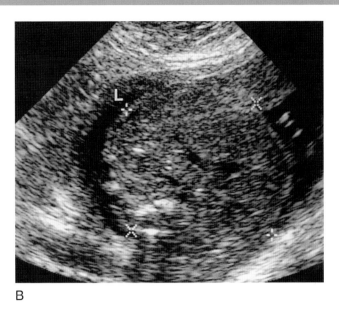

B

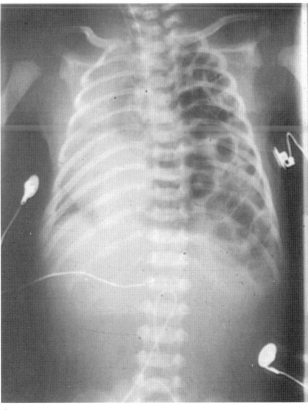

C

1. What is the diagnosis in this sonogram of a second-trimester fetus? Figure A is a coronal image of the fetal chest and abdomen (arrows = diaphragm; H = heart; L = left side of the fetus). Figure B is an axial image of the upper fetal abdomen (L = left side of the fetus).

2. Are there associated anomalies with this diagnosis?

3. What prenatal measurements help to predict survival?

4. What finding aids in distinguishing congenital diaphragmatic hernia (CDH) from cystic adenomatoid malformation (CAM)?

Congenital Diaphragmatic Hernia, Left-Sided Bochdalek

1. Left-sided diaphragmatic hernia (Bochdalek).

2. Yes (congenital heart disease and chromosomal anomalies).

3. Quantification of the contralateral lung area and an assessment of ventricular symmetry.

4. Paucity of abdominal contents. Also see plain x-ray of chest and abdomen (Fig. C).

References

Guibaud L, Filiatrault D, Garel L, et al: Fetal congenital diaphragmatic hernia: Accuracy of sonography in the diagnosis and prediction of the outcome after birth. *AJR* 166:1195–1202, 1996.

Hubard AM, Adzick NS, Crombleholme TM, Haselgrove JC: Left-sided congenital diaphragmatic hernia: Value of prenatal MR imaging in preparation for fetal surgery. *Radiology* 203:636–640, 1997.

Cross-Reference

Ultrasound: THE REQUISITES, 2nd ed, pp 422–424.

Comment

CDH can occur laterally (Bochdalek's hernia) or medially (Morgagni's hernia). Abdominal contents (e.g., stomach, bowel, liver, mesenteric fat) can herniate into the thorax. Pulmonary hypoplasia and pulmonary hypertension result from compression of the ipsilateral and contralateral lung. Associated malformations include congenital heart disease and chromosomal anomalies.

Left-sided Bochdalek's hernias, as shown in this case, are much more common. Ultrasound reveals cystic and solid structures in the left hemithorax. Coronal views (see Fig. A) are particularly useful for demonstrating a supra-diaphragmatic stomach or bowel. If herniated, the stomach will not be identified in the abdomen on a standard axial view (see Fig. B). Shift of the heart and mediastinum are common. Polyhydramnios is associated with this diagnosis and has a worse prognosis if it occurs early in the gestation period. Herniation of the left lobe of the liver carries a poor prognosis because of difficulty in postnatal surgical repair. It may be difficult to distinguish hyperechoic herniated contents from the ipsilateral lung.

The contralateral residual lung area has been shown to correlate with the outcome. If the contralateral lung area is equal to or greater than half of the hemithorax, the survival rate is often higher. Another assessment of the contralateral lung volume is its ratio to head circumference. Disproportion of the cardiac ventricles is a predictor of a poor outcome.

Notes

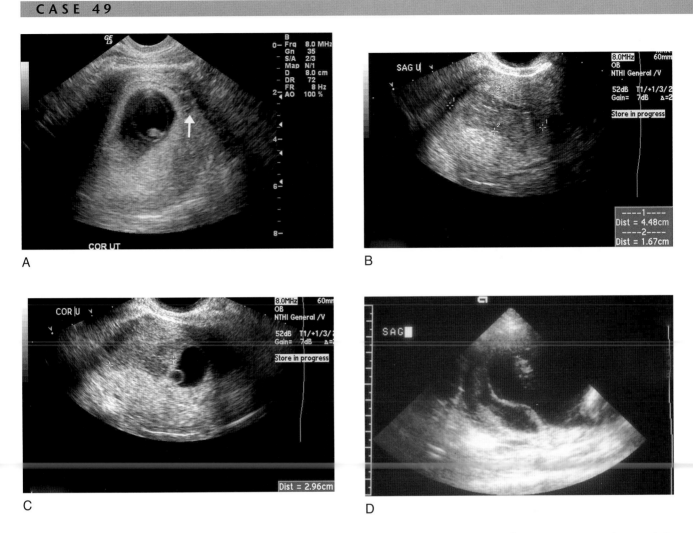

A

B

C

D

1. Figures A, B, and C are first-trimester scans of a gestational sac. Figure A is of one patient, and B and C are sagittal and coronal images of a second patient. Figure D is a sagittal image of a third-trimester pregnancy. What is the finding, and what is the usual presentation of these pregnant women?

2. What is the overall spontaneous abortion rate if this abnormality is present?

3. What is the spontaneous abortion rate in normal (uncomplicated) pregnancies with a living fetus seen by ultrasound at less than 12 weeks?

4. What three factors influence the outcome in cases such as the one shown here?

Subchorionic Hemorrhage

1. Hemorrhage. Vaginal bleeding.

2. Nine percent.

3. Two percent.

4. Hemorrhage volume, gestational age, and maternal age.

Reference

Bennet GL, Bromley B, Lieberman E, Benacerraf BR: Subchorionic hemorrhage in the first-trimester pregnancies: Prediction of pregnancy outcome with sonography. *Radiology* 200:803–806, 1996.

Dogra V, Paspulati, Bhatt S: First trimester bleeding evaluation: *Ultrasound Q* 21:69–85, 2005.

Cross-Reference

Ultrasound: THE REQUISITES, 2nd ed, pp 349–351, 493–494.

Comment

The differential diagnosis of a pregnant woman who presents with vaginal bleeding in the first trimester includes spontaneous abortion (miscarriage), ectopic pregnancy, anembryonic pregnancy, molar pregnancy, and subchorionic hemorrhage.

Early in the gestation, a hemorrhage is often within the endometrial canal but may be subchorionic. Approximately 20% of women with first-trimester bleeding have a subchorionic hematoma. Later in the pregnancy, if the hemorrhage has not been decompressed by vaginal bleeding, it is often identified below the amniochorionic membrane (subchorionic if over the placenta or submembranous if anywhere else). On ultrasound, a first-trimester hemorrhage appears as a crescentic or oval-shaped fluid collection adjacent to the gestational sac in the endometrial canal (see Figs. A, B, C). It is important not to confuse an unfused amniotic membrane (chorionic-amniotic separation) with this diagnosis, a normal finding that may be seen up to 16 weeks' gestation. In the second and third trimesters, a hemorrhage appears as a crescentic or ovoid-shaped mass projecting into the amniotic space (see Fig. D).

The echogenicity varies with the age of the hemorrhage. The bleed is anechoic acutely, becomes heterogeneous in the subacute stage, and eventually resumes an anechoic appearance when chronic. Follow-up studies are imperative to confirm a decrease in size and progressive liquification (becoming anechoic).

Studies have shown that the spontaneous abortion rate is increased in these patients from a baseline of 2% to 9% when a subchorionic hemorrhage is identified early in the gestation. The outcome depends on the size (volume) of the hemorrhage (see Fig. A of the first patient compared with Figs. B and C of the second), the gestational age of the fetus, the degree of separation of the chorionic sac by the hemotoma (a higher degree confers up to a three-fold increase in risk of spontaneous abortion), and the maternal age. The prognosis is worse for larger hemorrhages, fetuses of 8 weeks' gestational age or younger, and women 35 years of age or older.

Notes

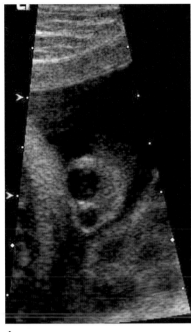

A

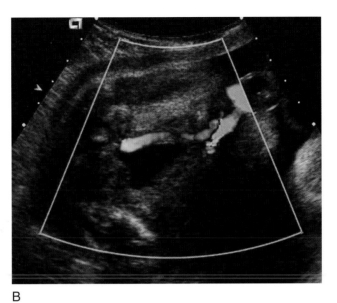

B

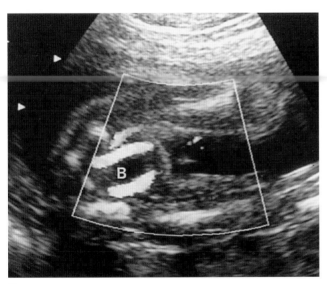

C

1. In Figure A, what is the finding in the transverse image of the umbilical cord? What is the significance of the Doppler images of Figures B and C? What is the clinical significance when the fetus has no other anomaly?

2. What central nervous system (CNS) anomalies have been associated with this finding?

3. What is the most common associated chromosomal anomaly?

4. What is shown by the color Doppler axial image of the fetal pelvis of another fetus (Fig. C)?

Single Umbilical Artery (Two-Vessel Umbilical Cord)

1. Two-vessel umbilical cord. Only one internal iliac artery is seen with color Doppler imaging adjacent to the fetal bladder (Fig. B). In the absence of fetal malformations, there is no clinical significance to this finding.

2. Holoprosencephaly, hydrocephalus, and cerebellar dysgenesis.

3. Trisomy 18.

4. Bilateral internal iliac arteries.

References

Budorick NE, Kelly TF, Dunn JA, Scioscia AL: The single umbilical artery in a high-risk patient population *J Ultrasound Med* 20:619–627, 2001.

Dudiak CM, Salomon CG, Posniak HV, et al: Sonography of the umbilical cord. *Radiographics* 15:1035–1050, 1995.

Nyberg DA, Mahony BS, Luthy D, Kapur R: Single umbilical artery: Prenatal detection of concurrent anomalies. *J Ultrasound Med* 10:247–253, 1991.

Cross-Reference

Ultrasound: THE REQUISITES, 2nd ed, pp 456–457, 491–492.

Comment

The presence of a single umbilical artery (a two-vessel umbilical cord) is a marker for concurrent fetal anomalies in 20% to 50% of singleton gestations in which it is detected. Fetal echocardiography is recommended in cases of isolated single umbilical arteries. Ultrasound reveals two vessels on cross-sectional imaging of the cord: a single umbilical artery, which may be as large as the adjacent umbilical vein (see Fig. A). When a two-vessel umbilical cord is suspected, however, care must be taken to evaluate the entire cord, especially that part close to the fetal insertion. In the development of the cord, part of it may be two vessels and part may consist of three vessels. If three vessels are detected in any part, more commonly occurring closer to the fetus, then the cord is considered to have three vessels. Color Doppler imaging of the fetal pelvis can often help to confirm the presence or absence of two internal iliac arteries (one on each side of the bladder) (Fig. C) supplying the two umbilical arteries.

The importance of the ultrasound examination is to exclude additional anomalies. Marginal and velamentous cord insertions have been associated with a single umbilical artery. Interestingly, infants with a single umbilical artery and no other congenital or chromosomal anomalies have an increased risk of an inguinal hernia.

CNS-associated anomalies include holoprosencephaly, hydrocephalus, and cerebellar dysgenesis. Various complex cardiac malformations, gastrointestinal abnormalities (omphalocele and congenital diaphragmatic hernia), and musculoskeletal and genitourinary anomalies have also been described. Trisomy 18 is the most common chromosomal anomaly; trisomy 13, Turner's syndrome, and triploidy are also associated.

Notes

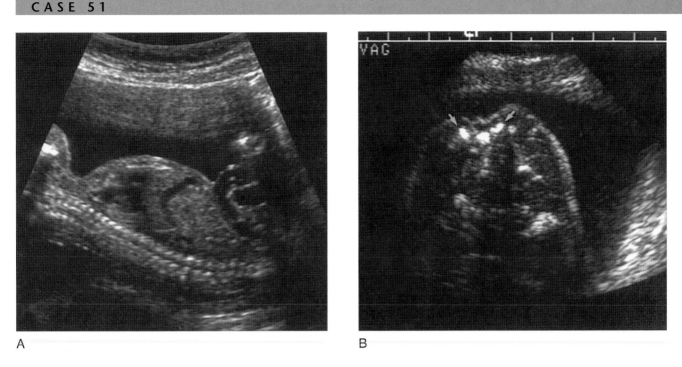

A   B

1. What does the transvaginal scan (Fig. B, axial view of lower lumbar spine) demonstrate in this case that was not apparent on the initial transabdominal image (Fig. A, sagittal image of fetus in breech position) and why?

2. What percentage of these fetuses with this disorder have a karyotype abnormality?

3. Other than gestational age, what factor correlates with the degree of ventriculomegaly in these fetuses?

4. Where is α-fetoprotein (AFP) produced, and when do fetal serum AFP levels peak?

Myelomeningocele

1. Spinal dysraphism due to a myelomeningocele; the spine is not adequately evaluated in Figure A.

2. Thirteen percent to 17%.

3. The severity of the posterior fossa defect.

4. Fetal liver and yolk sac; 12 to 13 weeks' gestation.

Reference

Aaronson OS, Hernanz-Schulman M, Bruner JP, Reed GW: Myelomeningocele: Prenatal evaluation—comparison between transabdominal US and MR imaging. *Radiology* 227:839–843, 2003.

Babcook CJ, Goldstein RV, Filly RA: Prenatally detected fetal myelomeningocele: Is karyotype analysis warranted? *Radiology* 194:491–494, 1995.

Sepulveda W, Corral E, Ayala C, Be C, et al: Chromosomal abnormalities in fetuses with open neural tube defects: Prenatal identification with ultrasound. *Ultrasound Obstet Gynecol* 23:352–356, 2004.

Thomas MT: The lemon sign. *Radiology* 228:206–207, 2003.

Cross-Reference

Ultrasound: THE REQUISITES, 2nd ed, pp 402–406, 404, 410.

Comment

Imaging of the entire fetal spine is essential, especially the lumbosacral region. In this case, the fetus was in a relatively poor position for complete evaluation—breech presentation with the spine down (see Fig. A). The lumbosacral region could at best be only partially imaged. Because the lower spine was close to the lower uterine segment, a transvaginal examination that is usually limited to first-trimester evaluation allowed complete visualization of the lumbosacral spine and in a better plane or section (see Fig. B). The posterior elements are abnormally splayed outward (arrows), and the overlying posterior soft tissues are absent.

A careful survey of the fetal spine is essential with prenatal ultrasound. The lemon sign, which means the frontal bones lose their normal convex contour and appear flattened or inwardly scalloped, has a strong association with spina bifida. The exact pathogenesis of this association is unknown. Each vertebral body should have three ossification centers. The two posterior ossification centers must be parallel or converge. Divergence can be detected in axial and coronal planes in a myelomeningocele. A fluid-filled mass is usually seen overlying the defect (see Case 17, Fig. C). Associated musculoskeletal findings include clubfoot and scoliosis or kyphosis. Movement of the lower extremities of the fetus does not correlate with postnatal motor function. Findings in prenatal ultrasound and MR imaging are equally accurate for the assignment of lesion level in a fetus with a myelomeningocele.

A significant number of fetuses with open neural tube defects are chromosomally abnormal. Karyotype abnormalities occur in 13% to 17% of fetuses with spina bifida. In 20% of these cases, a prenatal sonogram shows only spina bifida. The presence of a neural tube defect should prompt a careful search for other anomalies which, if present, significantly raise the likelihood of a karyotype abnormality.

Notes

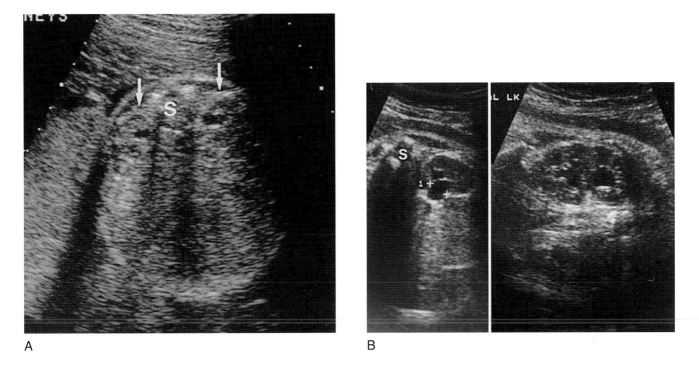

A

B

1. Is there an abnormality in either of these middle second-trimester fetuses? Figure A (fetus 1) is an axial view of both kidneys (arrows). Figure B (fetus 2) shows axial (on the reader's left) and coronal views of the left kidney; + signs in the axial view measure the renal pelvis at 11 mm; S = spine.

2. What are the upper limits of normal for the fetal renal pelvis on prenatal ultrasound?

3. What chromosomal anomaly may present with pyelectasis as one of the findings?

4. Name five potential etiologies for fetal renal pyelectasis.

Hydronephrosis

1. Fetus 2 (see Fig. B) is abnormal, showing pelvocaliectasis. Fetus 1 (see Fig. A) shows normal mild pyelectasis, without caliectasis.

2. Four millimeters or less before 23 weeks' gestation; 7 mm after 23 weeks.

3. Down syndrome (trisomy 21).

4. Vesicoureteral reflux, ureterocele with ureterovesical junction obstruction, ureteropelvic junction obstruction, urethral atresia, and posterior urethral valves.

References

Anderson N, Traci C-E, Allan R, et al: Detection of obstructive uropathy in the fetus: Predictive value of sonographic measurements of renal pelvic diameter at various gestational ages. *AJR* 164:719–723, 1995.

Kaefer M, Peters CA, Retik AB, Benacerraf BB: Increased renal echogenicity: A sonographic sign for differentiating between obstructive and nonobstructive etiologies of in utero bladder distension. *J Urol* 158:1026–1029, 1997.

Roth JA: Prenatal hydronephrosis. *Curr Opin Pediatr* 13: 138–141, 2001.

Cross-Reference

Ultrasound: THE REQUISITES, 2nd ed, pp 453, 460–461, 463, 465.

Comment

A number of studies have proposed upper limits of normal for fetal renal pelves throughout the gestation period. Prior to 23 weeks, the normal renal pelvis can measure up to 4 mm (3 to 5 mm in range). After 23 weeks, many use 7 mm as a cutoff point, but the upper limit of normal in some series is up to 10 mm. The incidence of fetal hydronephrosis is 1:100 to 1:500 maternal-fetal ultrasound studies.

The differential diagnosis of dilated renal pelves includes vesicoureteral reflux, ureteropelvic junction obstruction, posterior urethral valves, duplicated renal collecting system, megaloureter, and ureterocele. Approximately 25% of all fetuses with Down syndrome have pyelectasis. Once pyelectasis is detected, it becomes important to attempt to determine if the cause is an obstruction. Obstructed collecting systems show a greater increase in diameter than do nonobstructed kidneys throughout pregnancy. Therefore, the presence of caliectasis and interval increase are important indicators of an obstruction.

Associated findings that support an obstructive etiology include ureteral dilatation, bladder wall thickening, and oligohydramnios. Increased echogenicity of the kidneys is a confirmatory finding that reflects a long-term obstruction leading to irreversible damage–secondary renal dysplasia.

Notes

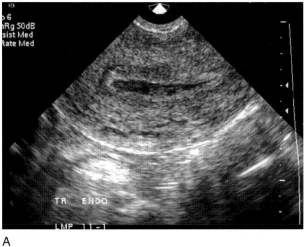

A

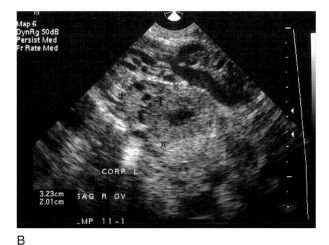

B

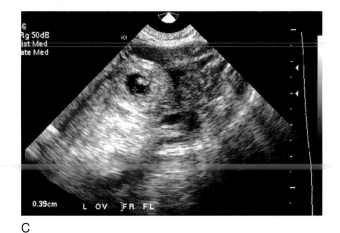

C

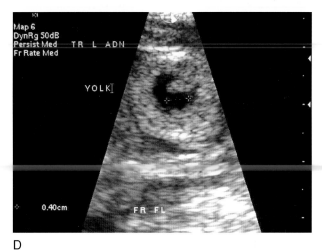

D

E

1. In a woman with a positive result on a pregnancy test, what is the diagnosis for these images of the uterus (Fig. A) and adnexa? Figure B is right intraovarian; C, D, and E are left and extraovarian.

2. How early does trophoblastic tissue produce β-human chorionic gonadotropin (hCG)?

3. Is the decidual reaction usually normal in the setting of an ectopic pregnancy?

4. What are the sonographic findings following methotrexate therapy to treat an ectopic pregnancy?

Ruptured Ectopic Pregnancy

1. Ruptured ectopic pregnancy.

2. Eight days after conception.

3. No; it is often thinner than would be seen with an intrauterine pregnancy.

4. An adnexal mass may persist for more than 3 months, even when the β-hCG level is zero.

References

Dogra V, Pasoulati RM, Bhatt S: First trimester bleeding evaluation: *Ultrasound Q* 21:69–85, 2005.

Fleischer AC, Pennell RG, McKee MS, et al: Ectopic pregnancy: Features at transvaginal sonography. *Radiology* 174:375–378, 1990.

Frates MC, Doubilet PM, Durfee SM, et al: Sonographic and Doppler characteristics of the corpus luteum: Can they predict pregnancy outcome? *J Ultrasound Med* 20:821–827, 2001.

Frates MC, Laing FC: Sonographic evaluation of ectopic pregnancy: An update. *AJR* 165:251–259, 1995.

Mostafa A: Ectopic pregnancy versus corpus luteum cyst revisited; best Doppler predictors. *J Ultrasound Med* 22: 1181–1184, 2003.

Nyberg DA, Hughes MP, Mack LA, Wang KY: Extrauterine findings of ectopic pregnancy at transvaginal US: Importance of echogenic fluid. *Radiology* 178:823–826, 1991.

Stein MW, Ricci ZJ, Novak L, Roberts, JH: Sonographic comparison of the tubal ring of ectopic pregnancy with the corpus luteum. *J Ultrasound Med* 23:57–62, 2004.

Cross-Reference

Ultrasound: THE REQUISITES, 2nd ed, pp 363–364, 367.

Comment

An ectopic pregnancy can involve any portion of the fallopian tube. The most common location is the isthmic portion; interstitial ectopics (in the thinnest part of the fallopian tube, adjacent to the uterus) are much less common but extremely important to detect because of the high risk of severe hemorrhage if a rupture occurs.

Transvaginal sonography enables detection of several findings that correlate with the presence of an ectopic pregnancy. Sonographic abnormalities can be seen with a β-hCG as low as 30 to 60 mIU/mL. Seventy percent of all unruptured ectopic pregnancies will have a "tubal ring," a 1- to 3-cm mass with a central hypoechoic area surrounded by concentric hyperechoic tissue. A tubal ring may be detected even if the tube is ruptured. Intraperitoneal fluid is seen in 63%; echogenic fluid suggests a hemoperitoneum. Twenty percent of patients with a ruptured tube, however, have no fluid or only a trace of detectable fluid. An extrauterine gestational sac can also be seen. If a corpus luteum cyst is present, it is only contralateral to the site of the ectopic gestation in up to one third of cases and on the same side as the ectopic pregnancy in many cases. Gray scale and Doppler characteristics of the corpus luteum cyst have shown no apparent relationship to first trimester pregnancy outcome. The presence of an extraovarian adnexal mass is the most common sonographic finding in an ectopic pregnancy. Sonographic signs to distinguish an ectopic pregnancy from a corpus luteum cyst include decreased wall echogenicity compared with the endometrium and an anechoic texture, which suggest a corpus luteum cyst. Most importantly, the corpus luteum is intraovarian, and intraovarian ectopics are exceedingly rare. Therefore, if the mass is intraovarian, it is almost always the corpus luteum.

Methotrexate is being administered with increasing frequency for the treatment of ectopic pregnancy. At our institution, a tubal ring greater than or equal to 2.5 cm is a contraindication to methotrexate and requires laparoscopy or laparotomy for treatment; similarly, signs of a ruptured ectopic or clinical instability would require surgery. Following methotrexate administration, an adnexal mass may transiently enlarge with increased Doppler flow. It is not unusual for the mass to persist for more than 3 months, even after the β-hCG level has declined to zero.

Notes

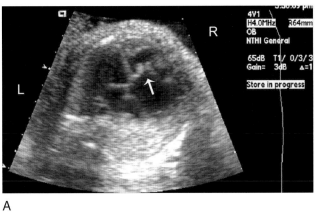

A

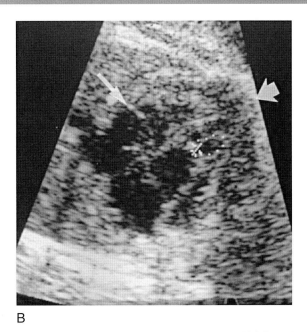

B

1. Figure A shows a four-chambered view of a late second-trimester fetal heart. What is the diagnosis? (Arrow points to the valve.)

2. Does the tricuspid valve regurgitate in this anomaly?

3. What is the maternal drug that results in this fetal anomaly?

4. What is the significance of the size of the fossa ovalis in this diagnosis?

Ebstein's Anomaly

1. Ebstein's anomaly.

2. Yes.

3. Lithium.

4. A small fossa ovalis has a worse prognosis.

References

Pavlova M, Fouron J-C, Susan P, et al: Factors affecting the prognosis of Ebstein's anomaly during fetal life. *Am Heart J* 135:1081–1085, 1998.

Weil SR, Huhta JC: Sonographic differential diagnosis of fetal cardiac abnormalities. *Semin Ultrasound CT MR* 14:298-317, 1993.

Cross-Reference

Ultrasound: THE REQUISITES, 2nd ed, pp 416–417.

Comment

Ebstein's anomaly results from displacement of a dysplastic tricuspid valve into the right ventricle, with consequent massive enlargement of the right atrium and atrialized right ventricle. Maternal lithium ingestion during pregnancy is a risk factor. The mortality rate of the neonate has been quoted to be as high as 85% in the perinatal period, which is considerably higher if the neonate presents with cyanosis.

Fetal ultrasound demonstrates a severely enlarged heart. The right atrium or atrialized right ventricle or both are greatly dilated (see Fig. A). The true residual right ventricle (see Fig. B) is small. The tricuspid valve is regurgitant, and tricuspid and pulmonic stenoses may also be present. The ductus arteriosus should be examined because ductal flow from the aorta to the pulmonary artery predicts postnatal ductal dependence for adequate pulmonary flow as a result of right-to-left shunting of desaturated blood.

Follow-up examinations are performed to measure the size of the chambers throughout the gestation period and to evaluate for decompensation revealed by hydrops fetalis. The true size of the right ventricular cavity is one factor that dictates the ability of the heart to compensate for increased pulmonary blood flow postnatally. Interestingly, left ventricular output affects whether such a fetus will reach term without problems. Because the fetal cardiac chambers run in parallel (rather than in a series as the postnatal heart functions) and because of communications between the great vessels and cardiac atria, the left ventricle may be able to compensate for right ventricular dysfunction.

Notes

Fair Game

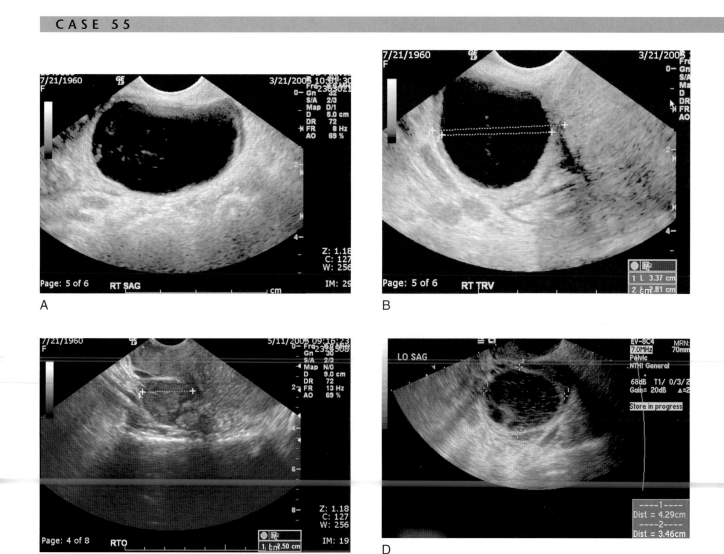

A

B

C

D

1. A 40-year-old woman presents with right adnexal pain. Is a hemorrhagic corpus luteum an unusual cause of pelvic pain? See Figures A and B, the sagittal and transverse transvaginal images of the right ovary. Figure C is a follow-up study 6 weeks later. Figures D and E are from a second patient with similar symptoms.

   Figures F and G are of an asymptomatic postmenopausal patient with no pelvic pain with Figure G as a follow-up image of the right ovary 3 months later. How would you report on that finding of a simple ovarian cyst less than 3 cm in diameter in a postmenopausal woman?

2. What is a corpus luteum?

3. Are these complex ovarian functional cysts usually smaller than 2 cm in diameter?

4. What is the classic ultrasonic appearance of a corpus luteum?

5. Are simple ovarian cysts uncommon in postmenopausal women?

6. In following patients with postmenopausal simple ovarian cysts over 2 years, about what percentage of cysts have disappeared?

7. How would you describe ovarian cysts that can be safely followed in postmenopausal women?

8. In reference to question 7, what is a normal resistive index (RI) for a simple ovarian cyst?

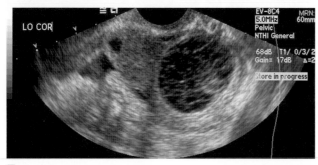

E

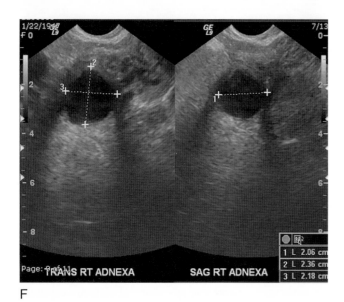

F

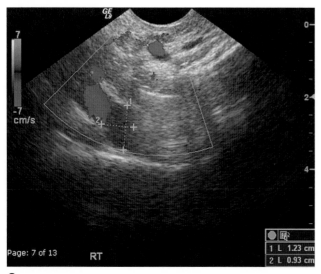

G

Ovarian Cyst

1. No. Simple adnexal cysts <5 cm can be safely followed by ultrasound in postmenopausal women because they are most likely benign.

2. Physiologic complex cyst formed after the release of an oocyte.

3. No, they can vary from 2.5 to 10 cm cubed.

4. Spongelike, lacelike, or reticular/spider-web appearance.

5. No, they are present in 15% to 20% of asymptomatic postmenopausal women.

6. About 50%.

7. Simple ovarian cysts less than 3 cm in diameter.

8. >0.4.

References

Bailey CL, Ueland FR, Land GL, DePriest PD et al: The malignant potential of small cystic ovarian tumors in women over 50 years of age. *Obstet Gynecol Surv* 53:544–546,1998.

Levine D, Gosink BB, Feldsman MR, et al: Simple adnexal cysts: The natural history in postmenopausal women. *Radiology* 184:653–659,1992.

Patel MD, Feldstein VA, Filly RA: The likelihood ratio of sonographic findings for the diagnosis of hemorrhagic ovarian cysts. *J. Ultrasound Med* 24:607–614, 2005.

Swire MN, Castro-Aragon I, Levine D: Various sonographic appearances of the hemorrhagic corpus luteum cyst. *Ultrasound Q* 20:45–58, 2004.

Timor-Tritsch IE, Goldstein SR: The complexity of a "complex mass" and the simplicity of a "simple cyst." *J Ultrasound Med* 24:255–258, 2005.

Cross-Reference

Ultrasound: THE REQUISITES, 2nd ed, pp 560–561, 563, 567, 568, 570–571.

Comment

Simple ovarian cysts of premenopausal women are usually physiologic follicles or dominant follicles, typically not larger than 3 cm in diameter. They do not cause pain unless there is a torsion, which is rare and has specific findings for diagnosis. A large simple cyst may be followed into the next cycle to check for physiologic change.

Ovarian cysts have been of more concern in postmenopausal women than in their premenopausal counterparts. It is important to detect any ovarian neoplasm, occurring more commonly in the older age group, as early as possible because with ovarian malignancies there is usually widespread disease before symptoms occur.

Simple ovarian cysts are not uncommon in post-menopausal women. In a study, these cysts are present in 15–17% of asymptomatic postmenopausal patients. In followup of cysts over 2 years in that study, approximately 53% of these simple cysts disappeared, 28% remained stable, 11% enlarged by 3 mm or more, and 3% decreased by 3 mm or more. The study recommended that simple adnexal cysts less than 3 cm (Fig. F) which have a normal resistive index (RI) <.4 in patients with a normal cancer antigen 125(CA 125) level are likely benign and can be safely followed by ultrasound. A more recent investigation of asymptomatic postmenopausal women that used 10 cm as maximum cyst diameter also showed that many of their ovarian cysts resolved spontaneously. Of those patients with unilocular cysts, 49% resolved within 60 days and 51% persisted. No cancers were detected in the examined ovaries after surgery in the patients with persistent cysts. Of the postmenopausal women with complex ovarian cysts, 55% resolved in 60 days and 45% persisted. Malignant ovarian tumors were found in this group. Data from this investigation leads to the suggestion that postmenopausal women with simple unilocular cysts <5 cm in diameter can be followed with ultrasound at 5 to 6 month intervals. However, complex ovarian cysts, even if small, are associated with a significant risk for malignancy and should be removed.

A hemorrhagic corpus luteum (called a cyst in some publications) is a common cause of pelvic pain. It is a physiologic cyst that forms upon release of the oocyte. The corpus luteum may rupture, resulting in a hemorrhagic cyst that may or may not be symptomatic. These cysts vary in size from 2.5 to 10 cm^2; the wall ranges in depth from 2 to 22 mm. The cyst composition causes posterior through transmission. However, the internal echo pattern varies, depending on the stage of the hemorrhage; this is best appreciated by transvaginal ultrasound scanning. See Figures A, B, D, and E. A classic appearance of hemorrhage is a spongelike, lacelike, or reticular pattern. See Figures D and E. Fibrin strands and/or a retracting clot were found in 90% of hemorrhagic cysts in a recent large series. Color flow Doppler sonography can show a typical "ring of fire." Four to 12 week follow-up studies show resolution of these complex cysts. See Figure C obtained 6 weeks after Figures A and B. The differential diagnosis of a complex, hemorrhagic ovarian cyst includes ectopic pregnancy, adnexal torsion, neoplasm, pelvic inflammatory disease, endometrioma, and degenerating fibroid.

If the complex ovarian cyst is not typical for corpus luteum or is larger than 3 cm, a follow-up ultrasound is recommended. This repeat study is often planned after a 6-week interval so that the patient's cyst is reimaged during a different phase of her menstrual cycle. If the patient is postmenopausal, a hemorrhagic cyst is abnormal. This mass is usually an indication for surgery.

Notes

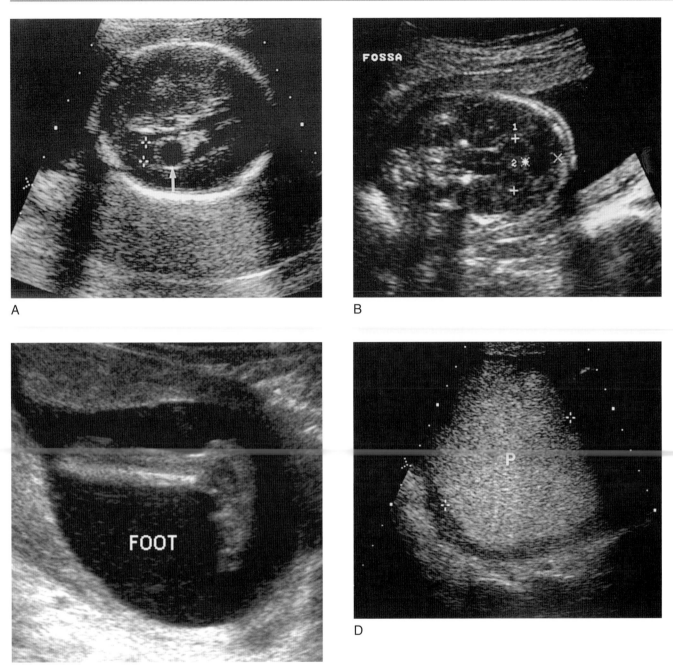

A

B

C

D

1. In this 28-week-old fetus, what are the two fetal head abnormalities detected by the arrow in Figure A and the x in Figure B? What is the likely chromosomal anomaly? Figure A is an axial image with + signs measuring the ventricular atrium. Figure B is a slanted axial image used to evaluate the posterior fossa (+ sign = the cerebellum).

2. What percentage of cases of this entity have choroid plexus cysts?

3. What limb anomaly is suggested in Figure C of the fetal leg and foot?

4. Which abnormality is denoted by the measurement (+ signs) of the placenta (P) in Figure D?

Trisomy 18

1. Figure A; the arrow points to a choroid plexus cyst. Figure B; x's denote an enlarged cisterna magna. Trisomy 18 (Edward's syndrome).

2. Choroid plexus cysts are present in 25% to 30% of cases of trisomy 18.

3. Rocker-bottom foot deformity.

4. Enlarged placenta.

Reference

Bronsteen R, Lee W, Vettraino IM, et al: Second-trimester sonography and trisomy 18: *J Ultrasound Med* 23:233–240, 2004.

Bronsteen R, Lee W, Vettraino IM, et al: Second-trimester sonography and trisomy 18: The significance of isolated choroid plexus cysts after an examination that includes the fetal hands. *J Ultrasound Med* 23:241–245, 2004.

Nyberg DA, Kramer D, Resta R, et al: Prenatal sonographic findings of trisomy 18: Review of 47 cases. *J Ultrasound Med* 2:103–113, 1993.

Nyberg DA, Souter VL: Sonographic markers of fetal trisomies. *J Ultrasound Med* 20:655–674, 2001.

Cross-Reference

Ultrasound: THE REQUISITES, 2nd ed, pp 395–397.

Comment

Trisomy 18 occurs second to trisomy 21 (Down syndrome) in terms of frequency of autosomal trisomies. Neonates with this disorder do not usually live longer than one week. In one series, the median survival rate was three days. Affected mothers have a bimodal age distribution of 25 to 29 years and 35 to 39 years of age; the prevalence increases with advanced maternal age.

More than 130 associated malformations have been described. Ultrasound can detect abnormalities in 80% of cases, and even a higher percentage of cases if imaging is performed after 24 weeks. Intrauterine growth restriction is seen in almost 90% of cases after 24 weeks. In the setting of polyhydramnios, symmetric intrauterine growth restriction should raise concern regarding the presence of trisomy 18.

Cardiac anomalies are present in almost 90% of cases. The most common malformations are atrial septal defect, ventriculoseptal defect, persistent ductus arteriosus, and dysplastic valves. Noncardiac malformations include cystic hygroma and bowel containing omphalocele.

Central nervous system malformations include a "strawberry-shaped" calvarium, which is believed to result from a hypoplastic frontal lobe of the brain. Choroid plexus cysts are present in 25% to 50% of cases (see Fig. A). However isolated choroid plexus cysts do not suggest trisomy 18. Between 80% and 90% of fetuses with trisomy 18 and choroid plexus cysts will have at least one other malformation facilitating diagnosis by prenatal ultrasound. Other central nervous system findings include meningomyelocele and an enlarged cisterna magna (see Fig. B). The cisterna magna measured from the posterior margin of the vermis to the inside margin of the occiput (x's) should not be more than 10 mm. If present, cisterna magna enlargement is frequently not detected until after 24 weeks' gestation. An enlarged cisterna magna without other abnormalities is often normal.

Both upper and lower limb anomalies may be present. Clenched fists, rocker-bottom feet (see Fig. C), and clubbed feet are associated findings. Decreased fetal movement and overlapping of fingers are attributed to generalized muscle spasticity.

The placenta can be enlarged. A measurement taken at its midpoint, perpendicular to its insertion, should normally be less than 4 cm (see Fig. D, + signs).

Notes

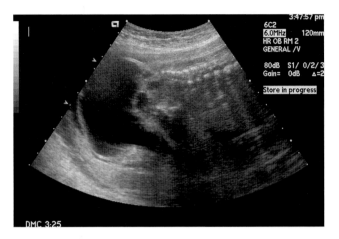

1. What is the differential diagnosis of the abnormality shown in the sagittal image of the lower fetal spine?

2. What spinal finding would aid in the distinction?

3. What abdominal finding would aid in the distinction?

4. Does an elevated α-fetoprotein (AFP) level contribute to the distinction?

Myelomeningocele Versus Sacrococcygeal Teratoma

1. Myelomeningocele versus sacrococcygeal teratoma.

2. Splaying or distortion of the posterior elements is compatible with a myelomeningocele.

3. Hydronephrosis may be seen with a sacrococcygeal teratoma (SCT).

4. No.

Reference

Hedrick HL, Flake Awm, Crombleholme TM, et al: Sacrococcygeal teratoma: Prenatal assessment, fetal intervention, and outcome. *J Pediatr Surg* 39:430–438, 2004.

Sheth S, Nussbaum SR, Sanders RC, et al: Prenatal diagnosis of sacrococcygeal teratoma: Sonographic-pathologic correlation. *Radiology* 169:131–136, 1988.

Thomas, M: The lemon sign. *Radiology* 228:206–207, 2003.

Westerburg B, Feldstein Vam, Sandberg PL, et al: Sonographic prognostic factors in fetuses with sacrococcygeal teratoma. *J Pediatr Surg* 35:322–325, 2000.

Cross-Reference

Ultrasound: THE REQUISITES, 2nd ed, pp 402–406, 408–410.

Comment

This case illustrates a myelomeningocele. The differential considerations include this and a sacrococcygeal teratoma.

Findings associated with a myelomeningocele include splayed or distorted posterior elements of the spine, hydrocephalus, banana-shaped cerebellum, and lemon-head deformity (frontal bones lose their normal convex contour and appear flattened or inwardly scalloped) of the calvarium (Chiari's malformation). SCT may result in displacement of the bladder and hydronephrosis owing to an anterior (presacral) component. Hydronephrosis is a poor prognostic indicator. An elevated AFP level may be present in both cases because immature components (yolk sac tumor components) of an SCT may secrete AFP.

Sacrococcygeal teratomas (especially when solid and highly vascularized.) as opposed to myelomeningoceles put the patient at risk for cardiac compromise and sometimes hydrops fetalis from high-output cardiac failure. Fetuses with this teratoma may require amnioreduction, cyst aspiration, and surgical debulking.

Notes

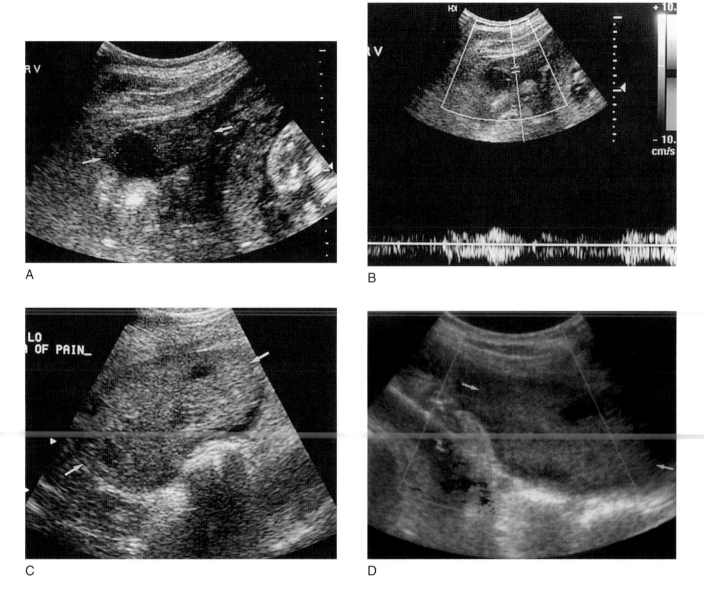

A

B

C

D

1. What is the abnormality in this 20-year-old pregnant patient with cyclical left-sided pelvic pain? Figures A and B display the right ovary. Figure B indicates a spectral Doppler signal from the soft tissue of that ovary (arrows = ovary; + signs = a simple follicle). Figures C and D illustrate the left ovary (arrows = ovary). Figure D provides a color Doppler evaluation.

2. What is the typical age (stage of life) of a patient with this diagnosis?

3. List three risk factors for this condition.

4. Is Doppler analysis a reliable aid in the diagnosis of this entity?

Ovarian Torsion

1. Left ovarian torsion.

2. Premenopausal.

3. Ovarian mass, ovarian hyperstimulation syndrome, and pregnancy.

4. No.

References

Albayram F, Hamper UM: Ovarian and adnexal torsion: Spectrum of sonographic findings with pathologic correlation. *J Ultrasound Med* 20:1083–1089, 2001.

Di Salvo DN: Sonographic imaging of maternal complications of pregnancy. *J Ultrasound Med* 22:69–89, 2003.

Lee EJ, Kwon HC, Joo HJ, et al: Diagnosis of ovarian torsion with color Doppler sonography: Depiction of the twisted vascular pedicle. *J Ultrasound Med* 17:83–89, 1998.

Stark JE, Siegel MJ: Ovarian torsion in prepubertal and pubertal girls: Sonographic findings. *AJR* 163:1479–1482, 1994.

Vijayaraghavan SB: Sonographic whirlpool sign in ovarian torsion. *J Ultrasound Med* 23:1643–1649, 2004.

Cross-Reference

Ultrasound: THE REQUISITES, 2nd ed, pp 567, 569, 576, 578, 579.

Comment

Ovarian torsion is a cause of acute abdominal pain in women requiring rapid diagnosis and treatment. Torsion occurs most commonly in women of reproductive years; a nonadherent ipsilateral adnexal mass is present in 50% to 81% of cases, most commonly a benign teratoma. Nonetheless, torsion of the normal ovary can occur in prepubertal females because of adnexal mobility. Ovarian torsion is slightly more common on the right side. Risk factors include the presence of an adnexal mass, ovarian hyperstimulation syndrome, and pregnancy. Ovarian torsion during pregnancy is facilitated by the presence of a corpus luteum during the first trimester. A large cyst that develops after ovulation induction can also be an inciting factor. The pain is classically cyclical and grows worse with each cycle, although constant or vague pain may be the presenting symptom.

The appearance of ovarian torsion has been described with ultrasound, computed tomography, and magnetic resonance imaging. With ultrasound, the findings vary, depending on the age of the patient. However, an enlarged ovary or mass should be present as the lead point of the torsion (see Fig. C). The appearance of an ovary in torsion is variable, depending on whether an underlying mass is present and the degree of hemorrhage or necrosis resulting in cystic and hyperechoic components. Free fluid is present in up to two thirds of cases.

Color and pulsed Doppler ultrasound have been shown to be unreliable in the definitive diagnosis of ovarian torsion. Whereas an enlarged abnormal-appearing ovary with no arterial or venous flow may indicate torsion (see Fig. D), arterial and venous flow have been demonstrated in surgically proven cases of ovarian torsion. Torsion can be intermittent. Therefore, the persistence of blood flow depends on the degree of torsion. Arterial flow with no diastolic component or absence of venous flow can be seen early. Venous thrombosis may precede arterial occlusion.

The twisted vascular pedicle is defined as the rotation site of the ovarian pedicle and has been imaged with ultrasound. The pedicle is located either adjacent to the ovary/ovarian mass or between the ovary and the uterus, where vessels usually run in a straight course. A positive whirlpool sign in the twisted vascular pedicle has been reported as the most definitive sign of ovarian torsion. In cases in which flow is still identified in the twisted pedicle, the ovary is viable at surgery and the pedicle is untwisted. The condition of no flow in the twisted pedicle and flow in the artery alone but not the vein has been predictive of nonviability of the ovary.

Notes

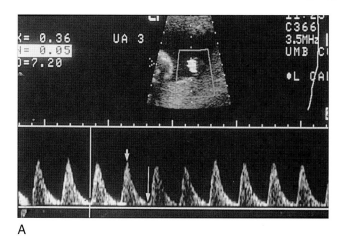

A

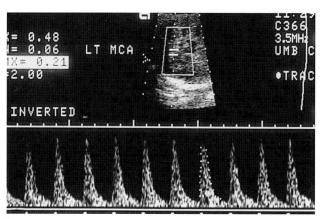

B

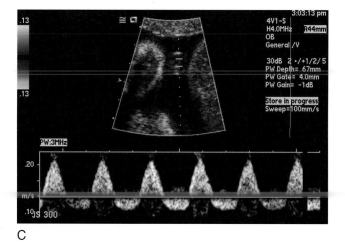

C

1. What does decreased, absent, or reversed diastolic flow in the umbilical artery indicate ?

2. What is the purpose of measuring the flow of the middle cerebral artery (MCA) (Fig. B)?

3. How is the umbilical artery impedance measured?

4. What is the normal pattern of the umbilical artery Doppler image as gestation progresses?

Umbilical Artery Doppler

1. Placental insufficiency and possibly a fetal abnormality.

2. To determine whether a compensatory, brain-sparing fetal response has occurred as a result of decreased umbilical artery diastolic flow.

3. As a ratio of peak systolic velocity (short arrow) divided by end-diastolic velocity (long arrow) (systolic/diastolic [S/D] ratio) (see Fig. A).

4. Increasing diastolic flow (lower ratio).

References

Alfirevic Z, Neilson JP: Fetus-placenta-newborn: Doppler ultrasonography in high-risk pregnancies: Systematic review with meta-analysis. *Am J Obstet Gynecol* 172:1379–1387, 1995.

Sepulveda W, Shennan A, Peek MJ: Reverse end-diastolic flow in the middle cerebral artery: An agonal pattern in the human fetus. *Am J Obstet Gynecol* 174:1645–1647, 1996.

Spinillo A, Montanari L, Bergante C, et al: Prognostic value of umbilical artery Doppler studies in unselected preterm deliveries *Obstet Gynecol* 105:613–620, 2005.

Valcamonico A, Danti L, Frusca T, et al: Absent end-diastolic velocity in umbilical artery: Risk of neonatal morbidity and brain damage. *Am J Obstet Gynecol* 170:796–801, 1994.

Cross-Reference

Ultrasound: THE REQUISITES, 2nd ed, pp 335–337.

Comment

Doppler ultrasound imaging has become an important component in the prenatal evaluation of high-risk pregnancies. The umbilical artery waveform can indicate abnormal fetal-placental blood flow by demonstrating elevated placental impedance. An abnormal umbilical artery waveform is associated with a higher incidence of adverse fetal outcome.

Indications for measuring the umbilical artery waveform include the presence of oligohydramnios and intrauterine growth restriction. A waveform should be obtained from the fetal end of the cord and also from the middle and the maternal end of the cord. The S/D ratio (peak systolic velocity/end-diastolic velocity) at each of these three points is averaged and compared with a chart of normal values for each gestational age (see Fig. A). With increasing gestational age, the S/D ratio should decrease, reflecting decreasing impedance.

If the impedance increases, the diastolic flow will decrease and can be absent (see Fig. A) or reversed in the umbilical artery (see Fig. C). Absence or reversal of diastolic flow has been associated with intrauterine growth restriction, fetal asphyxia, perinatal mortality, cerebral palsy, and long-term permanent fetal neurologic sequelae. In addition, there is a higher likelihood that the fetus has a chromosomal anomaly. Routine use of Doppler ultrasound of the umbilical artery to guide management (i.e., timing of delivery) has resulted in a lower incidence of antenatal admissions, labor induction, emergency cesarean section for fetal distress, perinatal death, and hypoxic fetal encephalopathy.

When fetal hypoxia results from decreased diastolic umbilical artery flow, the fetal circulation responds with a "brain-sparing" effect. The MCA index is measured either as the S/D ratio or as a pulsatility index (i.e., peak systole minus end-diastole divided by the area of one waveform; see Fig. B: the dotted lines outline one waveform). The MCA Doppler image is evaluated to determine if blood is being redistributed from other sources (e.g., mesenteric) to the intracranial structures. In this case, the MCA pulsatility index is normal, reflecting redistribution of blood to the brain (see Fig. B). If further decompensation occurs, the MCA pulsatility index actually *decreases* and diastolic flow to the brain increases.

Notes

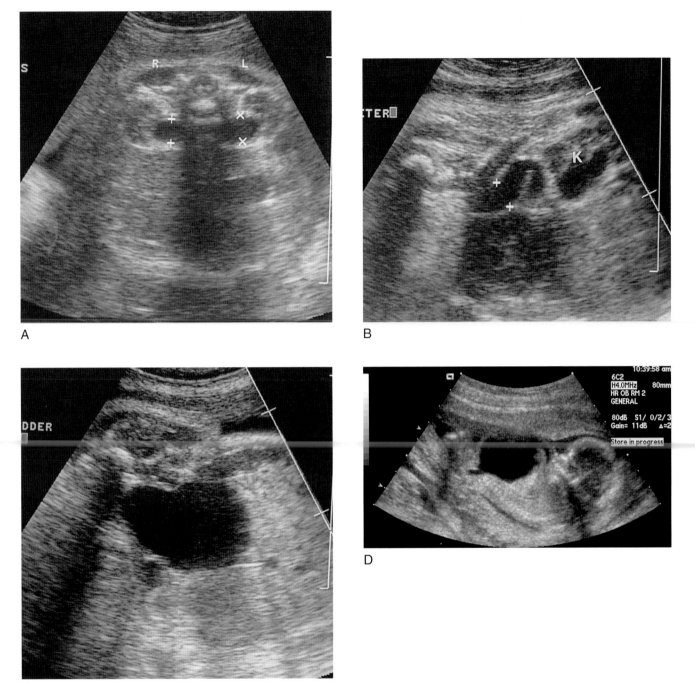

A

B

C

D

1. What are the findings and the differential diagnoses in the ultrasound images of this third-trimester fetus? Figure A is an axial view of the fetal kidneys (+ signs = renal pelves; R = right kidney; L = left kidney). Figure B is a coronal image of the lower abdomen (K = left kidney; + signs = ureter). Figure C is an oblique image of the fetal pelvis.

2. What two findings aid in confirming that dilatation of the renal collecting system is obstructive?

3. What is the classic appearance of the bladder with posterior urethral valves (PUVs)?

4. Does dilatation of the renal collecting system always indicate an obstruction?

Posterior Urethral Valves

1. Dilated urinary tract from the kidneys to the bladder. The differential diagnoses are posterior urethral valves (male), urethral agenesis (female), prune-belly syndrome, and megacystis-megaureter syndrome.

2. Bladder wall thickening and echogenic (hyperechoic) kidneys.

3. Keyhole.

4. No.

References

Hutton KAR, Thomas DFM, Davies BW: Prenatally detected posterior urethral valves: Qualitative assessment of second trimester scans and prediction of outcome. *J Urol* 158:1022–1025, 1997.

Kaefer M, Peters CA, Retik AB, Benacerraf BB: Increased renal echogenicity: A sonographic sign for differentiating between obstructive and nonobstructive etiologies of in utero bladder distension. *J Urol* 158:1026–1029, 1997.

Montemarano H, Bulas DI, Rushton HG, Selby D: Bladder distension and pyelectasis in the male fetus: Causes, comparisons, and contrasts. *J Ultrasound Med* 17:743–749, 1998.

Cross-Reference

Ultrasound: THE REQUISITES, 2nd ed, pp 459–460, 463–464, 468.

Comment

Detection of an enlarged fetal bladder immediately raises suspicion for an obstructive etiology. The fetus should be imaged over time to determine if the bladder will empty; the bladder fills and empties every 15 to 45 minutes. Bladder dilatation can be caused by obstructive etiologies (e.g., posterior urethral valves in males, urethral atresia in females) or nonobstructive etiologies (e.g., prune-belly syndrome, megacystis-megaureter syndrome). Dilatation of the pelvicaliceal system (hydronephrosis) and ureter (hydroureter) can be caused by obstructive etiologies (e.g., posterior urethral valves, urethral atresia, ectopic ureterocele) or by nonobstructive etiologies (e.g., prune-belly syndrome, megacystis-megaureter syndrome, vesicoureteral reflux).

Determining fetal gender is important in cases of urinary tract obstruction. In a male fetus, the most likely diagnosis in this case is an obstructive uropathy secondary to PUVs, which occurs exclusively in males (see Figs. A to C). A keyhole appearance of the urinary bladder is classic for PUVs (Fig. D). The presence of oligohydramnios, progressive bladder wall thickening, and dilated posterior urethra was most suggestive of PUVs, whereas the presence of a patent urachus was most suggestive of prune-belly syndrome in one study of male fetuses. The presence of pyelectasis and megacystis without additional amniotic fluid, bladder, urethral, or renal abnormalities was most suggestive of vesicoureteral reflux, ureterovesical junction obstruction, or nonrefluxing, nonobstructive megacystis-megaureter.

The timing of detection and the degree of obstruction have been shown to be predictors of outcome in fetuses with PUVs. An obstructed bladder detected before 28 weeks carries a poor prognosis. Obstruction of the urinary tract that results in dilatation detected at this early age often results in intrauterine death or poor renal function in those who survive. With moderate to severe upper tract dilatation, the prognosis is significantly worse than with isolated bladder distention or mild upper tract dilatation. Moderate to severe dilatation is defined as an anteroposterior diameter of the renal pelvis of 10 mm or greater with caliectasis. Detection of echogenic kidneys or cystic renal parenchymal changes indicate renal dysplasia, which also has a poor prognosis.

In utero decompression can be performed with vesicoamniotic shunting. However, this has not been shown to improve outcome. Nonetheless, detection of the posterior urethral valves and characterization of the degree of obstruction may be helpful in counseling parents about the prognosis.

Notes

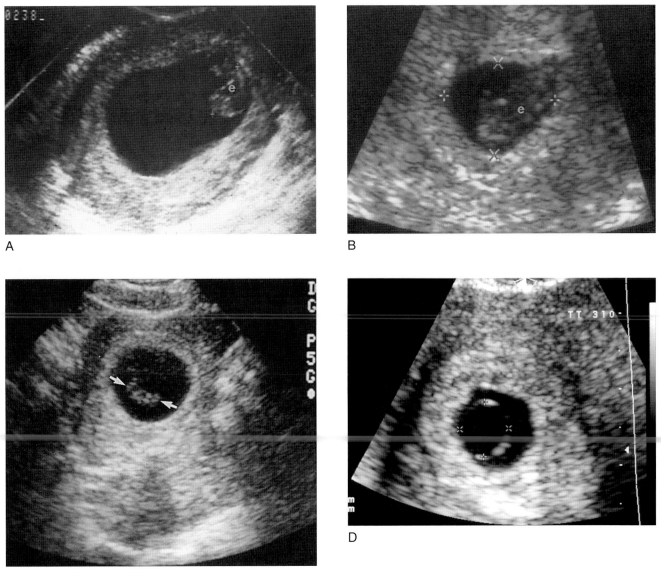

A

B

C

D

1. Which of these early pregnancies is normal? (Figs. A to E; e or arrows = embryos.) Why?

2. At what size of the gestational sac should you visualize (1) a yolk sac, and (2) a fetal pole transvaginally?

3. Can the detection of a yolk sac in the first trimester predict pregnancy as an outcome?

4. Does detection of an embryo less than 5 mm in size without a heartbeat indicate fetal demise?

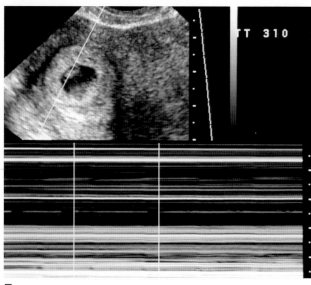

E

Early Intrauterine Gestational Sac

1. Figure C is normal. The normal gestational sac is about twice the length of the embryo with appropriate surrounding fluid. In the other two, the gestational sac is too large (see Fig. A) and too small (see Fig. B) for the embryo. Figure D has too large a yolk sac (larger than 9 to10.8 mm from published data); the cardiac tracing in Figure E shows the fetal demise of the embryo.

2. The yolk sac should be seen with an 8-mm sac; the fetal pole should be seen with a 16-mm sac. If they do not meet these criteria, follow-up is advised as long as the gestational sac appears to be normal. Normal intrauterine pregnancies (IUPs) are occasionally delayed, and an embryo is not detected until the gestational sac is approximately 20 mm.

3. No.

4. No.

References

Chiang G, Levine D, Swire M, McNamara A, et al: The intradecidual sign: Is it reliable for diagnosis of early intrauterine pregnancy? *AJR* 183:725–731, 2004.

Dogra V, Paspulati RM, Bhatt S: First trimester bleeding evaluation. *Ultrasound Q* 21:69–85, 2005.

Kurtz AB, Needleman L, Pennell RG, et al: Can detection of the yolk sac in the first trimester be used to predict the outcome of pregnancy? *AJR* 158:843–847, 1992.

Mara E, Foster GS: Spontaneous regression of a yolk sac associated with embryonic death. *J Ultrasound Med* 19:655–656, 2000.

McKenna KM, Feldstein VA, Goldstein RB, Filly RA: The empty amnion: A sign of early pregnancy failure. *J Ultrasound Med* 23:371–374, 2004.

Mehta RS, Levine D, Beckwith B: Treatment of ectopic pregnancy: Is a human chorionic gonadotropin level of 2000 ml U/ml a reasonable threshold? *Radiology* 205:569–573, 1997.

Stampone C, Nicotra M, Muttinelli C, Cosmi E: Transvaginal sonography of the yolk sac in normal and abnormal pregnancy. *J Clin Ultrasound* 24:3–9, 1996.

Cross-Reference

Ultrasound: THE REQUISITES, 2nd ed, pp 342, 347, 352, 353, 359.

Comment

Many ultrasound imaging criteria have been described to aid in distinguishing a normal IUP from an abnormal IUP or anembryonic gestation. A gestational sac with a mean sac diameter of 16 mm or more without an embryo is a sonographic sign of anembryonic gestation. It is essential to know the quantitative β-human chorionic gonadotropin (β-hCG) level when evaluating any early pregnancy as well as which international standard (IS) is being performed in your laboratory. There are three different tests: the first, second, and third IS. The first IS is twice the second IS. The third IS is 1.8 times the second IS (similar to the first).

Data have suggested that an intrauterine sac should be visible by 1000 mIU/mL using the first and third IS. Accordingly, in cases where the β-hCG level is 1000 to 2000 mIU/mL and no IUP is seen with transvaginal ultrasound, ectopic pregnancy becomes a concern. However, a recent study has shown that in cases where no definite IUP was visible by transvaginal ultrasound with a β-hCG of 2000 mIU/mL, normal pregnancies subsequently developed in one third of cases. It is essential to be careful when interpreting these studies, because methotrexate is being administered with increasing frequency by obstetricians if an ectopic pregnancy is suspected when no IUP is visible on ultrasound. Close follow-up should be considered if clinically appropriate.

Once an early sac is identified in the uterus, transvaginal scanning is often required to visualize a yolk sac or a small fetal pole. A yolk sac should be visible when the mean sac diameter (MSD) is 8 mm; the fetal pole should be visible when the MSD is 16 mm. However, follow-up should be recommended, as a normal IUP may be identified later even when these criteria are not met (some embryos are not visualized until the MSD exceeds 18 mm). If a fetal pole is seen, fetal heart motion is usually detected when the pole is equal to or greater than 5 mm. The size of the fetal pole in relation to the sac is also predictive of outcome. If the fetal pole is too small for the sac (see Fig. A) or too large for the sac (see Fig. B), fetal demise often results. Visualization of an amnion (and the yolk sac) but not an embryo (empty amnion) is associated with pregnancy loss.

The yolk sac (actually the secondary yolk sac) becomes visible before the fetal pole. An abnormal or absent yolk sac is associated with poor pregnancy outcome. However, the presence of a normal-appearing yolk sac is not consistently predictive of a normal early pregnancy. A large yolk sac, 9 to 10.8 mm, is a sign of possible impending fetal demise, and close follow-up is indicated. Also normal yolk sacs are smooth, spherical, lucent, and not calcified. However, transient abnormally shaped yolk sacs have resulted in normal pregnancies.

Notes

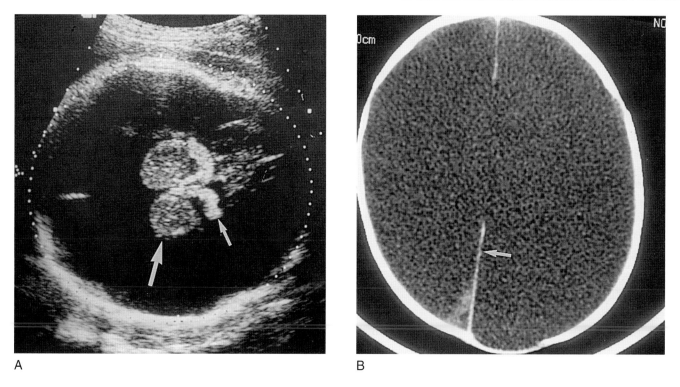

A   B

1. From this axial ultrasound image of a third-trimester fetus (Fig. A), what is the most likely diagnosis? Name the labeled structures.

2. Name the structure labeled in the neonatal computed tomography (CT) scan of the head (Fig. B, arrow). What diagnosis does it exclude?

3. Would ventricular shunting be indicated in this case?

4. What is the presumed etiology of this disorder?

CASE 62

Hydranencephaly

1. Hydranencephaly. Large arrow = thalamus; small arrow = choroid plexus.

2. Falx; alobar holoprosencephaly.

3. No; shunting is indicated for noncommunicating or obstructive hydrocephalus.

4. Bilateral internal carotid artery (ICA) infarctions. Infection has also been associated.

Reference

Greene MF, Benaceraff BR, Crawford JM: Hydranencephaly: US appearance during in utero evolution. *Radiology* 156:779–780, 1985.

Cross-Reference

Ultrasound: THE REQUISITES, 2nd ed. pp 382–383.

Comment

Hydranencephaly is caused by massive bilateral cortical destruction with *ex vacuo* enlargement of the already formed lateral ventricles. Leptomeninges surround fluid replacing the cerebral cortex. Remaining structures include the brainstem, thalami, cerebellum, and choroid plexus; the choroid plexus continues to make cerebrospinal fluid, accounting for the associated macrocephaly.

The etiology of hydranencephaly is believed to be the result of a bilateral supraclinoid ICA infarct. In addition to the proposed etiology of an ICA infarct, infection is believed to be the cause in some cases. Associated infections include toxoplasmosis, herpes virus, equine virus, and cytomegalic virus inclusion disease.

A prenatal ultrasound distinction from marked hydrocephalus is essential but often difficult to make. Identification of a thin mantle of residual cerebral cortex confirms that hydrocephalus is the etiology. The presence of the falx (arrow in Fig. B) and separate thalami (large arrow in Fig. A) distinguish hydranencephaly from alobar holoprosencephaly. The face is normal in hydranencephaly, as opposed to the various facial anomalies associated with holoprosencephaly. Polyhydramnios is usually present in conjunction with hydranencephaly as well as the other associated central nervous system malformations.

The disorder usually leads to death in the first few days of life; rarely, a child lives several months or longer. Postnatal CT is helpful in evaluating suspected hydranencephaly. Massive subdural effusions may mimic hydranencephaly on postnatal CT scans.

Notes

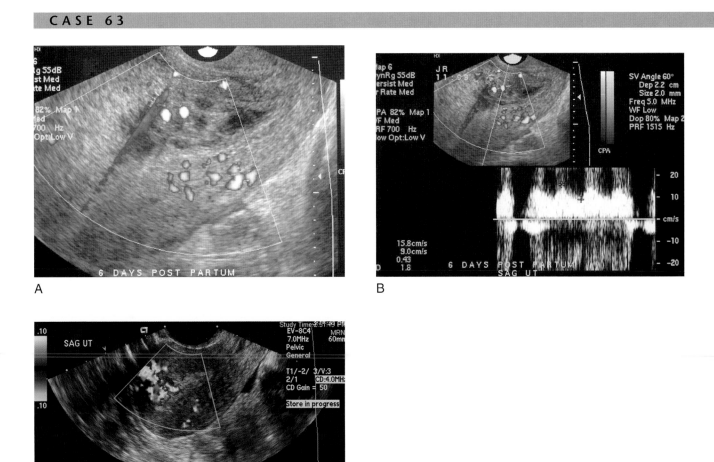

A

B

C

1. A 24-year-old woman presents with persistent abnormal vaginal bleeding postpartum. Figure A is a sagittal transvaginal image showing Doppler flow; Figure B also shows the spectral tracing. Figure C is the sagittal transvaginal Doppler image of a second patient with the same symptoms. The endometrial thickness is greater than 5 mm in both patients. What is your most likely diagnosis and why?

2. Can a molar pregnancy (hydatidiform mole) present with a similar appearance?

3. What is the normal endometrial thickness following a miscarriage (spontaneous abortion) or a dilatation and curettage?

4. How can Doppler ultrasound help in the evaluation of the uterine findings (see Fig. B)? Figure B displays a split-screen image of the same patient; the upper half shows the uterus with a pulsed Doppler cursor in the endometrium, and the lower half shows the spectral waveform (arrow = peak systole; arrowhead = end-diastole).

Retained Products of Conception

1. Retained products of conception (POCs). Hyperechoic focal soft tissue distending the endometrial canal with Doppler ultrasound confirming trophoblastic tissue by the arterial low impedance waveform.

2. Unlikely, because the amount of tissue is small; furthermore, the tissue does not have good through-transmission.

3. The endometrial thickness should be no greater than 5 mm.

4. Doppler color flow if present may help in distinguishing retained POCs from decidua and hemorrhage but the presence of an endometrial mass in the proper clinical context is more sensitive for retained products of conception.

References

Achiron R, Goldenberg M, Lipitz S, et al: Transvaginal duplex Doppler ultrasonography in bleeding patients suspected of having residual trophoblastic tissue. *Obstet Gynecol* 81:507–511, 1993.

Durfee SM, Fratews MC, Luong A, Benson CB: The sonographic and color Doppler features of retained products of conception. *J Ultrasound Med* 24:1181–1186, 2005.

Hertzberg BS, Bowie JD: Ultrasound of the postpartum uterus: Prediction of retained placental tissue. *J Ultrasound Med* 10:451–456, 1991.

Kaakaji Y, Nghiem HV, Nodell C, Winter TC: Sonography of obtstetric and gynecologic emergencies: Part 1, obstetric emergencies. *AJR* 174:841–849, 2000.

Kurtz AB, Shlaansky-Goldberg RD, Choi HY, et al: Detection of retained products of conception following spontaneous abortion in the first trimester. *J Ultrasound Med* 10:387–395, 1991.

Sadan O, Golan A, Girtler O, Lurie S, et al: Role of sonography in the diagnosis of retained products of conception. *J Ultrasound Med* 23:371–374, 2004.

Cross-Reference

Ultrasound: THE REQUISITES, pp 540–541

Comment

Retained POCs present with bleeding, uterine tenderness, and fever in the first 10 days following incomplete pregnancy loss, spontaneous or elective abortion, or full-term pregnancy. Complications of a delayed diagnosis may include peritonitis, septic and hypovolemic shock, disseminated intravascular coagulopathy, and, rarely, osseous endometrial metaplasia.

On ultrasound examination, retained POCs may be difficult to distinguish from intrauterine decidua, hemorrhage, and endometrium. Following a spontaneous abortion or after a dilatation and curettage, an endometrial stripe of less than 5 mm in thickness is an excellent but not absolute predictor of the absence of a retained POC. Any endometrial collection or endometrial thickening greater than 5 mm suggests retained POCs. The endometrial contents may appear as hypoechoic or hyperechoic solid material, with or without a mass; heterogeneous fluid with solid material; or a solid mass with calcification. A hyperechoic mass (>15 mm) that expands the endometrial canal is the best predictor (see Fig. A). A recent study determined that an endometrial mass is the most sensitive finding for retained POCs; if no mass or fluid is seen and the endometrial thickness is less than 10 mm, retained POCs are very unlikely. The presence of color flow on Doppler was not helpful in that series. In other studies it has been more helpful. Retained trophoblastic tissue has low-resistance arterial flow, which is uncommonly seen with endometritis. A more recent publication found the reliance on common signs and symptoms to diagnose retained products of conception, as well as the use of sonography, associated with an unacceptably high false-positive rate.

The differential diagnosis should also include a molar pregnancy (hydatidiform mole), which may present with vaginal bleeding. On ultrasound examination, this tissue may be hyperechoic, as in this case; however, owing to the multiple fluid-filled spaces, the tissue will have good through-transmission. The uterus is usually very enlarged.

Active trophoblastic tissue from any source will give arterial waveforms with elevated diastolic flow (low impedance) (see Fig. B). When detected, it distinguishes retained POCs from decidua and hemorrhage. However, similar waveforms can be seen with a hydatidiform mole. If doubt remains between POCs and a molar pregnancy, evaluation of the serum β-human chorionic gonadotropin levels should be diagnostic because a molar pregnancy will have persistently elevated levels whereas POCs will have low levels that often continue to fall.

Notes

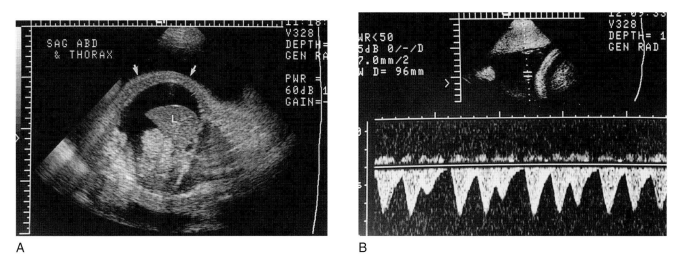

A

B

1. What are the findings in this third-trimester fetus and what is the diagnosis (Fig. A)? Figure A is a sagittal image of the fetal body. The thorax lies toward the reader's right. L = liver; arrows = the anterior abdominal wall.

2. Can Doppler ultrasound imaging of the umbilical artery establish a cause for the appearance of this fetus (Fig. B)?

3. What is believed to be one of the earliest findings if this presents in the first trimester?

4. What is the outcome?

Nonimmune Fetal Hydrops

1. Ascites and skin thickening. Fetal hydrops.

2. Yes; nonimmune hydrops caused by fetal tachyarrhythmia (trigeminy).

3. Increased nuchal translucency.

4. Poor; mortality is higher than 70%.

References

Jauniaux E: Diagnosis and management of early non-immune hydrops fetalis. *Prenat Diagn* 17:1261–1268, 1997.

Santolaya J, Jaffe R, Warsof SL: Antenatal classification of hydrops fetalis. *Obstet Gynecol* 79:256–259, 1992.

Cross-Reference

Ultrasound: THE REQUISITES, 2nd ed, pp 414–415, 419–422.

Comment

Fetal hydrops (hydrops fetalis) is a condition of fluid accumulation in the fetal pleural, peritoneal, and pericardial spaces as well as skin edema and placentomegaly (see Fig. A). At present, isoimmunization related to blood group incompatibilities of the mother and fetus has become a relatively rare cause, and most cases are classified as nonimmune hydrops.

There are approximately 80 different causes of nonimmune hydrops. In the first trimester, this is usually attributable to a chromosomal defect (e.g., trisomy 21, 18, or 13 or Turner's syndrome) in which lymphatic obstruction causes hydrops. Some believe that increased nuchal translucency is the first manifestation of fluid accumulation due to hydrops. This can be detected as early as 9 weeks, with a nuchal translucency of more than 3 mm. In cases diagnosed during the first trimester, karyotypically normal fetuses have demonstrated resolution of the hydrops later in the gestation. However, the outcome of these fetuses remains unfavorable. If diagnosed before 20 weeks, the two most common indicators of hydrops include generalized skin thickening and placental enlargement.

Structural anomalies account for many cases of hydrops diagnosed after 15 weeks. Common causes include cardiac malformations and cardiac arrhythmias (see Fig. B, tachyarrhythmia), which can be intermittent and not appreciated on any one examination. Other nonimmune cases include cystic hygroma with diffuse lymphatic obstruction and any mass that obstructs venous return to the heart. Teratomas, particularly sacrococcygeal, may lead to hydrops, which is believed to be caused by high outflow through the tumor. The high-output heart failure associated with a vein of Galen arteriovenous malformation or severe anemia are additional causes. Finally, maternal-fetal infection, such as the TORCH (*t*oxoplasmosis, *o*ther infections, *r*ubella, *c*ytomegalovirus, *h*erpes) group and parvovirus can result in hydrops. There is a long list of causes of hydrops, for which we refer you to Nyberg's *Diagnostic Ultrasound of Fetal Anomalies*.

The early detection of fetal hydrops is often difficult. This, however, is important clinically because by the time that fluid is detected within body cavities and marked skin thickening is noted, the fetus is often significantly compromised. Work on fetuses at risk for immune hydrops has shown that the length of the liver (from the dome of the right hemidiaphragm to the distal tip) increased as the first sign of impending hydrops in moderate to severe cases. It has not been determined whether this is a uniform finding, and its use in nonimmune hydrops has not been fully worked out.

At present, the outcome of a fetus with full-blown sonographic signs of fetal hydrops is generally poor, and mortality is higher than 70%.

Notes

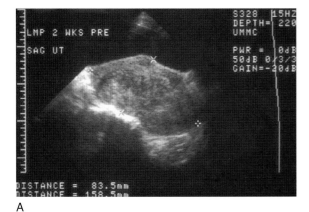

A

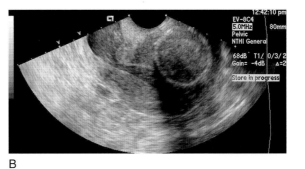

B

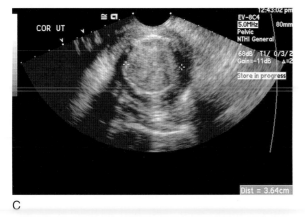

C

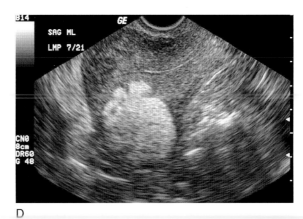

D

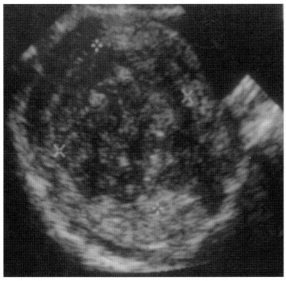

E

1. These are images from four women with uterine enlargement and palpable uterine masses. Two cases are fibroid tumors, one a lipoleiomyoma and one a leiomyosarcoma. Can you tell them apart?

2. What accounts for the increased echogenicity in the lipoleiomyoma (Fig. B)?

3. What is the incidence of uterine sarcomas?

4. How is a leiomyosarcoma of the uterus distinguished from a leiomyoma?

CASE 65

Uterine Masses

1. Figures A, B, and C show solid hypoechoic masses that are myometrial fibroids. (Fig. A has a coarse heterogeneous echotexture and greatly distorts the uterine contour; B and C have calcified rims.) Figure D is a very echogenic well-defined fibroid containing fat, a lipoleiomyoma. Figure E, which is a large heterogeneous solid mass, could have been a fibroid but was a leiomyosarcoma at pathologic examination.

2. Multiple closely packed boundary interfaces of multiple tissue types.

3. One percent to 3% of all uterine malignancies.

4. It frequently cannot be distinguished.

References

Becker E, Lev-Toaff AS, Kaufman EP, Halpern MD, et al: The added value of transvaginal sonohysterography over transvaginal sonography alone in women with known or suspected leiomyoma. *J Ultrasound Med* 21:237–247, 2002.

Cacciatore B, Lehtovirta P, Wahlstrom T, Ylostalo P: Ultrasound findings in uterine mixed müllerian sarcomas and endometrial stromal sarcomas. *Gynecol Oncol* 35:290–293, 1989.

Carter JR, Ruhr DM, Okagaki T, Fowler JM: Uterine lipoleiomyoma: A rare tumor. *J Ultrasound Med* 12:491–492, 1993.

Wallach EE, Viahos NF: Uterine myomas: An overview of development, clinical features, and management. *Obstet Gynecol* 104:393–406, 2004.

Cross-Reference

Ultrasound: THE REQUISITES, 2nd ed, pp 546, 549–555.

Comment

The four uterine masses depicted in this case have different histologic features. Figure A shows a typical uterine leiomyoma, the most common solid pelvic tumor in women, although this first example is of the type with a coarse heterogeneous echotexture which, if large enough, often distorts the endometrial stripe. Figures B and C are examples of fibroids with calcified rims. These benign masses of smooth muscle are actually monoclonal proliferations of muscle cells. Uterine leiomyomas have a genetic basis, and their growth is related to genetic predisposition, hormonal influences, and various growth factors. They can be found in subserosal, myometrial, submucosal, or intracavitary locations. On ultrasound, a simple leiomyoma is hypoechoic and solid with some attenuation of the sound beam. The echogenicity may be heterogeneous owing to the presence of calcification, necrosis, hemorrhage, or hyalinization. It is important to describe the relationship with the endometrial lining, and follow-up studies are often performed to evaluate for a change in size. Sonohysterography is an important adjunct to transvaginal sonography in symptomatic women with known myomas, especially before surgical or medical therapy.

The mass in Figure D is a rare lipoleiomyoma. This benign subtype of leiomyoma contains lipid. The presence of multiple closely packed (multiple) boundary interfaces in the tumor accounts for the homogeneous increased echogenicity on ultrasound. It is important when imaging an exophytic lipoleiomyoma to be certain that the mass arises from the myometrium because the appearance is similar to that of an ovarian dermoid.

The fourth case is a uterine leiomyosarcoma (see Fig. E). This rare uterine malignancy can be indistinguishable from a leiomyoma on ultrasound and computed tomography imaging. A rapid increase in size of a leiomyoma should raise concern regarding a leiomyosarcoma. In addition, leiomyosarcomas are usually necrotic and large. The leiomyosarcoma is the most common type of uterine myometrial malignancy. The mixed mesodermal tumor is less common. A characteristic ultrasound appearance of the mixed mesodermal tumor has been described. A heterogeneous myometrial echotexture can be seen with hyperechoic areas and anechoic areas, which may be large and irregularly shaped, scattered throughout the myometrium. Although in general uterine sarcomas have the worst prognosis of uterine masses, the mixed mesodermal tumor also has a very poor prognosis.

Notes

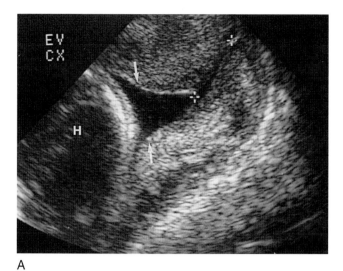

A

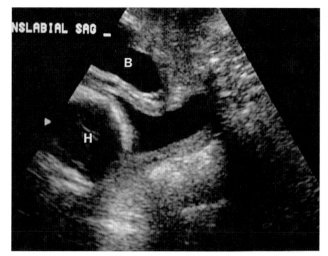

B

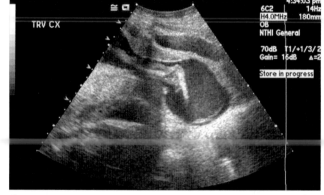

C

1. Which abnormality is demonstrated in this third-trimester pregnancy by the sagittal image of the lower uterine segment? Figure A is transvaginal (+ signs = closed endocervical length of 2.2 cm). Figure B is a sagittal translabial image. H = fetal head; B = urinary bladder. Are the findings on either image more severe and why? The most extreme condition is shown in Fig. C.

2. What is cervical funneling?

3. Does the shape of the funnel have any significance?

4. Which is more accurate for measuring the cervix: ultrasound or a digital examination?

5. Who is at increased risk of developing an incompetent cervix?

6. What is the best technique for measuring the cervical length?

7. Which maneuver is most reliable to dilate a closed but incompetent cervix: coughing, standing, or transfundal pressure?

Incompetent Cervix

1. Incompetent cervix with funneling. Figures A and B show an incompetent cervix. Figure B is worse, because it shows complete incompetence with bulging membranes. Figure C shows prolapse of the amniotic sac into the vagina.

2. Opening of the internal os. Figure A (arrows).

3. Yes; V-shaped is worse.

4. Ultrasound.

5. Women who have a history of preterm labor or preterm delivery.

6. Transvaginal imaging.

7. Transfundal pressure.

References

Gomez R, Galasso M, Romero R, et al: Ultrasonographic examination of the uterine cervix is better than cervical digital examination as a predictor of the likelihood of premature delivery in patients with preterm labor and intact membranes. *Am J Obstet Gynecol* 171:956–964, 1994.

Hertzberg BS, Livingston, DM, DeLong PJ, et al: Ultrasonographic evaluation of the cervix: Transperineal versus endovaginal imaging. *J Ultrasound Med* 20:1071–1078, 2001.

Iams JD, Goldenberg RL, Meis PJ, et al: The length of the cervix and the risk of spontaneous premature delivery. *N Engl J Med* 334:567–572, 1996.

Kaakaj Y, Nghiem HV, Nodell C, Winter TC: Sonography of obstetric and gynecologic emergencies: Part 1, obstetric emergencies. *AJR* 174:641–649, 2000.

Roman AS, Rebarber A, Pereira L, et al: The efficacy of sonographically indicated cerclage in multiple gestations. *J Ultrasound Med* 24:763–768, 2005.

Cross-Reference

Ultrasound: THE REQUISITES, 2nd ed, pp 327, 502–509.

Comment

It is well established that cervical shortening is associated with preterm delivery. Although many observers believe that an endocervical length between 2.5 and 3 cm is the lower limit of normal, there is a continuum. A normal cervical length is 3 cm or more; 2 to 3 cm is borderline; and less than 2 cm is definitely abnormal (see Figs. A and B).

The lower uterine segment can be imaged using a transabdominal, translabial, or transvaginal technique. Distension of the urinary bladder compresses the lower uterine segment, which can create the false appearance of a long cervix and the false appearance of a funneled cervix (dilatation of the internal os). Therefore, translabial and transvaginal ultrasound are more accurate techniques when performed with an empty urinary bladder. Results of one large recent study showed that endovaginal images were frequently superior to transperineal ones. Transperineal measurements of cervical length can be significantly shorter than endovaginal measurements, especially before 20 weeks' gestation; therefore short cervical lengths at transperineal sonography before 20 weeks should be confirmed by endovaginal sonography. Ultrasound is more accurate than the digital examination, particularly for the detection of funneling. The degree of dilatation of the internal os, which defines incompetence, has been quoted as greater than 3 to 6 mm. Cervical incompetence is a common cause of pregnancy failure in the second trimester; it is painless dilatation of the cervix. The length of the funnel has prognostic value. V-shaped funneling has been shown to be more predictive of preterm delivery than U-shaped funneling. In addition to cervical shortening, a change in cervical length between examinations (particularly a change of 6 mm or more) has a small association with preterm labor. A recent study of patients with multiple gestations, with short cervical lengths, determined that sonographically indicated cerclage was not associated with a lower incidence of spontaneous preterm delivery compared with conservative management.

Transvaginal scanning with an empty bladder is the most consistently accurate technique to evaluate the cervix. The vaginal probe is inserted into the anterior fornix of the vagina, withdrawn slightly, and then advanced only enough to obtain a clear image. This action decreases the pressure on the cervix, which can artificially increase the length.

Notes

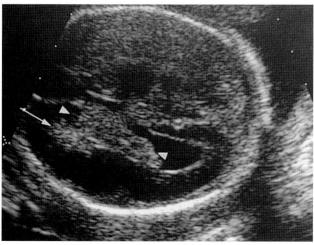

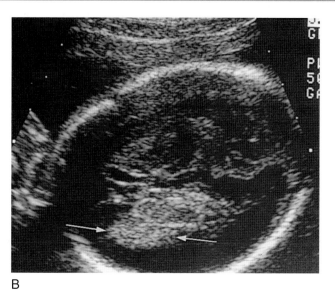

A

B

1. Which abnormality is shown in these axial images of a late second-trimester fetal brain (arrows and arrowheads)?

2. Is there a difference in prognosis if this occurs intraventricularly or intraparenchymally?

3. What is the most common cause of this abnormality?

4. At what time in the gestation is this diagnosis usually detected?

Intracranial Hemorrhage

1. Intracranial hemorrhage.

2. Yes.

3. Direct maternal abdominal trauma in the third trimester.

4. Third trimester.

Reference

Brown MA, Sirlin CB, Farahmand N, et al: Screening sonography in pregnant patients with blunt abdominal trauma. *J Ultrasound Med* 24:175–181, 2005.

Ghi T, Simonazzi G, Perolo A, et al: Outcome of antenatally diagnosed intracranial hemorrhage: Case series and review of the literature. *Ultrasound Obstet Gynecol* 22:108–109, 2003.

Vergani P, Strobelt N, Locatelli A, et al: Clinical significance of fetal intracranial hemorrhage. *Am J Obstet Gynecol* 175:536–543, 1996.

Cross-Reference

Ultrasound: THE REQUISITES, 2nd ed, p 399.

Comment

Fetal hemorrhage is included in the differential diagnosis of an intracranial fetal mass. In the neonate, changes in cerebral blood pressure and perinatal asphyxia contribute to the development of cerebral hemorrhage. However, in the fetus, the intracerebral pressure is regulated and protected from fluctuations in the maternal blood pressure, which suggests that an alternative pathophysiology might be associated with a cerebral hemorrhage. The most common cause is secondary to direct maternal abdominal trauma in the third trimester. Sonography is an effective screening modality to determine the sequelae of the trauma. Most hemorrhages are detected after 23 weeks and are possibly related to the fact that the germinal matrix vascular connections to subependymal venous networks develop after 20 weeks.

Prenatal cerebral hemorrhage can occur in the ventricle (arrowheads in Fig. A), parenchyma (arrows in Figs. A and B), or subdural or subarachnoid space. The prognosis is poor with subdural and parenchymal hemorrhages but better in cases of isolated intraventricular hemorrhage. Higher degrees of ventricular dilatation (>15 mm) also worsen the prognosis.

On ultrasound, hemorrhage appears as a hyperechoic (either homogeneous or heterogeneous) mass. Intraventricular hemorrhage may present as an irregular, enlarged choroid plexus. The ventricular diameter and any parenchymal abnormality must be evaluated and closely followed. Fetal intracranial hemorrhage is generally accurately identified and categorized by antenatal sonography. Magnetic resonance imaging may be helpful in the characterization and delineation of the hemorrhage.

Notes

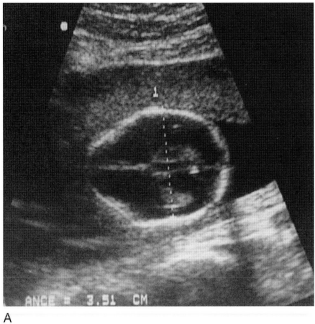

A

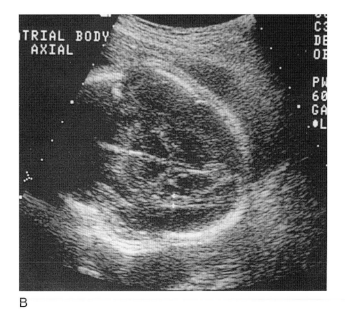

B

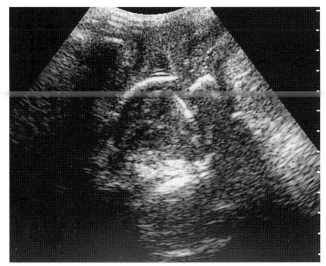

C

1. Which entity is associated with a "strawberry-shaped skull"?

2. What are the most common central nervous system (CNS) malformations associated with a "lemon head" (Fig. A)?

3. Which syndrome can be associated with a "cloverleaf skull" (Fig. B)?

4. What is Spalding's sign (Fig. C)?

Calvarial Abnormalities

1. Trisomy 18.

2. Myelomeningocele with associated Chiari II malformation; encephalocele.

3. Thanatophoric dwarf.

4. Overlapping fetal skull bones occurring in a second- or third-trimester fetal death.

References

Ball RH, Filly RA, Goldstein RB: The lemon sign: Not a specific indicator of meningomyelocele. *J Ultrasound Med* 3:131–134, 1993.

Nicolaides KH, Salvesen DR, Snijders RJ, Gosden CM: Strawberry-shaped skull in fetal trisomy 18. *Fetal Diagn Ther* 7:132–137, 1992.

Shiroyama Y, Ito H, Yamashita T, et al: The relationship of cloverleaf skull to hydrocephalus. *Childs Nerv Syst* 7:382–385, 1991.

Cross-Reference

Ultrasound: THE REQUISITES, 2nd ed, pp 404, 406, 477, 479–480.

Comment

Evaluation of the fetal skull begins with a measurement of the biparietal diameter (BPD). This is used to calculate the mean estimated gestational age if the first study is performed at 12 weeks of gestation or later. For follow-up examinations, the gestational age is always dictated by the first study, and the BPD, abdominal circumference, and femur length are measured to assess for interval growth. Beyond measuring the BPD, the shape of the fetal skull should be evaluated. Several syndromes have been associated with skull abnormalities.

The "lemon head" (Fig. A) (seen before 24 weeks' gestational age) is a well-known finding in Chiari II malformation: myelomeningocele with a small posterior fossa and a banana-shaped cerebellum. However, one series demonstrated that a lemon-shaped head can be seen in fetuses with other CNS malformations, including encephalocele, Dandy-Walker malformation, and agenesis of the corpus callosum. In addition, a few cases with unrelated anomalies presented with a lemon-shaped head (umbilical vein varix with a two-vessel cord and fetal hydronephrosis); if the deformity is mild, it may be a normal variant.

A "strawberry-shaped" calvarium can be seen in trisomy 18. Although not present in all cases, it is considered to be secondary to hypoplasia of the frontal lobes of the brain. Choroid plexus cysts may also be present. Limb anomalies include rocker-bottom feet, clubbed feet, and overlapping fingers.

A cloverleaf skull or "*kleeblattschädel*" can be seen in some cases of thanatophoric dwarfism, where it is associated with a narrow, bell-shaped thorax and shortened telephone receiver–shaped femurs. However, as shown in Figure B, it can also be caused by an isolated craniosynostosis. Additionally, several rare syndromes may involve a cloverleaf skull deformity, including infants with atypical Apert's syndrome, the syndrome of marfanoid phenotype with craniosynostosis (Shprintzen-Goldberg syndrome), and Pfeiffer's syndrome type 2. Furthermore, the shape of the skull can cause both communicating and noncommunicating hydrocephalus.

Spalding's sign describes overlapping skull bones seen with fetal death. The bone collapse results from autolysis. This is demonstrated in Figure C of a fetal demise.

Notes

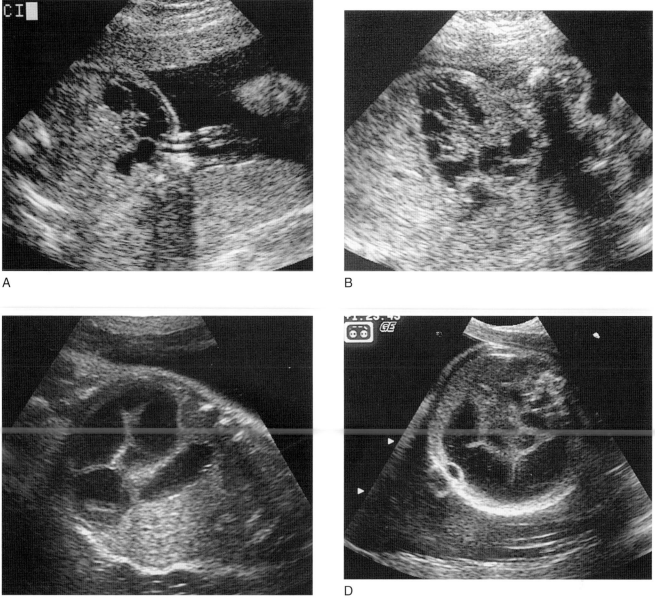

A

B

C

D

1. Which cystic abnormalities are shown in these axial abdominal images of a middle second-trimester fetus (Figs. A and B)?

2. How is small bowel obstruction defined?

3. What is the differential diagnosis of dilated fetal small bowel?

4. How does one distinguish large from small bowel obstruction?

Small Bowel (Jejunoileal) Obstruction

1. Dilated small bowel.

2. Persistent loops that are greater than 7 mm in diameter and greater than 15 mm in length.

3. Bowel atresia and stenosis, volvulus, Ladd's bands, and meconium ileus.

4. The ascending and descending colon are peripherally located and show no evidence of peristalsis. Although some of the dilated loops of obstructed small bowel may appear to be peripheral, most do not, and commonly peristalsis is present.

References

Corteville JE, Gray DL, Langer JC: Obstetrics: Bowel abnormalities in the fetus: Correlation of prenatal ultrasonographic findings with outcome. *Am J Obstet Gynecol* 175:724–729, 1996.

Hertzberg BS: Sonography of the fetal gastrointestinal tract: Anatomic variants, diagnostic pitfalls and abnormalities. *AJR* 162:1175–1182, 1994.

Cross-Reference

Ultrasound: THE REQUISITES, 2nd ed, pp 436–439.

Comment

Small bowel obstruction occurs in the jejunum and ileum combined as frequently as it does in the duodenum. The incidence of jejunal obstruction is equal to that of ileal obstruction, with the latter being more commonly distal. Small bowel atresia is the most common cause of fetal small bowel obstruction. Atresia can occur in multiple sites and results from in utero vascular compromise. Cystic fibrosis accounts for 18% to 36% of cases of obstruction.

A large prospective series showed that ultrasound is more sensitive for the prenatal detection of small bowel obstruction than for large bowel obstruction. Overall, the diagnosis of small bowel obstruction is made in utero less than 50% of the time. Ultrasound may demonstrate dilatation of small bowel loops, which should not measure more than 7 mm in diameter and 15 mm in length (see Figs. A to D). Other findings include an unusual bowel pattern, ascites (which may be the only finding), polyhydramnios (more common with high obstructions and after 24 weeks), or a cystic abdominal mass (dilated bowel loop). Hyperperistalsis suggests that this cystic mass is in the small bowel. Whereas a dilated colon is usually peripheral, obstructed small bowel can appear to be partially peripheral, as shown in Figures C and D demonstrating a jejunal obstruction.

Fetuses with cystic fibrosis may develop meconium ileus (an ileus owing to thick meconium). This usually obstructs the ileum and causes proximal small bowel dilatation. It may be accompanied by echogenic bowel and polyhydramnios.

Meconium peritonitis occurs from perforation of the small bowel. Although it may result from bowel obstruction due to cystic fibrosis, it is more commonly associated with small bowel atresia and secondary perforation. Complications of meconium peritonitis include meconium pseudocyst formation, which is also part of the differential diagnosis of a cystic abdominal or pelvic mass. Ascites, typically complicated, and calcification also occur.

Notes

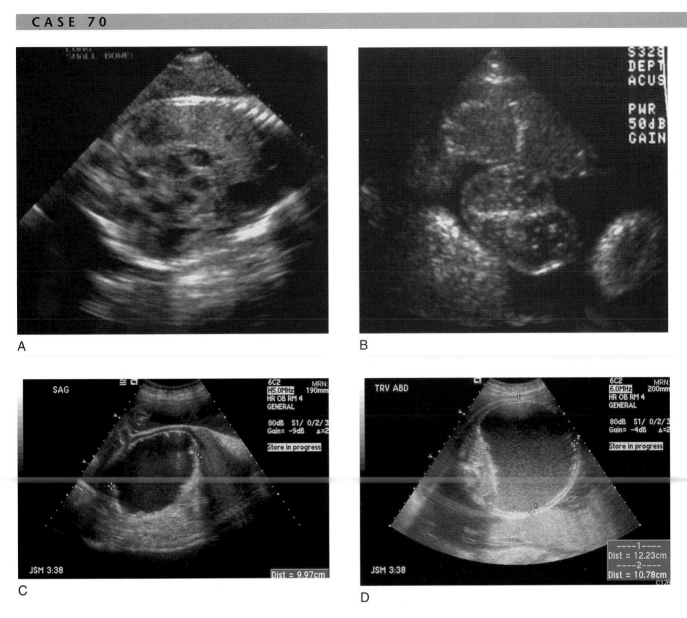

A

B

C

D

1. What is shown in Figure A (coronal abdomen view), Figure B (axial scrotum view), and Figures C and D (sagittal and transverse axial mid-abdomen views)?

2. What is the most common etiology of these findings?

3. What is the most common cause of meconium peritonitis?

4. What is the significance of peritoneal calcifications?

Cystic Fibrosis

1. Figure A: dilated, obstructed small bowel; Figure B: complex scrotal ascites; Figures C and D: meconium pseudocyst.

2. Meconium peritonitis due to a small bowel perforation.

3. Small bowel atresia.

4. It reflects perforation of the bowel and meconium peritonitis in a patient *without* cystic fibrosis (CF).

References

Foster MA, Nyberg DA, Mahoney BS, et al: Meconium peritonitis: Prenatal sonographic findings and their clinical significance. *Radiology* 165:661–665, 1987.

Rypens FF, Avni EF, Abehserva MM, et al: Areas of increased echogenicity in the fetal abdomen: Diagnosis and significance. *Radiographics* 15:1329–1344, 1995.

Scotet V, DeBraekeleer M, Audrezet M-P, et al: Prenatal detection of cystic fibrosis by ultrasonography: A retrospective study of more than 346,000 pregnancies. *J Med Genetics* 39:443–448, 2002.

Cross-Reference

Ultrasound: THE REQUISITES, 2nd ed, pp 439, 440–441.

Comment

CF, the commonest severe autosomal recessive disease that affects children in white populations and is caused by mutations in a gene that encodes a protein called CFTR, most commonly initially presents with gastrointestinal abnormalities. The enzyme deficiencies of the exocrine glands result in thickened meconium which can obstruct the small bowel or colon. The most common gastrointestinal disorder in CF is meconium ileus, an obstruction of the small bowel with meconium. Occasionally, the abnormality is in the large bowel. Although meconium ileus occurs in only 10% to 15% of infants with CF, almost all cases result from CF.

On prenatal ultrasound, the small bowel in CF may appear to have an increased echogenicity, although this is not present in approximately 40% of cases. In addition, increased bowel echogenicity is not specific to CF, as it can be a sign of chromosomal anomalies. Obstruction of the small bowel by meconium may be detected as locally dilated bowel. This is usually seen after 26 weeks. Polyhydramnios may be present.

Meconium peritonitis results when an obstructed bowel perforates. Findings on prenatal sonograms include fetal ascites, which is usually complex and echogenic, intra-abdominal calcifications (linear or clumped), bowel dilation, and polyhydramnios. The differential diagnosis in a newborn includes several etiologies, such as small bowel atresia, meconium ileus, volvulus, internal hernia, intussusception, or congenital band. The presence of peritoneal calcifications reflects an etiology other than CF because the enzyme deficiency in CF prevents calcification.

The incidence of CF has been reported to be from 15% to 40% in cases of meconium peritonitis. However, a study by Foster and associates demonstrated that a large percentage of cases of meconium peritonitis detected prenatally with ultrasound are due to other etiologies, including small bowel atresia, stenosis, or volvulus.

Notes

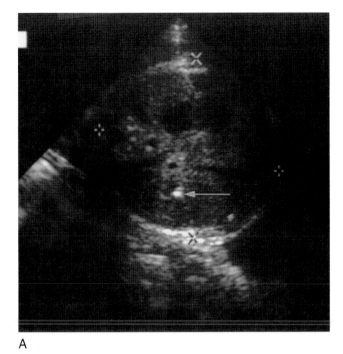

A

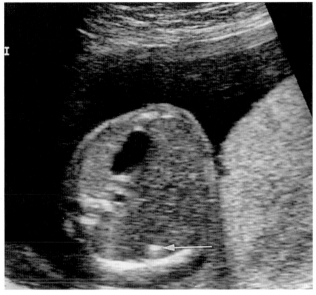

B

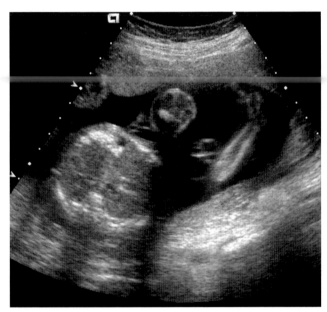

C

1. Three fetal upper abdominal second-trimester studies (axial images) are shown. What do the arrows identify in cases A and B and is seen very prominently anteriorly in Figure C ?

2. What is the cause of fetal intrahepatic calcification?

3. What neonatal liver tumor(s) might contain calcification?

4. What actions should be taken when fetal hepatic calcification is detected?

C A S E 7 1

Fetal Liver Calcifications

1. Figures A and B show intrahepatic calcification. Figure C shows perihepatic calcification.

2. Differential diagnoses include idiopathic, ischemic hepatic necrosis, intrauterine infection, neoplasm if associated with a mass, and rarely portal vein calcification.

3. Hepatoblastoma and metastatic neuroblastoma.

4. Exclude other anomalies and TORCH (*t*oxoplasmosis, *o*ther infections, *r*ubella, *c*ytomegalovirus infection, and *h*erpes simplex) infection; do follow-up scans.

Reference

McNamara A, Levine D: Intraabdominal fetal echogenic masses: A practical guide to diagnosis and management. *RadioGraphics* 25:633–645, 2005.

Stein B, Bromley B, Michlewitz H, et al: Fetal liver calcifications: Sonographic appearance and postnatal outcome. *Radiology* 197:489–492, 1995.

Cross-Reference

Ultrasound: THE REQUISITES, 2nd ed, pp 431–433.

Comment

Hepatic calcifications can arise from various etiologies (see Figs. A and B). These include ischemic hepatic necrosis, intrauterine infection such as cytomegalic virus and toxoplasmosis, a hepatic mass, or rarely calcification in the portal vein. Perihepatic calcifications (see Fig. C) on the liver surface are usually peritoneal from meconium peritonitis. The location, size, and distribution are major factors for management of these calcifications.

Detection of hepatic calcification warrants a careful search for associated anomalies. A wide spectrum of associated abnormalities has been reported, including intrauterine growth restriction, Hirschsprung's disease, cardiac anomalies, stippled epiphysis, sacral agenesis, and Dandy-Walker variant. If the hepatic calcifications are single, there is usually no underlying abnormality; when no other fetal morphologic abnormalities are detected in follow-up ultrasound studies and infection screening test results are negative, the prognosis is promising.

Notes

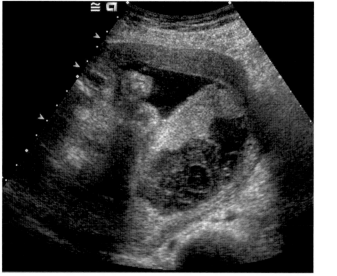

A

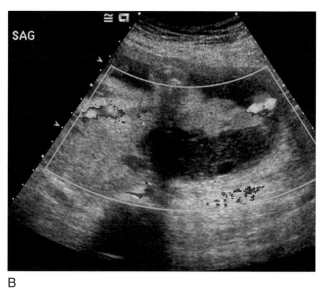

B

1. Which abnormality is shown in this prenatal sonogram of a third-trimester pregnancy?

2. How is the lucent area in Figure D of Case 49 different from that in Figures A and B in this case?

3. How do most women present with this fetal abnormality?

4. What is the incidence of fetal death from this condition?

Placental Abruption

1. Placental abruption (retroplacental bleeding).

2. The lucent area in Figure D Case 49 is subchorionic. In the present case the hemorrhage is retro-placental.

3. Most women have pain or bleeding.

4. Twenty percent to 35% perinatal mortality.

References

Eastman NJ, Hellman LM (eds): *Williams Obstetrics*, 13th ed. Stamford, CT, Appleton-Century-Crofts, 1966, pp 625–632.

Glantz C, Purnell L: Clinical utility of sonography in the diagnosis and treatment of placental abruption. *J Ultrasound Med* 21:837–840, 2002.

Harris RD, Cho C, Wells WA: Sonography of the placenta with emphasis on pathological correlation. *Semin Ultrasound CT MR* 17:66–89, 1996.

Kaakaji AY, Nghiem HV, Nodell C, Winter TC: Sonography of obstetric and gynecologic emergencies: Part 1, obstetric emergencies. *AJR* 174:641–649.

Nyberg DA, Cyr DR, Mack LA, et al: Sonographic spectrum of placental abruption. *AJR* 148:161–164, 1987.

Townssend RR, Laing FC, Brooke Jeffrey Jr R: Placental abruption associated with cocaine abuse. *AJR* 150: 1339–1340, 1988.

Cross-Reference

Ultrasound: THE REQUISITES, 2nd ed, pp 494–495.

Comment

Hemorrhage around the placenta is classified according to its location. Many hemorrhages occur in a subchorionic location. Hemorrhage located between the placenta and the uterine wall is called retroplacental. If the hemorrhage extends from the retroplacental region lateral to the placenta, it is called marginal. Intraplacental hemorrhage may accompany a retroplacental bleed. A retroplacental hemorrhage that separates the placenta from the uterine wall prematurely is called an abruption, which can be partial or complete.

Placental abruption often presents with pelvic/uterine pain and bleeding. Vaginal hemorrhage occurs with large retroplacental hematomas when the peripheral margins of the placenta are disrupted and the fetal membranes are stripped from the decidua basalis. The fetal prognosis relates to the volume of hemorrhage and the degree of placental separation. The bleed, even if extensive, can decompress if vaginal bleeding is present. If the hemorrhage remains confined to the retroplacental region ("concealed"), the outcome can be worse for the fetus and the mother. This may result in complete placental separation and fetal death, as well as a consumptive coagulopathy in the mother. Risk factors for developing an abruption include maternal hypertension, cigarette smoking, alcohol consumption, cocaine abuse, trauma, and premature rupture of the membranes.

Ultrasound can demonstrate many of these hemorrhages; a hypoechoic or hyperechoic (depending on the stage) retroplacental collection will be seen, elevating the placenta from the uterine wall. However, if the bleed is entirely isoechoic to the placenta, it may not be apparent. Sonography is generally not sensitive for the detection of placental abruption. Once an abruption is diagnosed, an assessment of fetal well-being and follow-up ultrasound imaging are important.

Notes

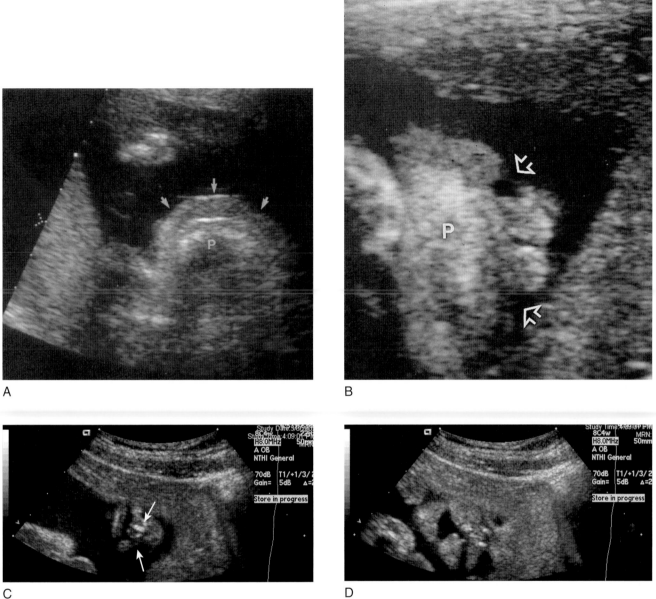

A

B

C

D

1. Fetus A (Fig. A) shows a normal upper lip (small arrows) and hard palate (P). What are the facial abnormalities identified by the open arrows in fetus B (Fig. B)? P = hard palate; and those in Figures C and D (coronal images of the face)?

2. Name a facial abnormality that may be associated with a bilateral anomaly.

3. What is the ultrasound classification of the spectrum of this anomaly?

4. Does the classification correlate with the outcome?

Cleft Lip and Palate

1. Fetus B has a bilateral cleft lip. Fetus C has a midline cleft lip and palate.

2. Premaxillary protrusion.

3. Type 1: Cleft lip alone; type 2: unilateral cleft lip and palate; type 3: bilateral cleft lip and palate; type 4: midline cleft lip and palate; and type 5: facial defects associated with amniotic bands or limb-body-wall complex.

4. Yes, types 4 and 5 are associated with other anomalies and a fatal outcome.

References

Babcook CJ, McGahan JP, Chong BW, et al: Evaluation of fetal midface anatomy related to facial clefts: Use of US. *Radiology* 201:113–118, 1996.

Kazan-Tannus JF, Levine D, McKenzie C, et al: Real-time magnetic resonance imaging aids prenatal diagnosis of isolated cleft palate. *J Ultrasound Med* 24: 1533–1540, 2005.

Mernagh JR, Mohide PT, Lappalainen RE, Fedoryshin JG: US assessment of the fetal head and neck: A state-of-the-art pictoral review. *RadioGraphics* 19:S229–S241, 1999.

Nyberg DA, Sickler GK, Hegge FN, et al: Fetal cleft lip with and without cleft palate: US classification and correlation with outcome. *Radiology* 195:677–684, 1995.

Cross-Reference

Ultrasound: THE REQUISITES, 2nd ed, pp 387, 388, 480.

Comment

Cleft lip, with or without cleft palate, is the most common facial anomaly and is associated with cleft palate in 80% of cases. Isolated cleft lip has a better prognosis. The incidence is 1 in 1000 births. When it occurs unilaterally, with or without a cleft palate, it is more commonly seen on the left side. In the setting of bilateral cleft lip and palate, a premaxillary protrusion may be present and was detected in 85% of one series. This soft tissue mass arising from the upper lip occurs when the maxilla is anteriorly displaced.

Nyberg described an ultrasound classification for cleft lip and palate:

Type 1: Cleft lip alone.
Type 2: Unilateral cleft lip and palate.
Type 3: Bilateral cleft lip and palate.
Type 4: Midline cleft lip and palate (see Fig. C).
Type 5: Facial defects associated with amniotic bands or a limb-body-wall complex.
Types 4 and 5 were associated with higher mortality.
The poor prognosis of type 4 clefts relates to concurrent anomalies or trisomies, particularly trisomy 13. Type 5 clefts have associated defects of the torso, limb, or cranium as part of the limb-body-wall complex.

Although an evaluation of the palate is not part of the standard prenatal ultrasound scans, it is important because ultrasound can reliably demonstrate the normal facial structures of the lip and hard palate in axial and coronal planes and exclude most cases of cleft lip and palate. The defect of cleft lip and palate is recognized because of the gap in the upper lip seen on coronal views of the nose and lips. Detection of hard palate anomalies is more reliable before 24 weeks of gestation. Small type 1 and 2 defects may be missed, particularly with a sagittal view. Soft palate abnormalities, when isolated, may also escape detection. Fetal magnetic resonance imaging is increasingly being used for fine assessment of complicated sonographic images.

Notes

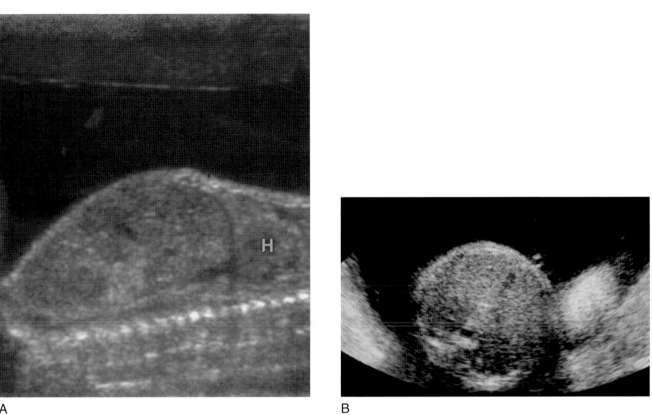

A

B

1. What are the two abnormal findings identified in this early third-trimester fetal examination? (Fig. A is a sagittal image of the left side of fetus; H = heart; Fig. B is a transverse image through the upper abdomen.)

2. What is the differential diagnosis of absence of the fetal stomach?

3. Does polyhydramnios help to distinguish the etiology?

4. Does gastric nonvisualization occur in all cases of this condition?

Esophageal Atresia

1. Absence of the fetal stomach and polyhydramnios.

2. Esophageal atresia, congenital diaphragmatic hernia, oligohydramnios, situs abnormality, and impaired swallowing (i.e., central nervous system abnormality, facial cleft, neuromuscular disorder, neck/chest mass, narrow chest).

3. No; it is seen with many of these conditions.

4. No; the stomach may be very small and unchanging.

References

Hertzberg BS: Sonography of the fetal gastrointestinal tract: Anatomic variants, diagnostic pitfalls and abnormalities. *AJR* 162:1175–1182, 1994.

McKenna KM, Goldstein RV, Stringer MD: Small or absent fetal stomach: Prognostic significance. *Radiology* 197: 729–733, 1995.

Cross-Reference

Ultrasound: THE REQUISITES, 2nd ed, pp 434–437.

Comment

The fetal stomach is seen as a fluid-filled structure in the left upper quadrant by 14 or 15 weeks (and often earlier) in almost all fetuses. Most observers feel that the stomach should always be identified by 19 weeks. Occasionally, nonvisualization of the stomach is a transient normal finding, due to physiologic emptying of the stomach. Rescanning serially over 60 minutes or re-examining at a later date is expected to demonstrate a fluid-filled stomach in normal cases.

Absence of the fetal stomach or a persistently small fetal stomach (<1 cm in size), which persists in the second or third trimester, carries a poor prognosis because of associated conditions. Swallowing dysfunction can be caused by a facial cleft, central nervous system or neuromuscular disorders, a neck/thoracic mass, or a narrow chest due to skeletal dysplasia. The stomach may be located in the thorax (diaphragmatic hernia) or right abdomen (situs abnormality). In true nonvisualization of the stomach, oligohydramnios may be the cause due to decreased amniotic fluid for the fetus to swallow.

Esophageal atresia is often accompanied by nonvisualization of the fetal stomach. However, in some fetuses with a tracheoesophageal fistula, and rarely in those with isolated esophageal atresia, fluid may cross the fistula or gastric secretions may accumulate and minimally distend the stomach (<1 cm in size). In these cases, the stomach will not become more prominent.

Only 50% of fetuses with esophageal atresia are detected in utero either by nonvisualization of the stomach or by polyhydramnios; both are seen in this case

(see Figs. A and B). When seen, they are more commonly identified after 24 weeks. The late onset of findings is a little puzzling and may be due to the failure on the part of the examiner to appreciate a very small stomach as potentially abnormal earlier in the pregnancy and the slow accumulation of amniotic fluid that may not increase to levels above normal until later in the pregnancy. Nevertheless, the presence of polyhydramnios or oligohydramnios with nonvisualization of the stomach has a worse prognosis than nonvisualization of the stomach with the presence of a normal amount of amniotic fluid. Karyotype abnormalities are also associated with esophageal atresia, including trisomies 18 and 21.

Detection of a small fetal stomach or persistent nonvisualization of the stomach necessitates a careful evaluation for associated anomalies. The fetal mortality depends on the presence or absence of associated abnormalities; the incidence is very high in cases of esophageal atresia because it is part of the VACTERL (*v*ertebral, *a*nal, *c*ardiac, *t*racheoesophageal, *r*enal, and *l*imb) syndrome. The prognosis is better if no other anomalies are associated and the amniotic fluid volume is normal; in one such series 96% of the cases survived.

Notes

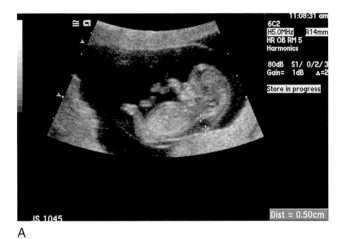

A

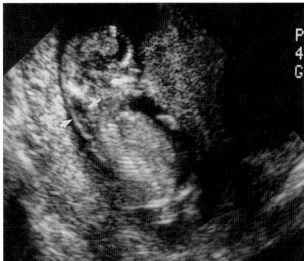

B

C

1. Which of these late first-trimester embryos/fetuses are abnormal and why (see cursors and small arrows)?

2. What is the significance of a septated nuchal lucency?

3. What chromosomal anomalies have been associated with nuchal lucencies?

4. What serum tests are now being combined with nuchal translucency measurements to yield a first-trimester screening tool for chromosomal anomalies?

C A S E 7 5

Nuchal Skin Measurement: First Trimester

1. Figures A and B: Increased nuchal translucency. Arrowhead in Figure C points to normal amnion. Plus sign markings in Figure A show the increased nuchal translucency.

2. Septated nuchal lucency has a higher risk of chromosomal abnormalities.

3. Trisomies 13, 18, 21, Turner's syndrome (XO), XXX, and translocations.

4. Maternal serum free β-human chorionic gonadotropin (hCG) and pregnancy-associated plasma protein A.

References

Bonilla-Musoles F, Raga F, Villalobos A, et al: First-trimester neck abnormalities: Three-dimensional evaluation. *J Ultrasound Med* 17:419–425,1998.

Fong KW, Toi A, Salem SW, et al: Detection of fetal structural abnormalities with US during early pregnancy. *RadioGraphics* 24:157–174, 2004.

Spencer K, Souter V, Tul N, et al: A screening program for trisomy 21 at 10-14 weeks using fetal nuchal translucency, maternal serum free beta-human chorionic gonadotropin and pregnancy-associated plasma protein-A. *Ultrasound Obstet Gynecol* 13:231–237, 1999.

Taipale P, Hiilesmaa V, Salonen R, Ylostalo P: Increased nuchal translucency as marker for fetal chromosomal defects. *N Engl J Med* 337:1654–1658, 1997.

van Vugt JMG, Van Zalen-Sprock R, Kostense PJ: First-trimester nuchal translucency: A risk analysis on fetal chromosome abnormality. *Radiology* 200: 537–540, 1996

Wapner R, Thom E, Simpson JL, et al: First trimester screening for trisomies 21 and 18. *NEJM* 349: 1405–1413, 2003.

Cross-Reference
Ultrasound: THE REQUISITES, 2nd ed, pp 394–395.

Comment

The nuchal region of the embryo/fetus refers to the soft tissue posterior to the cervical spine or occipital bone. Increased nuchal thickening or translucency are associated with chromosomal anomalies, most commonly Down syndrome, but also trisomies 13 and 18, Turner's syndrome, and translocations.

In the first and early second trimester, the nuchal translucency is usually measured in the sagittal plane, either transabdominally or transvaginally. A translucency thickness of more than 3 mm from 10 to 14 weeks' gestation is considered abnormal. This measurement should include only the anechoic region between two hyperechoic (echogenic) lines. Three-dimensional ultrasonography has been useful. Figures A and B show increased nuchal translucency in two first-trimester fetuses with Down syndrome. It is important to realize that this finding may be limited to this very narrow gestational window. After 14 weeks, the finding may resolve, but the risk for a chromosomal abnormality remains increased.

At the present time, screening for chromosomal anomalies is performed with a maternal serum triple screen between 15 and 20 weeks. This includes analysis of maternal β-hCG, estriol, and α-fetoprotein. This test alone has only 60% sensitivity for Down syndrome (slightly higher when maternal age is considered), with a high false-positive rate leading to amniocentesis of normal pregnancies. A newer screen includes maternal serum free β-hCG and pregnancy-associated plasma protein A as well as a measurement of the nuchal translucency and consideration of maternal age, and is usually conducted between 11 to 14 weeks of gestation. Studies have shown that a combination of the nuchal translucency and serum markers like these results in a sensitivity of 80% to 90% for detecting Down syndrome, with only a 5% false-positive rate.

Notes

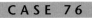

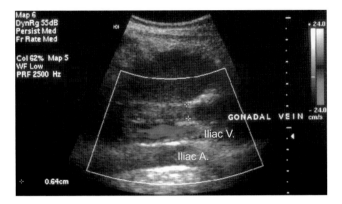

1. An ultrasound examination of the right lower quadrant was performed in a woman 3 days postpartum because of pain (coronal paraovarian area on the right). What do the +markings show? What is the diagnosis?

2. On which side does this condition usually occur?

3. What predisposes a woman to this entity?

4. Can pulmonary embolism complicate ovarian vein thrombosis?

Ovarian Vein Thrombosis

1. Dilated vein filled with thrombus and no Doppler flow apparent. Ovarian vein thrombosis.

2. Right side.

3. Ovarian vein thrombosis can occur after an ectopic pregnancy, abortion, or full-term delivery.

4. Yes.

References

Brown DL: Pelvic ultrasound in the postabortion and postpartum patient. *Ultrasound* 121:27–37, 2005.

Dunnihoo DR, Gallaspy JW, Wise RB, Otterson WN: Postpartum ovarian vein thrombophlebitis: A review. *Obstet Gynecol Surv* 46:415–427, 1991.

Jacoby WT, Cohan RH, Baker ME, et al: Ovarian vein thrombosis in oncology patients: CT detection and clinical significance. *AJR* 155:291–294, 1990.

Martin B, Mulopulos GP, Bryan PJ: MRI of puerperal ovarian-vein thrombosis (Case Report). *AJR* 147: 291–292, 1986.

Shah AA, Buckshee N, Yankelevitz DF, Henschke CI: Assessment of deep venous thrombosis using routine pelvic CT. *AJR* 173:659–653, 1999.

Twickler DM, Setiawan AT, Evans RS, et al: Imaging of puerperal septic thrombophlebitis: Prospective comparison of MR imaging, CT and sonography. *AJR* 169:1039–1043, 1997.

Cross-Reference

Ultrasound: THE REQUISITES, 2nd ed, p 237.

Comment

Ovarian vein thrombosis (OVT) is caused by an ascending infection following an ectopic pregnancy, abortion, vaginal delivery, or cesarean section. Patients usually are seen in the first week postpartum with fever, lower abdominal pain, or a tender mass. It occurs in less than 2% of postpartum patients. The right ovarian vein is thrombosed in most cases (80%), both veins in 15% of cases, with isolated left ovarian vein thrombus occurring in only 6% of cases. The differential diagnosis includes other right lower quadrant pathologies: appendicitis, tubo-ovarian abscess, pyelonephritis, ovarian torsion, endometritis, and hematoma of the broad ligament. OVT is also classically associated with pelvic inflammatory disease and gynecologic surgery.

Cross-sectional imaging modalities can often confirm the diagnosis. Computed tomography CT) usually shows well-defined tubular intraperitoneal masses, the dilated gonadal veins, with central low attenuation of thrombus extending from the pelvis to the infrarenal inferior vena cava. CT and magnetic resonance imaging (MRI) have been found comparable in the evaluation of OVT. Because the ovarian vein cannot be consistently identified by ultrasound, it is the least reliable modality. However, when detected, a thrombus of the ovarian vein has the typical appearance of a thrombus elsewhere (see figure). The signs include a hypoechoic or heterogeneous thrombus (depending on its age) distending the vein, with pain occurring directly over the region. The distended vein can appear mass-like. The two tubular spaces behind the thrombosed vein (see figure) are the normal more deeply positioned iliac artery and vein.

Knowledge of the anatomic position of the right ovarian vein, its oblique course adjacent and lateral to the psoas muscle, and its insertion into the inferior vena cava 4 cm below the right renal vein origin, help to improve its identification. Color Doppler imaging has been found helpful in evaluating the ovarian vein, inferior vena cava, and renal vein for thrombus propagation. Enlargement of the ipsilateral ovary is an important secondary finding.

MRI is accurate in detecting ovarian vein thrombosis, and a single case report suggests that MRI can differentiate acute from subacute thrombus, using the signal intensity of the clot.

Complications of ovarian vein thrombosis include right-sided hydronephrosis, pulmonary or septic emboli, Budd-Chiari syndrome, and hepatic infarction as well as renal vein or inferior vena cava thrombosis.

Notes

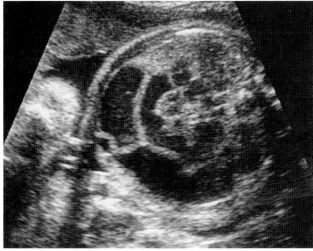
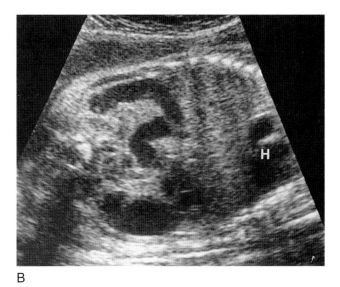

A   B

1. In this third-trimester fetus, what is the likely anatomic location of the bowel obstruction? Figure A is an axial image of the mid-fetal abdomen; Figure B is a coronal image of the fetal body (H = heart).

2. What is the differential diagnosis of a dilated fetal colon?

3. Would sacral agenesis aid in distinguishing the possible etiologies?

4. At what gestational age is colon dilatation due to anorectal atresia more likely to be diagnosed on prenatal ultrasound?

Large Bowel (Anorectal) Atresia

1. Distal colon.

2. Anorectal atresia, Hirschsprung's disease, and meconium plug syndrome.

3. Yes.

4. After 27 weeks.

Reference

Harris RD, Nyberg DA, Mack LA, Weinberger E: Anorectal atresia: Prenatal sonographic diagnosis. *AJR* 149:395–400, 1987.

Cross-Reference

Ultrasound: THE REQUISITES, 2nd ed, pp 436–439, 439.

Comment

Anorectal atresia is often one manifestation of a spectrum of anomalies as part of the VACTERL syndrome, which includes *v*ertebral, *a*norectal, *c*ardiovascular, *t*racheo-*e*sophageal, *r*enal, and *l*imb anomalies. In neonates, almost 75% of cases will have such associated malformations. Anorectal atresia can also be seen as part of the caudal regression syndrome. A careful search for associated anomalies is imperative, as one ultrasound series demonstrated other VACTERL anomalies in more than 90% of the fetuses with anorectal atresia. The differential diagnosis of dilated colon includes Hirschsprung's disease, anorectal atresia, and meconium plug syndrome; the latter two are associated with maternal diabetes.

The fetal bowel normally becomes more dilated with increasing gestational age. Normal fetuses have a mean colon diameter of 15 to 16 mm at term, and the upper limits of normal approach 20 mm. In anorectal atresia, the bowel dilatation is often greater than two standard deviations (SDs) above the mean for any given gestational age. A dilated colon is often peripheral in location (see Figs. A and B); however, some cases of small bowel dilatation can appear peripheral. Tracing the dilatation to the rectosigmoid colon in the pelvis (see Fig. B) aids in confirming that the obstructed bowel is colon. Peristalsis has been described in dilated large bowel loops but would be considered unusual (dilated small bowel loops more commonly show peristalsis).

One series showed that prenatal ultrasound detects less than 10% of cases of large bowel obstruction. The presence of dilated bowel in anorectal atresia correlates with the gestational age. The bowel does not dilate before 22 weeks but will often show progressive dilatation and can be detected after 27 weeks. The presence of a perineal fistula does not correlate with degree of bowel dilatation. Oligohydramnios and occasionally polyhydramnios have been reported, both probably related to the commonly present additional abnormalities.

Notes

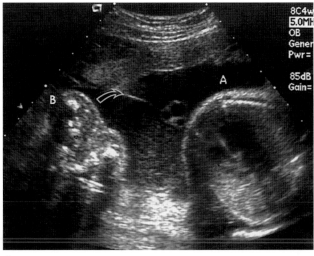

A

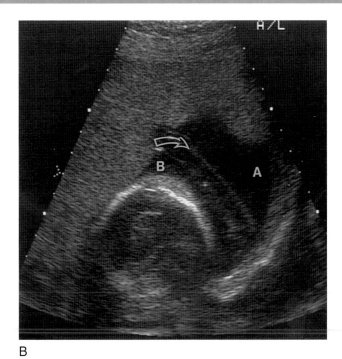

B

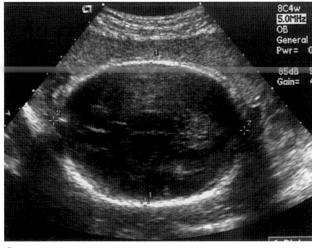

C

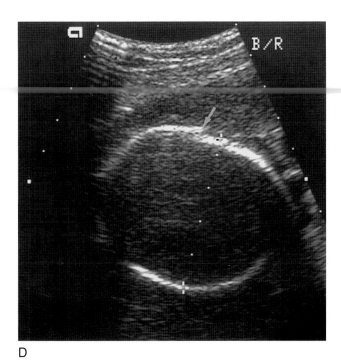

D

1. A woman with a known twin pregnancy presents at 24 weeks for a routine assessment of twin growth. Figures A and B show both fetuses (fetus A on the reader's right and fetus B on the reader's left) and the separating membrane (open arrow). Is this a dichorionic or monochorionic pregnancy and why?

2. Additional images of the fetal heads, are seen in Figure C (fetus A) and Figure D (fetus B). The arrow in Figure D denotes a calvarial suture line. What is the most likely diagnosis and why?

3. If there is fetal demise in a twin gestation, in which trimester is this most likely?

4. If one of the twins dies in a dichorionic pregnancy, is there increased risk of demise for the other fetus?

Second-Trimester Twin Gestation and Fetal Demise

1. Dichorionic pregnancy. The intervening membrane is well defined and more than 2 mm in thickness.

2. Demise of fetus B. Fetus B shows overlapping of calvarial sutures (see Fig. D, arrow) with poorly defined internal anatomy. Amniotic fluid surrounding fetus B appears decreased.

3. The first trimester.

4. Little to none. If the demise occurs late in the second and third trimester, labor can infrequently be induced, or the demised fetus may obstruct the delivery of the normal fetus.

Reference

Benson CB, Doubilet PM, David V: Prognosis of first-trimester twin pregnancies: polychotomous logistic regression analysis. *Radiology* 192:765–768, 1994.

Bromley B, Beracerraf B: Using the number of yolk sacs to determine amnionicity in early first trimester monochorionic twins: *J Ultrasound Med* 14:415–419, 1995.

Crow HC: Trouble with twins. *Appl Radiol* 25:19–24, 1996.

Feldstein VA, Filly RA: Complications of monochorionic twins: *Radiol Clin North Am* 41:709-27, 2003.

Richard JA, MacDonald PC, Gant F (eds): *Williams Obstetrics*, 17th ed. Norwalk, CT, Appleton-Century-Crofts, 1985, pp 212–217.

Cross-Reference

Ultrasound: THE REQUISITES, 2nd ed, pp 375, 516–521, 523–527.

Comment

In 80% of cases, twin gestations occur in their own separate sacs (dichorionic-diamniotic [Di-Di]) and therefore have separate environments. In the other 20%, the twins develop within the same monochorionic environment, either partially or completely. They then partially share the same environment and are diamniotic (monochorionic-diamniotic [Mono-Di]) or completely share the same environment and are monoamniotic (Mono-Mono), both with intermingled placental circulations. Sonographic identification of two yolk sacs in monochorionic twins has provided for the diagnosis of diamniotic twins early in the first trimester, before the amniotic membrane can be seen.

The rate of spontaneous abortion (miscarriage) in singleton pregnancies is approximately 20% to 25%. This rate is slightly higher in twin gestations. In a Di-Di pregnancy, a first-trimester loss of one of the twins may not be noticed. If incidentally detected by ultrasound, the demised twin will show an abnormal empty sac, a sac containing an embryo without heart motion, or an abnormal yolk sac. In these cases, if the pregnancies are followed, the demised twin will "vanish," leaving one developing gestational sac. In a monochorionic twinning, because of the shared circulation, the demised twin may adversely affect the living twin.

In the second and third trimesters, a spontaneous loss of one of the twins is uncommon. However, even in Di-Di twin pregnancies, the loss rate is slightly higher than in singleton pregnancies, partially because of the somewhat higher incidence of growth restriction. With monochorionic pregnancies, there are additional problems because of the shared placental circulation, which could lead to a twin-twin transfusion; late in the pregnancy if the pregnancy is monoamniotic, there is also the potential complication of demise caused by entangled umbilical cords.

When there is a loss of a twin in a Di-Di pregnancy in the second or third trimester, the demise should not adversely affect the living fetus (see Figs. A to D). The demised fetus will, of course, have no detectable heart motion. Because autolysis occurs within the first week, the demised fetus will lose its internal anatomy and will begin to collapse. The fetal head of the demised fetus B (see Fig. D) shows no demonstrable internal anatomy and overlapping of calvarial sutures (arrow), called the Spalding's sign. Additionally, there appears to be a decrease in the amount of amniotic fluid in the sac surrounding fetus B (see Figs. A and B), a finding also noted in fetal demise. The increased echogenicity of the fluid, however, is of uncertain significance.

The diagnosis of dichorionic pregnancy is important because it helps predict the risk to the remaining fetus. This can be determined by the following: different fetal genders, separate placentas, or a thick (1–2 mm), and well-defined membrane. The membrane is better defined in the first trimester, but when clearly seen in the second or third trimester it is indicative of a dichorionic pregnancy (see Figs. A and B).

The demised twin in the second and third trimesters does not "vanish." Instead, in a Di-Di pregnancy, the fetus may flatten and be pushed to one side but may still be visible even at term. This is called a fetus papyraceous (paper fetus). This fetus, although not directly impinging on the other fetus, may cause either spontaneous labor or, at term, may block the exit of the normal fetus. If the pregnancy is monochorionic, the shared placental circulation may create significant problems for the living remaining fetus, most likely owing to disseminated intravascular coagulopathy. This can cause in utero demise or destructive (embolic) changes in the surviving fetus.

Notes

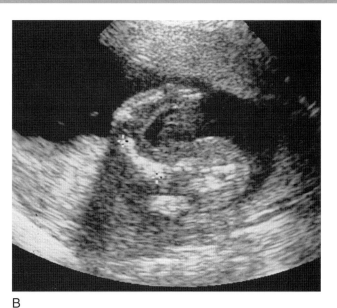

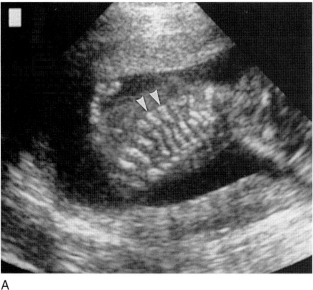

A

B

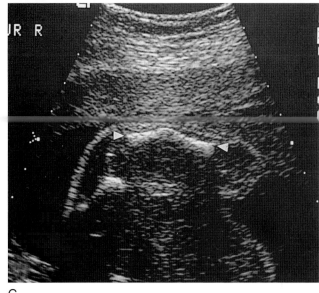

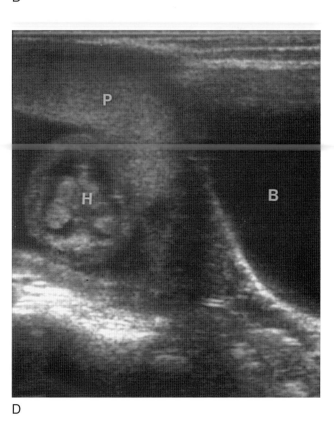

C

D

1. In this 22-week-old fetus (fetus A), which abnormalities are detected in the sagittal image of the fetal chest (Fig. A, arrows) and long axis image of one of the femurs? Figure B; + signs = femoral shaft. What is the most likely diagnosis, and what is the level of severity?

2. In another fetus (fetus B) at 35 weeks of age with the same disorder, what is seen in this image of one of its femurs? Figure C; arrowheads = the femoral shaft. If this is the only bone involved, is this case likely to be as severe as that of fetus A?

3. Can osteogenesis imperfecta (OI) be ruled out by a normal ultrasound examination?

4. What is the underlying biochemical abnormality in OI?

5. What is changed on comparing the fetal skull in the two images, Figures E and F?

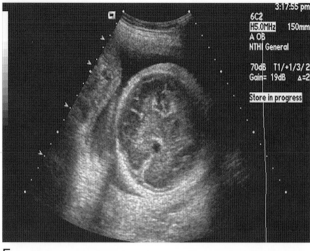

E

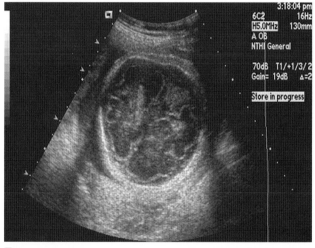

F

Osteogenesis Imperfecta

1. Rib fracture and bowed femur with grossly normal bone brightness. Osteogenesis imperfecta, severe.

2. Angled bone due to a healed fracture with normal bone brightness. No, less severe.

3. No.

4. OI is a connective tissue disorder with defective type I collagen.

5. Skull is being compressed transabdominally by the weight of the transducer in Figure E and is not compressed in F, when transducer pressure is discontinued.

Acknowledgment

Figures A and B for Case 79 courtesy of Beryl Benacerral, M.D.

References

Bulas DI, Stern HJ, Rosenbaum KN, et al: Variable prenatal appearance of osteogenesis imperfecta. *J Ultrasound Med* 13:419–427, 1994.

McEwing RL, Alton K, Johnson J, et al: First-trimester diagnosis of osteogenesis imperfecta type II by three dimensional sonography. *J Ultrasound Med* 22: 311–314, 2003.

Munoz C, Filly RA, Golbus MS: Osteogenesis imperfecta type II: Prenatal sonographic diagnosis. *Radiology* 174:181–185, 1990.

Parilla, BV, Leeth EA, Kambich MS, et al: Antenatal detection of skeletal dysplasias. *J Ultrasound Med* 22:255–258, 2003.

Pretorius DH, Rumack CM, Manc-Johnson ML, et al: Specific skeletal dysplasias in utero: Sonographic diagnosis. *Radiology* 159:237–242, 1986.

Sanders RC, Greyson-Fleg, RT, Hogge, WA, et al: Osteogenesis imperfecta and campomelic dysplasia: Difficulties in prenatal diagnosis. *J Ultrasound Med* 13:691–700, 1994.

Cross-Reference

Ultrasound: THE REQUISITES, 2nd ed, pp 476–478.

Comment

OI is a connective tissue disorder that is attributed to defective type I collagen. Various organ systems may be involved, including the eyes (sclerae), skin, teeth, and ears; however, the most widely recognized abnormalities involve the skeletal system. The outcome ranges from mild affliction (e.g., osteoporosis) to stillbirth or early neonatal death.

A classification system has been described using genetic, clinical, and radiographic criteria. Types I and IV are autosomal dominant and nonlethal. Type I has mildly fragile bones without significant deformity, whereas type IV presents with osteoporosis and fragile bones that bow. Types II and III are more severe. Type II can be autosomal dominant, in which most affected fetuses die, and type III presents as nonlethal autosomal recessive. Type II has demineralization and multiple fractures, whereas type III presents with fractures that result in deformed bones and spine.

The ultrasound diagnosis relies on the detection of fractures, unusual bowing of the long bones, and decreased bone brightness. If none of these is present, the diagnosis of OI cannot be made, even in the appropriate clinical and biochemical settings. Therefore, the lack of positive ultrasound findings cannot rule out an affected fetus.

The ultrasound criteria for the lethal type II OI centers not only on marked deformities or fractures but also on bone demineralization, particularly of the calvarium. Cranial compressibility with clear visualization of intracranial contents, especially the cerebral gyri, suggests the diagnosis of OI. See Figures E and F. Demineralization cannot be quantitated but is suggested by the lack of normal bone brightness. This is shown in a third affected fetus, fetus C (Fig. D). Figure D, an axial view of the head (H), shows normal internal anatomy, including the choroid plexus but no normal calvarial brightness. (P = placenta; B = urinary bladder.) The differential diagnosis of skull demineralization includes congenital hypophosphatasia and achondrogenesis, both of which may produce poor ossification of the spine, with less than three ossification centers characteristic of the latter. Note the change in the appearance of the fetal skull with slight pressure as seen in Figure E compared to Figure F. Three-dimensional sonography has been helpful in making this diagnosis.

Fractures can be multiple and involve long bones and ribs, which may also appear bowed or beaded, as in type III OI (fetus A, see Figs. A and B). A bowed femur is more difficult to measure for an accurate length. A "wrinkled appearance" has been used to describe the femur with multiple fractures. If the spine can be clearly imaged, the vertebral bodies may be flattened, called platyspondyly, caused by softening of the vertebral bodies. Polyhydramnios may be present.

Prenatal diagnosis of the nonlethal subtypes may be more difficult. Bowing or angulation at the point of a fracture may be seen, as in fetus B (see Fig. C). Normally, only the inner surface of the femur can appear mildly bowed. Any other long bone with bowing could be considered abnormal. Mineralization, identified on ultrasound as brightness, is usually normal. Limb length can be normal to moderately shortened.

Notes

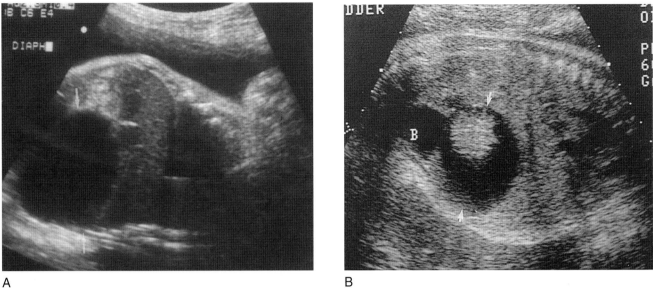

A

B

1. What is the most likely origin of the cystic abdominopelvic mass (arrow) shown in the third-trimester female fetus (Fig. A)? What is the cause?

2. Which fetal ovarian mass (arrows) can have cystic and solid components (Fig. B)? B = urinary bladder.

3. What are the potential complications of an ovarian cyst?

4. What endocrine syndrome has been described in association with fetal ovarian cysts?

Fetal Ovarian Cyst

1. Ovarian cyst; maternal hormones crossing the placenta.

2. Teratoma.

3. Rupture, torsion, hemorrhage, bowel obstruction, and dystocia.

4. Congenital hypothyroidism.

References

Crombleholme TM, Craigo SD, Garmel S, D'Alton ME: Fetal ovarian cyst decompression to prevent torsion. *J Pediatr Surg* 32:1447–1449, 1997.

Jafri SZH, Bree RL, Silver TM, Ouimette M: Fetal ovarian cysts: Sonographic detection and association with hypothyroidism. *Radiology* 150:809–812, 1984.

Cross-Reference

Ultrasound: THE REQUISITES, 2nd ed, pp 447, 464.

Comment

Small follicular ovarian cysts have been detected in one third of stillbirths and neonatal female deaths. Ovarian cysts are usually functional and histologically benign, induced by maternal hormones crossing the placenta. In females, ovarian cysts occur in association with long-standing hypothyroidism. This is a result of precocious sexual development. The pituitary secretes a nonspecific glycoprotein hormone as a result of hypothyroidism. Fetal ovarian cysts have been detected prenatally on ultrasound in the setting of congenital hypothyroidism.

On ultrasound, a simple ovarian cystic mass (see Fig. A) will be identified in the pelvis if small, or if large extending out of the pelvis into the abdomen. Polyhydramnios has been reported in 10% of cases, possibly caused by small bowel obstruction by large cysts. Bilateral cysts have been described. Fetal ovarian teratomas (see Fig. B) appear as cystic and solid masses of the ovary.

Complications include hemorrhage and bowel obstruction in addition to ovarian torsion. The cyst can rupture at delivery or cause dystocia due to abdominal distension if it is large.

Decompression has been recommended in the literature from large centers that perform in utero surgery, although this is controversial. It is recommended, however, when the cyst is larger than 4 cm, enlarges rapidly (>1 cm/wk), or can be shown to move around the fetal abdomen on serial ultrasounds. These signs are considered indicators of an increased risk of torsion. Fetal ovarian cysts can resolve spontaneously. Ultrasound is performed postnatally, and the cysts can be aspirated in the neonate if necessary.

Notes

A

B

1. What is the diagnosis in these early first-trimester transvaginal ultrasound scans of the uterus?

2. What is the incidence of *spontaneous* heterotopic pregnancy? The incidence has increased in high-risk groups to as high as 1 in 1600. What accounts for the rise?

3. What is the incidence of heterotopic pregnancy after assisted reproduction?

4. What are the treatment options?

CASE 81

Heterotopic Pregnancy

1. Heterotopic pregnancy: concomitant intrauterine and extrauterine pregnancies.

2. 1 in 7000. Assisted reproduction and pelvic inflammatory disease.

3. Up to 1 in 100.

4. Salpingectomy, salpingostomy, and direct infusion of potassium chloride into the ectopic gestation (salpingocentesis).

Acknowledgment

Figure B for Case 81 courtesy of Alda Cossi, M.D.

References

Botash RJ, Spirt BA: Ectopic pregnancy: Review and update. *Applied Radiology* 29:7–12, 2000.

Dialani V, Levine D: Ectopic pregnancy: A review. *Ultrasound Q* 20:105–117, 2004.

Doubilet PM, Benson CB, Frates MC, Ginsburg E: Sonographically guided minimally invasive treatment of unusual ectopic pregnancies. *J Ultrasound Med* 23:359–370, 2004.

Rojansky N, Schenker JG: Heterotopic pregnancy and assisted reproduction—an update. *J Assist Reprod Genet* 13:554–601, 1996.

Tal J, Haddad S, Gordon N, Timor-Tritsch I: Heterotopic pregnancy after ovulation induction and assisted reproductive technologies: A literature review from 1971-1993. *Fertil Steril* 66:1-12, 1996.

Cross-Reference

Ultrasound: THE REQUISITES, 2nd ed, pp 359, 366, 368, 576.

Comment

The occurrence of an intrauterine pregnancy with a simultaneous extrauterine gestation was once a rare phenomenon, with spontaneous incidence estimated at 1 in 30,000 pregnancies. Later investigations determined the spontaneous heterotopic pregnancy rate to be 1/ 7000. However, in recent years, several factors have led to an increase in the incidence of heterotopic pregnancy: assisted reproduction techniques (ARTs) as well as but also intrauterine contraceptive devices, pelvic inflammatory disease, and previous tubal surgery. In these high-risk groups, the incidence of heterotopic pregnancy has been estimated to be as high as 1 in 3000. For women undergoing ARTs, this complication occurs in 1% to 3%.

In cases where women have undergone ARTs, the diagnosis is often made with a screening ultrasound early in the gestation period while the woman is asymptomatic. Symptomatic patients present with abdominal pain in most cases; vaginal bleeding occurs in only 50%.

Improvements in ultrasound have resulted in an increased rate of detection for heterotopic pregnancies, particularly using transvaginal imaging. However, a preliminary transabdominal scan is essential to exclude any mass in a suprauterine location or the rare abdominal pregnancy. In a heterotopic pregnancy, in addition to the intrauterine gestation, ultrasound may demonstrate a live extrauterine gestation, an adnexal gestational sac, or an adnexal mass. The cases shown here demonstrate an intrauterine pregnancy with an intrauterine gestational sac and a yolk sac and similar findings in the right cornu of the uterus. Although the presence of an intrauterine gestation formerly excluded an ectopic pregnancy, in any woman with risk factors for heterotopic pregnancy, careful evaluation for an adnexal mass or complex fluid must be performed. It is important to keep in mind that a ruptured corpus luteum cyst can also result in a moderate amount of intraperitoneal hemorrhage.

Treatment options are aimed at salvaging the intrauterine pregnancy. Salpingectomy, salpingoscopic removal, and salpingocentesis (direct infusion of potassium chloride into the ectopic gestation) have all been performed. Sonographically guided injection of potassium chloride into the ectopic gestation or fetus is safe, ablating the ectopic pregnancy but also permitting the normal continuation of a concomitant intrauterine pregnancy. Also, with this option the uterus is preserved for future gestations. Oophorectomy is performed for the rare ovarian heterotopic pregnancy.

The outcome depends somewhat on the location of the heterotopic pregnancy. Cornual heterotopic pregnancies are particularly hazardous owing to hemoperitoneum, with a lower rate of survival for the intrauterine gestation. Overall, the intrauterine gestation survival rate is 60% to 70%.

Notes

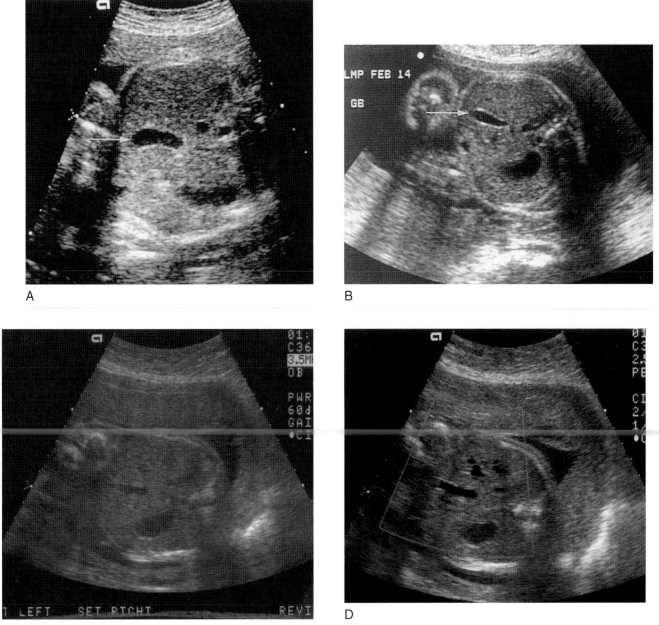

A

B

C

D

1. What are the most likely diagnosis and the differential diagnosis of the two fluid-filled structures in the upper abdomen of these middle second-trimester fetuses (Figs. A and B, axial images of the upper abdomen; L = liver)

2. What fluid-filled upper abdominal structure do these additional images (Figs. C and D; same fetus as in Fig. B) of the upper abdomen detect?

3. When is the gallbladder usually seen?

4. Does nonvisualization of the fetal gallbladder predict biliary atresia?

5. What is the diagnosis in Figure E regarding the fetal gallbladder?

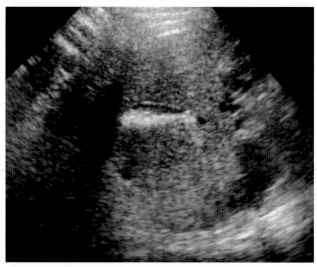

E

Fetal Gallbladder

1. Fetal gallbladder. Differential diagnosis includes a dilated or normal portal (intra-abdominal portion of the umbilical) vein and cystic abdominal masses (e.g., duplication, mesenteric cyst, choledochal).

2. The normal umbilical portion of the left portal vein.

3. Between 24 and 32 weeks.

4. No.

5. Cholelithiasis.

References

Blazer S, Zimmer EZ, Bronshtein M: Nonvisualization of the fetal gallbladder in early pregnancy: Comparison with clinical outcome. *Radiology* 224:379–382, 2002.

Brown DL, Teele RL, Doubilet PM, et al: Echogenic material in the fetal gallbladder: Sonographic and clinical observations. *Radiology* 182:73, 1992.

Hertzberg BS, Kliewer MA: Fetal gallstones in a contracted gallbladder: Potential to simulate hepatic or peritoneal calcification. *J Ultrasound Med* 17:667–670, 1998.

Hertzberg BS, Kliewer MA, Bowie JD, et al: Enlarged fetal gallbladder: Prognostic importance for aneuploidy or biliary abnormality at antenatal US. *Radiology* 208: 795–798, 1998.

Hertzberg BS, Kliewer MA, Maynor C, et al: Nonvisualization of the fetal gallbladder: Frequency and prognostic importance. *Radiology* 199:679–682, 1996.

McNamara A, Levine D: Intraabdominal fetal echogenic masses: A practical guide to diagnosis and management. *RadioGraphics* 25:633–645, 2005.

Cross-Reference

Ultrasound: THE REQUISITES, 2nd ed, p 431.

Comment

The fetal gallbladder can be seen in 82% to 100% of all second and third trimester prenatal ultrasound studies. It is seen more frequently between 24 and 32 weeks. Visualization declines later in the gestation period, perhaps due to gallbladder contractions near term. In fetuses in whom the gallbladder is not visualized, the outcome is usually normal, with no increased incidence of biliary tract anomalies or cystic fibrosis. A more recent study shows a gallbladder detection rate of 99.9% at 14 to16 weeks' gestation when the transvaginal ultrasound technique is used. Nonvisualization of the gallbladder in early pregnancy was associated with anomalies in 40% of patients.

The fetal gallbladder enlarges progressively through the gestation period. The average area is 8 mm^2 between 12 and 15 weeks and is as large as 91 mm^2 between 32 and 35 weeks. It plateaus at 30 to 36 weeks. "Cholecystomegaly," or gallbladder enlargement, is not associated with biliary tract abnormalities. Infants with trisomy 13 have an increased incidence of gallbladder enlargement; however, this is not a predictor of chromosomal anomalies on prenatal ultrasonography.

The gallbladder may extend directly anteriorly (see Figs. A and B) and can be mistaken for the normal umbilical portion of the left portal vein (see Figs. C and D). It should not be mistaken for an umbilical varix, which is a focal dilatation of the intra-abdominal umbilical vein just inside the abdominal wall; this can be distinguished by color Doppler imaging. A prominent gallbladder should not be mistaken for a cystic abdominal mass.

Fetal cholelithiasis (Fig. E) is a relatively common finding and is almost always a third trimester phenomenon. Many gallstones resolve spontaneously in utero or soon after birth. Those that persist rarely cause symptoms.

Notes

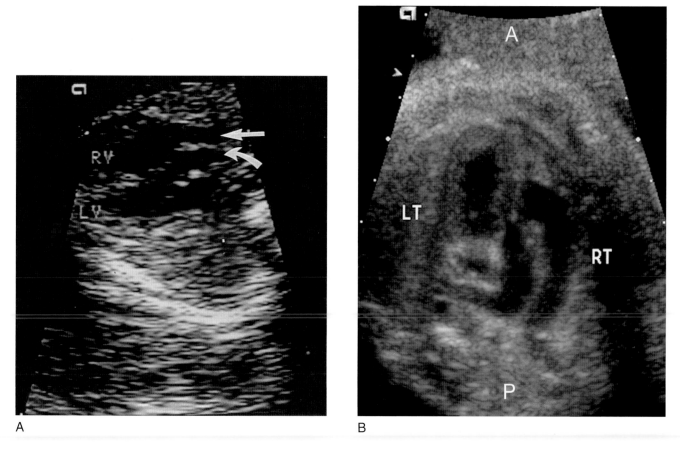

A   B

1. What is the abnormality shown in these images of the outflow tracts of the heart (Figs. A and B)? RV = right ventricle; LV = left ventricle; RT = right; LT = left; A = anterior; P = posterior.

2. What is the diagnosis?

3. Which great vessel is anterior in transposition of the great vessels (TGV)?

4. How do the ventricles appear on a four-chamber view in TGV?

C A S E   8 3

Transposition of the Great Vessels

1. Parallel great vessels.

2. Transposition of the great vessels.

3. Aorta.

4. Most commonly normal.

Acknowledgment
Figure A for Case 83 courtesy of Dennis Woods.

References

Allan LD: Sonographic detection of parallel great arteries in the fetus. *AJR* 168:1283–1286, 1997.

Benacerraf BR: Sonographic detection of fetal anomalies of the aortic and pulmonary arteries: Value of the four-chamber view vs. direct images. *AJR* 163:1483–1489, 1994.

Bonnet D, Coltri A, Butera G, et al: Detection of transposition of the great arteries in fetuses reduces neonatal morbidity and mortality. *Circulation* 99:916–918, 1999.

Vettraino IM, Lee W, Bronsteen RA, Comstock CH: Sonographic evaluation of the ventricular cardiac outflow tracts. *J Ultrasound Med* 24:566, 2005.

Cross-Reference
Ultrasound: THE REQUISITES, 2nd ed, pp 415–419.

Comment

TGV is the most common anomaly of great vessel position. The aorta is located anteriorly and arises from the right ventricle (see Fig. A; straight arrow = aorta). The pulmonary artery arises posteriorly from the left ventricle (see Fig. A; curved arrow = main pulmonary artery). The ventricles are in their normal position in D-TGV, with the aorta on the right of the pulmonary artery. In naturally corrected transposition, or L-TGV, the ventricles are also reversed, so that the aorta is located to the left of the pulmonary artery. Corrected TGV is associated with a number of other cardiac malformations, including ventricular septal defect, arrhythmias, and peripheral pulmonic stenosis, any of which contribute to neonatal morbidity.

On the prenatal sonogram, the four-chamber view is usually normal with TGV. Therefore, an evaluation of the outflow tracts is essential. The normal aorta arises posteriorly from the left ventricle and courses right and cranially, then posteriorly. The normal pulmonary artery originates from the anterior right ventricle and runs posteriorly, crossing over the origin of the aorta. A parallel relationship of the proximal aorta to the pulmonary trunk indicates TGV, as shown in this case. One should be aware that *more distally*, the aorta and pulmonary artery may run parallel for a short course. Prenatal detection of TGV by ultrasound has been shown to decrease the preoperative mortality of neonates with TGV.

The differential diagnosis of parallel great vessels is a double-outlet right ventricle. This cardiac anomaly is commonly associated with other systemic malformations.

Notes

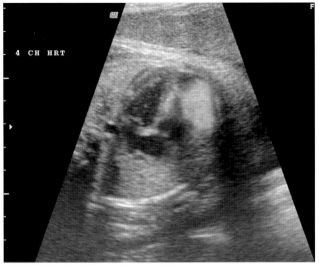

A

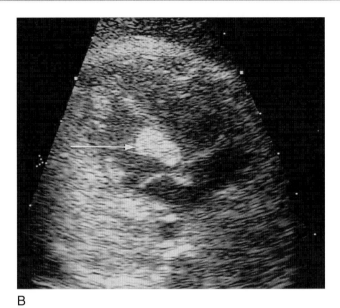

B

1. Images of two second-trimester fetal hearts are presented. What is the most common etiology for the intracardiac abnormalities on the axial four-chamber view?

2. What percentage of cardiac rhabdomyomas are associated with tuberous sclerosis?

3. What percentage of patients with tuberous sclerosis have cardiac rhabdomyomas?

4. What percentage of cardiac rhabdomyomas are multiple?

Cardiac Rhabdomyoma

1. Intracardiac rhabdomyomas.

2. Fifty percent to 78%.

3. Fifty percent to 60%.

4. Ninety percent.

Acknowledgment

Figure B for Case 84 courtesy of Dennis Woods.

References

Paladini D, Palmierie S, Russo MG, Pacileo G: Cardiac multiple rhabdomyomatosis: Prenatal diagnosis and natural history. *Ultrasound Obstet Gynecol* 7:84–85, 1996.

Seki I, Singh AD, Longo S: Pathologic case of the month: Congenital cardiac rhabdomyoma. *Arch Pediatr Adolesc Med* 150:877–878, 1996.

Uzon O, McGawley G, Wharton GA: Multiple cardiac rhabdomyomas: Tuberous sclerosis or not. *Heart* 77: 388, 1997.

Cross-Reference

Ultrasound: *THE REQUISITES*, 2nd ed, p 416.

Comment

The most common cardiac mass in the fetus, infant, and child is a rhabdomyoma. Ninety percent are multiple. The differential considerations (fibroma and myxoma) are much less common and occur as isolated masses. Of patients diagnosed with cardiac rhabdomyomas, 50% to 78% have tuberous sclerosis. Conversely, 50% to 60% of patients with tuberous sclerosis have cardiac rhabdomyomas. Tuberous sclerosis is an autosomal dominant syndrome with variable expression.

Cardiac rhabdomyoma can be detected on prenatal ultrasound. Single or multiple homogeneously hyperechoic masses are seen in the right or left ventricle; the case shown here demonstrates two masses in the right ventricle and one in the left. These arise from the intraventricular septum (Fig. B) or ventricular wall (Fig. A). The masses show a biphasic growth in utero, enlarging until 32 weeks' gestational age and subsequently shrinking in the first year of life. If detected, follow-up imaging is required to identify complications of arrhythmia, cardiac failure, and fetal hydrops.

Rhabdomyomas are histologically benign, and small rhabdomyomas that do not cause hemodynamic abnormalities regress in 80% of cases before 4 years of age. Complications of larger masses include intracardiac flow obstruction and arrhythmia. Such sequelae carry a poor prognosis.

Notes

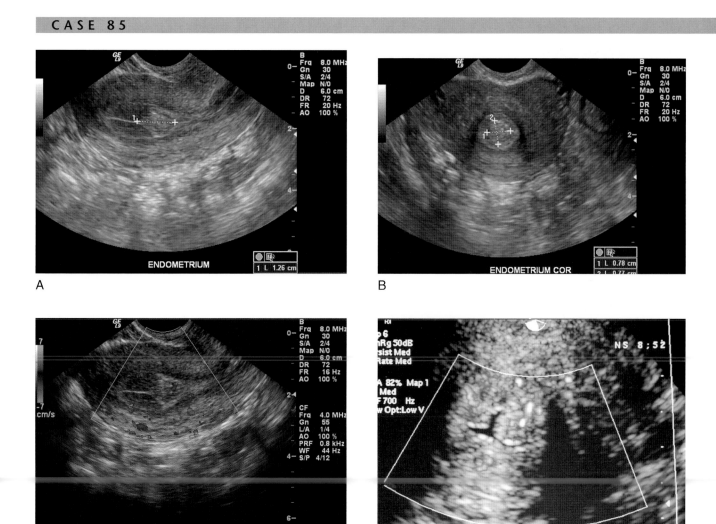

A

B

C

D

1. This 40-year-old woman presents with vaginal bleeding. Transvaginal sagittal and transverse ultrasound images of the uterus (Figs. A and B) show a well-defined spherical soft tissue mass of the endometrium. What are the differential diagnoses? How does color Doppler imaging help in arriving at a diagnosis (see Fig. C of the same patient and Fig. D from a second patient)?

2. In some cases fluid in the endometrial cavity or cervical canal can help show any mass that is present (Fig. D). What is the ultrasound procedure to place fluid into the endometrial cavity?

3. What accounts for the cystic (anechoic) spaces seen in some endometrial polyps on ultrasound?

4. What is the typical echogenicity of an endometrial polyp versus a submucosal or intracavitary myoma?

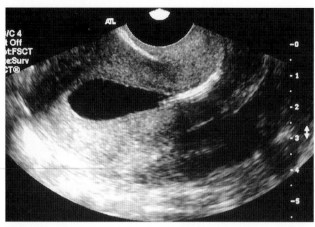

E

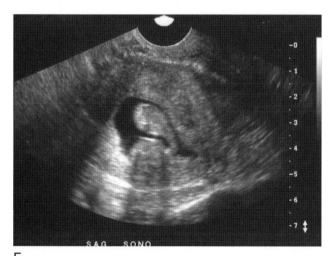

F

Endometrial Polyp

1. Polyp and submucosal fibroid. Color Doppler imaging shows any vascular stalk or grouping of small vessels.

2. Sonohysterogram.

3. Dilated glands.

4. Hyperechoic; hypoechoic.

References

Alcazar JL, Castillo G, Minguez JA, Galan MJ: Endometrial blood flow mapping using transvaginal power Doppler sonography in women with postmenopausal bleeding and thickened endometrium. *Ultrasound Obstet Gynecol* 21:583–588, 2003.

Alcazar JL, Galan MJ, Minguez JA, Garcia-Manero M: Transvaginal color Doppler sonography versus sono-hysterography in the diagnosis of endometrial polyps. *J Ultrasound Med* 23:743–748, 2004.

Guven MA, Bese T, Demirkiran F, et al: Comparison of hysterosonography and transvaginal ultrasonography in the detection of intracavitary pathologies in women with abnormal uterine bleeding. *Int J Gynecol Cancer* 14:57–63, 2004.

Laifer-Narin S, Ragavendra N, Parmenter EK, Grand EG: False-normal appearance of the endometrium on conventional transvaginal sonography: Comparison with saline hysterosonography. *AJR* 178;129–133, 2002.

Lev-Toaff AS, Toaff ME, Liu J-B, et al: Value of sonohysterography in the diagnosis and management of abnormal uterine bleeding. *Radiology* 201:179–184, 1996.

Cross-Reference

Ultrasound: THE REQUISITES, 2nd ed, pp 539, 541, 543–545.

Comment

Causes of dysfunctional uterine bleeding include complications of pregnancy, polyp, myoma, endometrial atrophy, hyperplasia, and endometrial cancer.

The appearance of the endometrium has been shown to have some correlation with the pathologic process, although there is overlap in appearances. As shown in this case, polyps are typically hyperechoic and can have small cystic spaces. Myomata are usually hypoechoic; they absorb sound and can be submucosal or completely intracavitary. Hyperplasia is often uniformly hyperechoic and can demonstrate cystic spaces. A heterogeneous thickened endometrium is a common appearance for endometrial cancer, which has been shown to manifest with a greater degree of endometrial thickening than one caused by benign processes. However the hyperplasia can be very thick.

Once a thickened endometrium is diagnosed, dilatation and curettage are often performed. However, because of sampling error, the pathologic diagnosis can be missed, particularly when only a portion of the endometrium appears to be thickened (see Fig. A). A thickened endometrial stripe on transvaginal ultrasound can be found to be normal, proliferative, or secretory endometrium, hyperplasia, polyp(s), or endometrial cancer. In a premenopausal patient a thickened endometrial stripe would be greater than about 1.6 cm; in a perimenopausal patient, about 1.3 cm, and in a postmenopausal patient, 0.5 cm, unless the patient is on hormone replacement therapy, in which case the cutoff is 0.8 to 1 cm. The increased thickness from the hormones is reversible. In many cases, a sonohysterogram (SHG) is useful (see Figs. E and F from another patient) and confirms the diagnosis of an endometrial polyp. The information can guide the gynecologist to the site of biopsy. Using an SHG, one can distinguish a polyp (as shown in this case) from a myoma and define the exact location of a myoma (intracavitary versus submucosal versus myometrial), which dictates whether surgery can be performed hysteroscopically. Therefore, many management decisions are aided by the findings on an SHG.

Notes

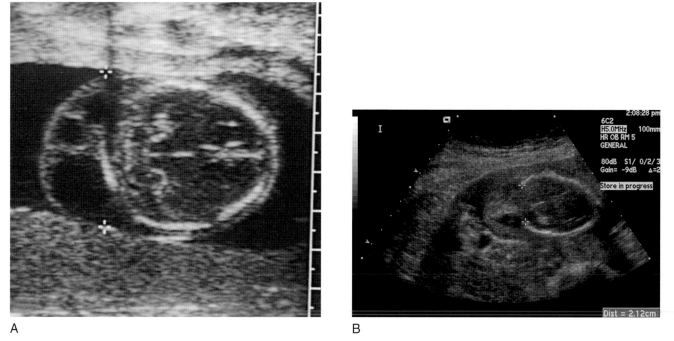

A

B

1. What are the diagnoses of the posterior neck masses shown in fetus A (Fig. A; + signs = mass) and fetus B (Fig. B; + signs = boundaries of abnormality arising through a bony defect)?

2. What findings will aid in distinction of the diagnosis?

3. Will the α-fetoprotein (AFP) level aid in identifying the diagnosis?

4. In which entity is karyotype testing warranted?

C A S E 86

Posterior Neck Mass

1. For fetus A (see Fig. A) the diagnosis is a cystic hygroma. For fetus B (see Fig. B) the diagnosis is an encephalocele.

2. For cystic hygroma, a "spoke-wheel" appearance of septations is pathognomonic (see Fig. A). For a cephalocele or an encephalocele, a cranial defect (note the defect in the occipital bone) and associated central nervous system (CNS) abnormalities such as dilated ventricles seen in Case 98, Figure A are associated findings.

3. Yes. Unlike other neural tube defects, AFP is usually normal in cephaloceles and encephaloceles. AFP levels can be elevated in a cystic hygroma or cervical meningomyelocele.

4. Both, as cephaloceles (and encephaloceles) and cystic hygromas are associated with abnormal karyotypes.

Reference

Bonilla-Musoles F, Raga F, Villalobos A, et al: First-trimester neck abnormalities: Three-dimensional evaluation. *J Ultrasound Med* 17:419–425, 1998.

Goldstein RB, LaPidus AS, Filly RA: Fetal cephaloceles: Diagnosis with US. *Radiology* 180:803–808, 1991.

Cross-Reference

Ultrasound: THE REQUISITES, 2nd ed, pp 406, 407–410.

Comment

A mass posterior to the fetal neck may arise from the soft tissues of the neck from nonfusion of the lymphatic vessels of the back and neck, as in the case of cystic hygroma (see Fig. A) or of the cervical spine, as in the case of a rare cervical meningomyelocele. A cephalocele (containing CSF) or encephalocele (containing CSF and brain) protrudes through a bone defect in the calvarium. The distinction may be difficult to make. Several findings have been elucidated to aid in determining the accurate diagnosis.

The appearance of the mass is important. Cephaloceles, cervical meningomyeloceles, and cystic hygromas can be entirely cystic. Cephaloceles contain no brain, but even in an encephalocele the CNS matter may not be apparent on ultrasound scans. If solid material or a definite cranial defect (see Fig. B, posterior) is identified, then an encephalocele can be confirmed. However, in many cases the cranial defect is difficult to visualize, or a dropout artifact creates a spurious defect. A cyst-within-a-cyst appearance has been described with an encephalocele and may represent a herniated, dilated fourth ventricle into the cephalocele.

The presence of septations (see Fig. A), particularly a "spoke-wheel appearance" or bullae, suggests a cystic hygroma. Most cephaloceles and cervical meningomyeloceles are midline defects, and cystic hygromas can be posterior or posterolateral. A cephalocele can rarely be caused by an amniotic band syndrome and is almost always asymmetric. Although cephaloceles usually have an acute angle between the mass and the skin line, a cystic hygroma usually forms an obtuse angle with the skin.

The presence of specific associated findings may aid in the diagnosis. CNS abnormalities, including ventriculomegaly, lemon-head deformity, beaked tectum, flattened basioccipital bone, and microcephaly, suggest a cephalocele or cervical meningomyelocele. Cystic hygroma can be complicated by serous effusions and subcutaneous edema (hydrops).

Notes

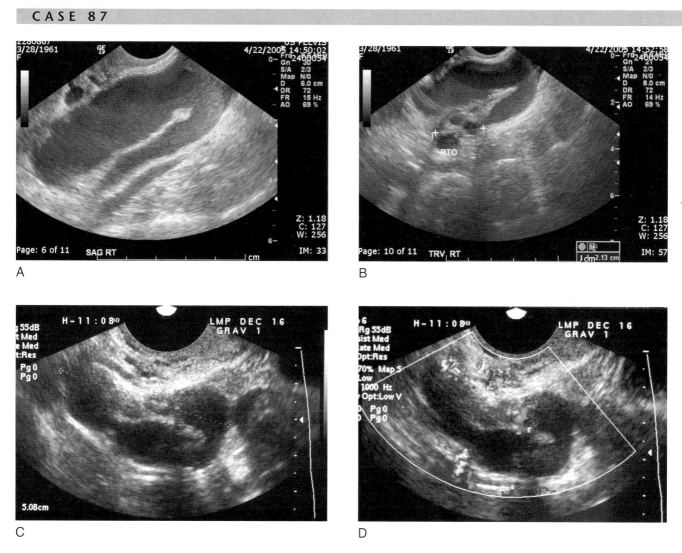

A

B

C

D

1. A 44-year-old woman has a complaint of pelvic pain. Figures A and B are transvaginal images (sagittal and transverse views) of the right adnexal areas. What are the findings and what is the most likely diagnosis? How does Doppler imaging help in the diagnosis in the case in Figures C and D?

2. Is a hydrosalpinx better detected by a transabdominal or transvaginal study?

3. Do clinicians often order an ultrasound examination in cases of pelvic inflammatory disease (PID)?

4. Are patients with PID at a greater risk for an ectopic pregnancy?

Pelvic Inflammatory Disease (Hydrosalpinx)

1. Dilated fallopian tube; diagnosis is hydrosalpinx from prior infection. Doppler imaging shows that the large tubular structure is not a vessel and has no flow.

2. Transvaginal study.

3. No.

4. Yes. Partially treated but abnormal fallopian tubes are a high risk factor for a tubal pregnancy.

Reference

Benjaminov O, Atri M: Sonography of the abnormal fallopian tube. *AJR* 183:737–742, 2004.

Horrow M: Ultrasound of pelvic inflammatory disease. *Ultrasound Q* 20:171–179, 2004.

Soper DE: Upper genital tract infection. In Copeland LJ (ed): *Textbook of Gynecology.* Philadelphia, WB Saunders, 1993, pp 517–559.

Cross-Reference

Ultrasound: THE REQUISITES, 2nd ed pp 573, 575–577.

Comment

Pelvic inflammatory disease (PID) includes endometritis, salpingitis, perio-ophoritis and tubo-ovarian abscess. It is usually due to a gynecologic infection (with *Chlamydia trachomatis* or *Neisseria gonorrhoeae*), but it may also be the result of direct extension from an inflamed appendix, diverticulitis, or other pelvic inflammatory conditions. The incidence of PID has increased in rate and in the number of hospitalizations. PID has also increased the rates of ectopic pregnancy and infertility. The economic consequences of PID are vast. More than 1 million women are treated for this disease in the United States each year, and more than 25% of these women are hospitalized annually with this diagnosis. As many as 150,000 women undergo surgical procedures for PID, some of which involve hysterectomies.

Typically, PID is clinically treated with antibiotics, and often an imaging study is not necessary. However, if the symptoms outlast or are worse than expected, an ultrasound examination is usually the first study to evaluate for the possibility of an abscess. A thickened fallopian tube is the main diagnostic feature of PID.

Figures A, B, C, and D show typically dilated fallopian tubes. When one tube is involved, it is almost always the same case with the other, even if not appreciated by imaging studies. Only in unusual cases of instrumentation or use of an intrauterine device is only one tube affected.

Although most cystic adnexal masses are ovarian in origin, an oval shape or an unusually complex mass should have several additional differential diagnoses, including infection, abscesses, and hydrosalpinges. If the hydrosalpinx contains internal echoes, it is probably infected (a pyosalpinx). On transabdominal study, it is not uncommon to see only an unusually oval-shaped mass. A transvaginal study is usually more definitive for detecting the true tubular nature of the mass.

Notes

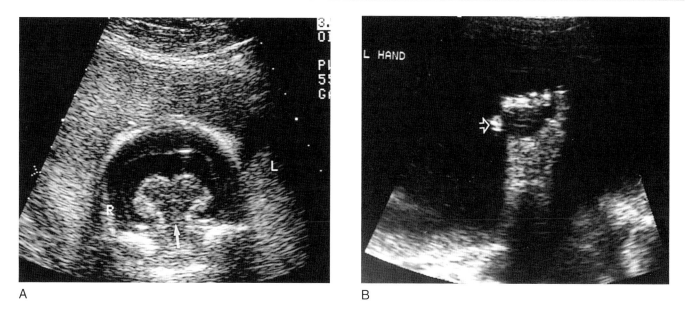

A   B

1. What is the most likely chromosomal anomaly associated with this second- trimester fetus? Figure A is a coronal image of the fetal head. Figure B is an image of the left hand.

2. What percentage of fetuses with this chromosomal anomaly has cardiac abnormalities?

3. What extremity malformations are associated?

4. Name three associated facial malformations.

Trisomy 13

1. Trisomy 13.

2. 50%.

3. Polydactyly and clubfoot.

4. Cleft lip/palate, cyclopia, and hypotelorism are among the facial malformations.

References

Hill LM: The sonographic detection of trisomies 13, 18, and 21. *Clin Obstet Gynecol* 39:831–850, 1996.

Lehman CD, Nyberg DA, Winter TC, et al: Trisomy 13 syndrome: Prenatal US findings in a review of 33 cases. *Radiology* 194:217–222, 1995.

Nyberg DA, Souter VL: Sonographic markers of fetal anomalies. *J Ultrasound Med* 20:655–674, 2001.

Cross-Reference

Ultrasound: THE REQUISITES, pp 384–385.

Comment

Trisomy 13 (Patau's syndrome) is a fatal chromosomal abnormality with many severe malformations associated. A high intrauterine spontaneous abortion rate compared with other trisomies accounts for its lower prevalence at birth. One large series reported that symmetric intrauterine growth restriction was present in almost half the cases; abnormal amniotic fluid was detected in almost one third, both oligohydramnios and polyhydramnios.

Malformations of the central nervous system are common. Neurologic malformations include holoprosencephaly (see Fig. A), microcephaly, enlarged cisterna magna, agenesis of the corpus calllosum, Dandy-Walker malformation, and hydrocephalus. Figure A shows a monoventrical with fused thalami (arrow) consistent with the most severe alobar form. Cleft lip/palate, cyclopia, and hypotelorism are among the facial malformations. Nuchal thickening, cystic hygroma, lymphangiectasia, and hydrops may be present.

The kidneys may be enlarged and are often hyperechoic (echogenic), with or without hydronephrosis. Omphalocele, bladder exstrophy, and echogenic (hyperechoic) bowel are additional abdominal abnormalities. Polydactyly (see Fig. B, open arrow = sixth digit), rocker-bottom or clubbed feet, and clenched/overlapping digits have been reported.

Cardiac defects can be seen in almost 50%. Hypoplastic left heart is common as well as ventriculoseptal defect. Single umbilical artery and papillary muscle calcification have also been reported in trisomy 13.

Notes

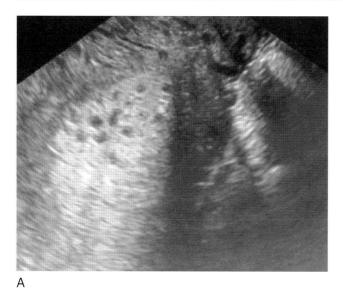

A

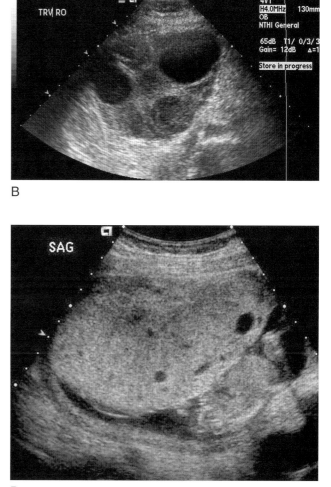

B

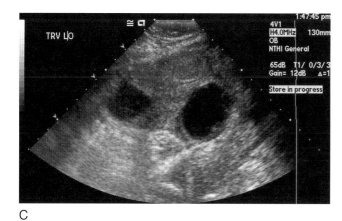

C

D

(Reprinted with permission from Doubilet P, Benson C: Atlas of Ultrasound and Obstetric Gynecology. Philadelphia, Lippincott Williams and Wilkins, 2003.)

1. What is the pathologic spectrum of disease associated with the entity in those patients with a positive serum β-human chorionic gonadotropin (hCG) reading? Figure A, a sagittal image of the uterus, is from one patient, a 30-year-old woman with continued bleeding after a dilation and curettage with a plateauing serum hCG level. Figures B and C show her ovaries. What is her diagnosis? Figure D is from a second patient and is a transabdominal image showing a placenta and portions of a fetus, Figures E and F are transvaginal images through the uterus (without and with Doppler imaging) from a third patient with a persistently elevated hCG serum level months following an 8-week fetal death.

2. What is the classic ultrasound appearance?

3. What risk does a partial mole carry?

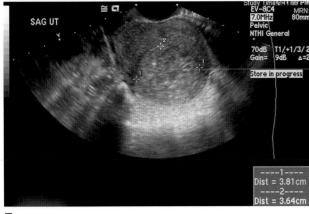

E

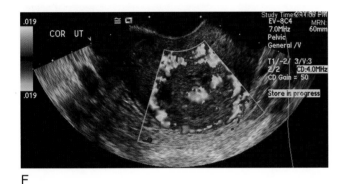

F

Gestational Trophoblastic Disease

1. Complete (Figs. A–C) and partial hydatidiform mole with fetus (Fig. D); invasive mole (Figs. E and F); and choriocarcinoma because of persistently elevated hCG.

2. "Snowstorm" of tiny vesicles (Fig. A) with increased through transmission expanding the endometrial canal.

3. Chromosomal anomalies.

References

Carter J, Fowler J, Carlson J, et al: Transvaginal color flow Doppler sonography in the assessment of gestational trophoblastic disease. *J Ultrasound Med* 12:595–599, 1993.

Di Salvo DN: Sonographic imaging of maternal complications of pregnancy. *J Ultrasound Med* 22:69–89, 2003.

Dogra V, Paspulati RM, Bhatt S: First trimester bleeding evaluation. *Ultrasound Q* 21:69-85, 2005.

Green CL, Angtuaco TL, Shah HR, et al: Gestational trophoblastic disease: A spectrum of radiologic diagnosis. *RadioGraphics* 16:1371–1384, 1996.

Wagner BJ, Woodward PJ, Dickey GE: Gestational trophoblastic disease: Radiologic-pathologic correlation. *RadioGraphics* 16:131–148, 1996.

Zhou Q, Lei X-Y, Xie Q: Sonographic and Doppler imaging in the diagnosis and treatment of gestational trophoblastic disease. *J Ultrasound Med* 24:15–24, 2005.

Cross-Reference

Ultrasound: THE REQUISITES, 2nd ed, pp 342, 355–357, 508-510.

Comment

Several pathologic entities comprise the spectrum of gestational trophoblastic disease, all of which begin with an initial fertilization that leads to a proliferative process with similarities to the normal trophoblast. These entities are a complete or partial hydatidiform mole (Figs.A, B, C, and D), which constitutes more than 80% of cases; an invasive mole (persistent local disease after treatment; Figs. E and F); or choriocarcinoma (1% to 2% of cases).

The ultrasound appearance of gestational trophoblastic neoplasms has been described as an enlarged uterus with an irregular shape in some cases. See the second patient, in whom the uterus was 12.2 cm long and very large for an 8-week gestation. The endometrium is classically expanded with a snowstorm appearance, which is caused by tiny vesicles that have increased through transmission (see Fig. A). If the vesicles enlarge, the appearance becomes more heterogeneous. Twenty-five percent to 65% of molar pregnancies have associated theca-lutein ovarian cysts. These cysts are due to the unusually high levels of hCG. Ultrasound documentation of extension into the myometrium is important; myometrial nodules reflect invasion. Transvaginal scanning is helpful in assessing myometrial extension, as is a demonstration of abnormal endometrial or myometrial flow with a high diastolic waveform, probably from decreased vessel tone. Color or power Doppler imaging can help to detect tumor invasion (Fig. F) by showing low-resistance arterial waveforms. Cystic vascular spaces may be seen in the myometrium when there is invasive hydatidiform mole or choriocarcinoma. Magnetic resonance imaging also may be helpful in assessing uterine invasion of gestational trophoblastic neoplasia. Heterogeneous, hypervascular masses can be seen that distort the zonal anatomy.

A partial mole (Fig. D) forms within the placenta of a coexistent fetus. The fetus is usually abnormal and has a high incidence of chromosomal anomalies. The differential diagnosis of this ultrasound appearance includes hydropic degeneration of the placenta. A partial mole may not have a recognizable coexistent fetus and thus sometimes cannot be distinguished from a complete mole on ultrasound imaging. Once this finding is detected, a careful ultrasound analysis and karyotype of the fetus should be performed because multiple abnormalities and triploidy are common. Unlike a complete mole, the partial mole does not have malignant potential.

Notes

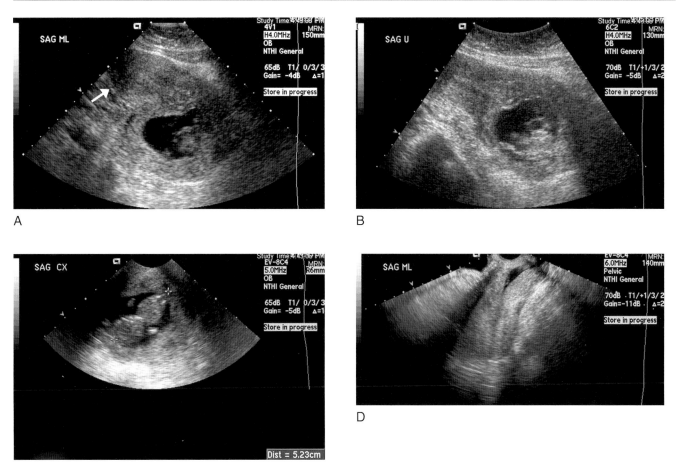

A

B

C

D

1. What are the most likely diagnoses of these gestational sacs in these two cases? Figures A, B, and C are sagittal images of the uterus; Figures B and C are coned-down views of the cervix in A. Figure D is a sagittal image of the second patient.

2. Why is the distinction between the two diagnoses so essential?

3. How is cervical ectopic pregnancy treated?

4. What accounts for the rising incidence of cervical ectopic pregnancies?

Cervical Ectopic Pregnancy

1. Figures A, B, and C show cervical implantation of the gestational sac (cervical ectopic pregnancy); Figure D shows an abortion in progress.

2. Treatment of a cervical ectopic pregnancy with dilatation and curettage can result in life-threatening hemorrhage.

3. With methotrexate, dilatation, and evacuation following uterine artery ligation, coils or ultrasound-guided potassium chloride injection.

4. In vitro fertilization.

References

Frates MC, Benson CB, Doubilet PM, et al: Cervical ectopic pregnancy: Results of conservative treatment. *Radiology* 191:773–775, 1994.

Ginsburg ES, Frates MC, Rein MS, Fox JH: Early diagnosis and treatment of cervical pregnancy in an in vitro fertilization program. *Fertil Steril* 61:966–969, 1994.

Rosenberg RD, Williamson MR: Cervical ectopic pregnancy: Avoiding pitfalls in the ultrasound diagnosis. *J Ultrasound Med* 11:365–367, 1992.

Cross-Reference

Ultrasound: THE REQUISITES, 2nd ed, pp 347, 359, 362.

Comment

Cervical implantation of an ectopic pregnancy is among the rarest of implantation sites and occurs in .15% or less than 1% of all ectopic pregnancies. Cervical ectopic pregnancies can arise after natural conception and are increasing in frequency with in vitro fertilization. Distinguishing this diagnosis from an abortion in progress is essential because simple dilatation and evacuation of a cervical ectopic pregnancy usually result in hemorrhage requiring a hysterectomy.

Patients with a cervical pregnancy usually present with bleeding, in one series between 5 and 8 weeks of gestation. Transvaginal sonography is the method of choice for the diagnosis of an early cervical pregnancy Ultrasound often demonstrates a normally shaped gestational sac in the lower uterine segment (as shown in Figure B), frequently with yolk sac and fetal heart activity. In an abortion in progress, the sac is malpositioned or abnormally shaped (as demonstrated by Figure D), usually without any recognizable fetal pole or fetal heart motion. There is often no clear decidual reaction around the sac. On a follow-up scan in 24 hours, an abortion in progress should show some change or the fetus should be expelled from the cervix, but a cervical ectopic pregnancy persists.

In cases where there is no gestational sac, a heterogeneous mass may be seen in the lower uterine segment with a cervical implantation. These cases are more problematic because the differential diagnosis would include other entities such as pedunculated degenerating myoma, abortion in progress, or vascularized retained products of conception (RPOC). Detection of high diastolic flow has been proposed as an indicator of cervical ectopic pregnancy; however, this can also be seen with RPOC and gestational trophoblastic disease.

Cervical ectopic pregnancies can be treated by several methods. Systemic and local methotrexate administration are common treatments. More recently, preliminarily embolization of uterine arteries followed by dilatation and evacuation has been shown to adequately control bleeding. Last, direct injection of the embryo or gestational sac with potassium chloride (KCl) can be performed under transvaginal ultrasound guidance. This procedure enables subsequent normal fertilization and pregnancy.

Notes

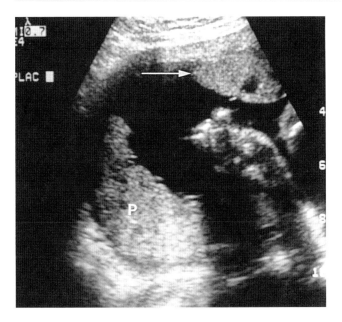

1. What is the abnormality (arrow) shown in this image of the uterus in a late second-trimester pregnancy? P = Placenta.

2. What is the etiology?

3. What is a possible perinatal complication?

4. What is a potential postnatal complication?

Succenturiate Lobe

1. Succenturiate lobe of the placenta.

2. Failure of normal villous atrophy.

3. Hemorrhage.

4. Retained placenta with hemorrhage or infection.

References

Hata K, Hata T, Aoki S, et al: Succenturiate placenta diagnosed by ultrasound. *Gynecol Obstet Invest* 25:273–276, 1988.

Nelson LH, Fishburne JI, Stearns BR: Ultrasonographic description of a succenturiate placenta. *Obstet Gynecol* 49(Suppl):79–80, 1977.

Cross-Reference

Ultrasound: THE REQUISITES, 2nd ed, p 488.

Comment

This case demonstrates a rare but important placental abnormality—the presence of a succenturiate lobe. This is defined as an accessory placental lobe that is removed from but in vascular continuity with the main placenta. Fetal vessels under the amniochorionic membranes connect this accessory lobe to the main placenta. This anomaly is reported to occur in up to 0.28% of pregnancies. The etiology is a regional failure of placental villi to atrophy.

Despite its rarity, this is a very important abnormality to detect on prenatal ultrasound. Sonography can detect and localize the accessory placenta. If it is not detected, several serious complications can ensue. Prenatally and during labor, the connecting vessels can rupture, leading to life-threatening fetal hemorrhage. A vaso previa (fetal hemorrhage) can develop at the time of labor and delivery if these vessels are over the internal cervical os. If the succenturiate lobe is not delivered, it can lead to postpartum maternal hemorrhage and infection. A succenturiate lobe should be suspected at the time of delivery if severed fetal vessels are present at the torn edge of the membranes of the placenta.

Notes

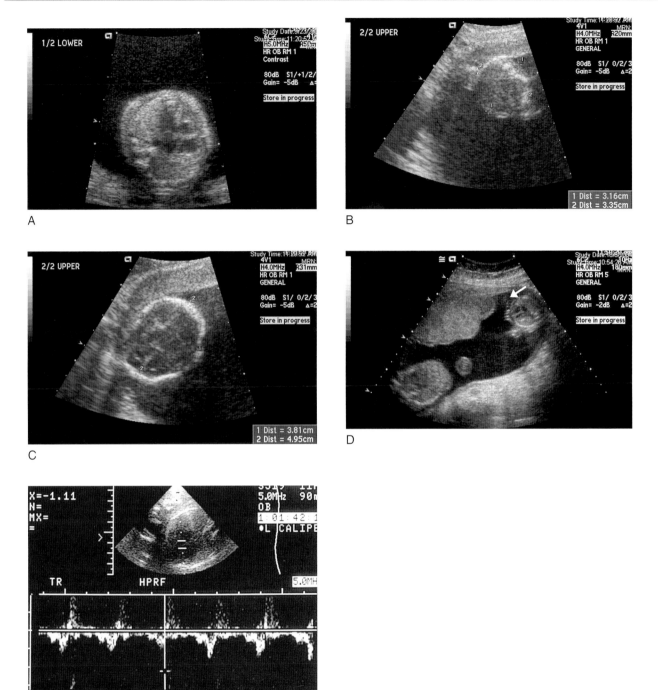

A

B

C

D

E

1. In this second-trimester twin pregnancy, fetus "one of two" is freely moving (Fig. A), and fetus "two of two" remains in a fixed position (Figs. B and C). Figure D shows both fetuses. The arrow points to the separating membrane. What is the most likely diagnosis?

2. What is the term used to describe the twin in this syndrome affected by oligohydramnios, and what is the most likely prognosis?

3. What are the ultrasound criteria used to define this syndrome?

4. In another twin pregnancy with the same syndrome, in the late third trimester, what is detected in the freely moving twin on this spectral Doppler ultrasound evaluation of the right atrium (Fig. E)?

Twin-Twin Transfusion

1. Twin-twin transfusion syndrome (TTT).

2. Adherence of the "donor" twin in its sac, called the "stuck twin syndrome." The prognosis is poor for the stuck twin.

3. Monochorionic placenta, same gender, marked growth discordance (>20%), polyhydramnios in the larger twin sac (see Fig. A) and oligohydramnios in the smaller twin sac.

4. Tricuspid regurgitation.

Reference

Bruner JP, Rosemond RL: Twin-twin transfusion syndrome: A subset of the twin oligohydramnios-polyhydramnios sequence. *Am J Obstet Gynecol* 169:925–930, 1993.

Duncombe GJ, Dickinson JE, Evans SF: Perinatal characteristics and outcomes of pregnancies complicated by twin-twin transfusion syndrome. *Obstet Gynecol* 101:1190–1196, 2003.

Moreira de Sa RA, Salomon LJ, Takahashi Y, et al: Analysis of fetal growth after laser therapy in twin-to-twin transfusion syndrome. *J Ultrasound Med* 24:1213–1219, 2005.

Cross-Reference

Ultrasound: THE REQUISITES, 2nd ed, pp 516, 521, 523–524.

Comment

The twin-twin transfusion (TTT) syndrome is a serious complication of monochorionic gestations and is a heterogeneous disorder in its clinical manifestations and progress. TTT is strictly defined by interconnecting placental vessels between the two twins, which result in umbilical arteriovenous shunting of blood from one twin to the other. When significant shunting occurs, one twin (donor) becomes small and develops anemia and oligohydramnios. The other twin (recipient) enlarges and develops polycythemia, volume overload, and heart failure as well as polyhydramnios. In the most severe form of TTT, the smaller twin can become stuck to the intervening membrane, with a very high mortality rate (see Fig. D). A high preterm birth rate typifies TTT.

Ultrasound criteria for the TTT include a monochorionic twinning (a monochorionic [fused] placenta), twins of the same gender, and a growth discordance between the twins of at least 20%. Polyhydramnios is often present in the larger sac and oligohydramnios in the smaller sac. Oligohydramnios may be so severe that the "stuck" fetus may be very difficult to identify.

The recipient twin is subject to several complications. Cardiomegaly results from biventricular hypertrophy and dilatation. Tricuspid regurgitation is often present (see Fig. E). If the donor twin dies, the recipient can suffer an embolic phenomenon through the arteriovenous connections, resulting in cerebral damage. Color Doppler ultrasound evaluation of the placenta has largely failed to identify the significant vascular connections. Laser therapy performed as laser coagulation of chorionic plate anastomoses has altered recipient growth patterns toward a decrease while not altering donor growth patterns. Less twin discordance has resulted.

Notes

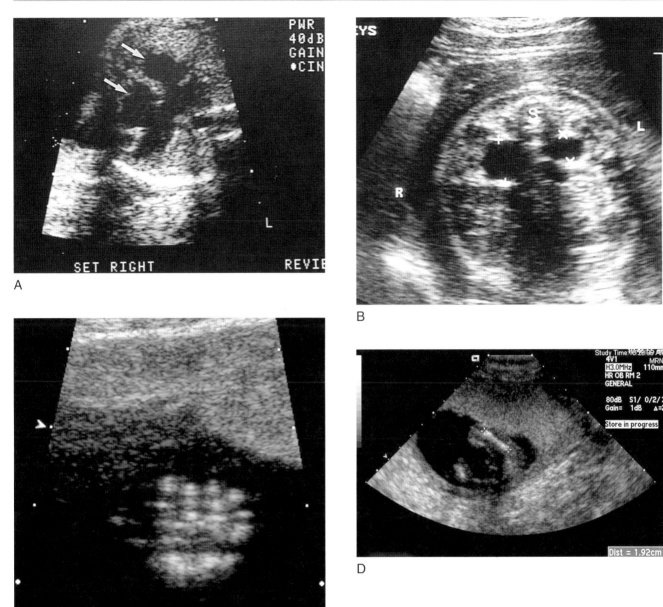

A

B

C

D

1. What is the finding in this axial image of the heart in this second-trimester fetus? (Fig. A; arrows = ventricles.) What is the most likely chromosomal anomaly?

2. What is the abnormality noted in this axial image of the fetal abdomen in the same fetus? (Fig. B; + sign = renal pelves; R= right; L = left.) Is your suspicion increased for the karyotype abnormality thought to be present?

3. What cardiac finding has recently been seen with higher frequency in this disorder?

4. What pelvic abnormality on prenatal ultrasound has been described in Down syndrome?

5. What is the significance of Figure C?

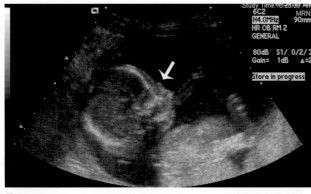

E

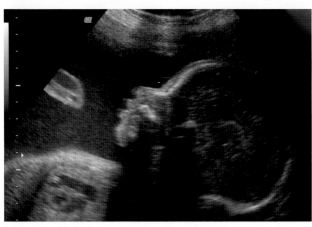

F

Trisomy 21 (Down Syndrome)—Advanced

1. Atrioventricular (AV) canal. Trisomy 21.

2. Pelviectasis. Yes.

3. Intraventricular echogenic focus.

4. Widening of the iliac angle.

5. Simian crease and polydactyl. Polydactyl, however, is not unique to trisomy 21.

References

Bromley B, Lieberman E, Shipp TD, Benacerraff BR: Fetal nose bone length: A marker for Down syndrome in the second trimester. *J Ultrasound Med* 22:162, 2003.

Goncalves LF, Espinosa J, Lee W, et al: Phenotypic characteristics of absent and hypoplastic nasal bones in fetuses with Down syndrome. *J Ultrasound Med* 23:1619–1627, 2004.

Kliewer MA, Hertzberg BS, Freed KS, et al: Normal fetal pelvis: Important factors for morphometric characterization with US. *Radiology* 215:453–457, 2000.

Nyberg DA, Souter VL: Sonographic markers of fetal trisomies. *J Ultrasound Med* 20:655–674, 2001.

Souter VL, Nyberg DA: Fetal aneuploidy screens take major step forward. *Diag Imag* 23:5–9, 2001.

Winter TC, Ostrovsky BA, Komarnski CA, Uhrich SB: Cerebellar and frontal lobe hypoplasia in fetuses with trisomy 21: Usefulness as combined US markers. *Radiology* 214:533–538, 2000.

Cross-Reference

Ultrasound: THE REQUISITES, 2nd ed, pp 417, 421, 480.

Comment

Various ultrasound findings have been described in trisomy 21. First-trimester ultrasound screening is based primarily on the nuchal translucency measurement (normal < or = 3.5 mm). Maternal serum biochemical markers are also used at this time, as is second-trimester ultrasound screening or genetic sonogram with maternal serum biochemical markers. A short humerus and femur (Figure D were three standard deviations below the norm for a fetus of this age), dilatation of the renal pelves (see Fig. B), and hyperechoic (echogenic) bowel can be seen. Hydrops fetalis and cystic hygroma have been associated with this trisomy. An echogenic focus in the ventricle of the heart, papillary muscle calcification, is seen more frequently in fetuses with Down syndrome. This calcification is present histologically in 15% to 17% of aneuploid fetuses versus 2% to 5% of normal fetuses. The significance of this finding is controversial, particularly if it is the only abnormality on a prenatal ultrasound. In a *high-risk* population, a statistically significant association of this abnormality with Down syndrome has been shown. Absence of the nasal bones is associated with the highest risk of Down syndrome. (Figure E with Figure F as a normal comparison.) A short nasal bone is associated with an increased likelihood of fetal Down syndrome in a high-risk population. Structural anomalies present later than in trisomy 13 and trisomy 18, not before 20 weeks.

Widening of the iliac angle in the pelvis correlates with the pelvic flaring that is characteristic of this syndrome. The iliac wing angle is measured on a transverse view of the pelvis, using the angle formed by the two iliac crests. The iliac angle is measured between 15 and 20 weeks, and the mean measurement is 75 degrees in Down syndrome versus 60 degrees in normal fetuses. However, the iliac angle varies with the level at which it is measured, and there is a large overlap between normal fetuses and those with Down syndrome. The iliac angle is strongly affected by the axial level and spine orientation.

The frontal lobe of the brain has been shown to be shorter and the cerebellum hypoplastic in Down syndrome fetuses compared with normal fetuses. The frontothalamic distance can be measured on prenatal ultrasound in the second trimester, from the calvarial table of the frontal lobe to the posterior margin of the thalamus. The cerebellum was measured as the maximal diameter from the lateral hemisphere to the lateral hemisphere. A simian crease can sometimes be seen in the hand.

Notes

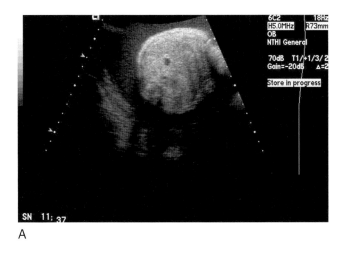

A

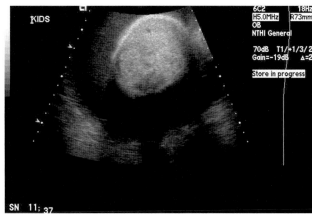

B

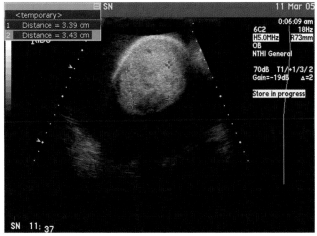

C

1. What is the predominant abnormality in Figures A and B?

2. What are the differential considerations for this finding?

3. What other organ is involved?

4. What is the constellation of findings associated with severe oligohydramnios, which may be seen in the most severe form of this disease in utero?

Autosomal Recessive Polycystic Kidney Disease

1. There are symmetrically enlarged and echogenic kidneys bilaterally.

2. Autosomal recessive polycystic kidney disease, autosomal dominant polycystic disease, glomerulocystic disease, Meckel-Gruber syndrome, renal vein thrombosis, diffuse cystic renal dysplasia, Jeune's syndrome, congenital nephrotic syndrome, Goldston's syndrome, Zellweger's syndrome.

3. The liver is typically also involved.

4. Potter facies consisting of low-set, flat ears, short snubbed nose, deep eye creases, and micrognathia. Oligohydramnios may also cause a clubbed foot deformity.

References

Blyth HM, Ockenden BG: A clinico-pathological and family study of polycystic disease of the kidneys and liver in children. *J Clin Pathol* 22:508, 1969.

Guay-Woodford LM, Desmond RA: Autosomal recessive polycystic kidney disease: The clinical experience in North America. *Pediatrics* 111:1072–1080, 2003.

Lonergan GJ, Rice RR, Suarez ES: Autosomal recessive polycystic kidney disease: Radiologic-pathologic correlation. *Radiographics* 20:837–855, 2000.

Ockenden BG, Blyth H: Polycystic disease of the liver and kidneys in childhood. *Arch Dis Child* 45:148, 1970.

Cross Reference

Ultrasound, THE REQUISITES, 2nd ed, pp 461–462.

Comment

Autosomal recessive polycystic kidney disease (ARPKD) is the most common inheritable cystic renal disease occurring in infancy. Clinical expression of this disease entity is variable in its penetrance and severity.

It is almost always characterized by kidney and liver involvement. Pathologic evaluation of diseased organs shows multiple cystic spaces that are a result of ectatic collecting ducts in the kidney and of biliary ducts in the liver. In addition, fibrosis occurs in the kidneys and the portal tracts.

ARPKD occurs 1 in 6000 to 1 in 55,000 live births in the United States. It affects both males and females equally and has no racial predominance. This disease accounts for 5% of cases per year of children with end-stage renal disease.

On prenatal ultrasound, ARPKD is characterized by nephromegaly, with kidneys that demonstrate a marked increase in echogenicity. Macroscopic cysts are not a typical finding. There may be associated olighydramnios in the most severe manifestations of the disease. The differential diagnosis of enlarged echogenic kidneys should also include autosomal dominant polycystic kidney disease (ADPKD), a entity distinct from ARPKD, glomerulocystic disease, bilateral renal vein thrombosis, Meckel-Gruber syndrome, congenital nephrotic syndrome, and other syndromes.

Although ARPKD is now considered more as a spectrum disease, Blyth and Ockenden have described four categories of the disease, which may overlap:

Category 1 is the perinatal type and the most prevalent and most severe form in which massive nephromegaly occurs in addition to oligohydramnios and resultant pulmonary hypoplasia. Liver involvement is minimal.

Category 2 is the neonatal type with enlarged kidneys but less renal impairment in the prenatal state and therefore fewer pulmonary complications. In this form renal failure is progressive, and death usually occurs in months rather than in weeks, as compared with in the perinatal category. Liver disease is mild in this group.

Category 3 is the infantile type and Category 4 is the juvenile type. These are characterized by a later expression of disease and have varying but more severe liver disease (portal hypertension and hepatic fibrosis). The renal failure is also progressive and still remains an important cause of death.

Treatment of this ARPKD is largely supportive, with most patients needing dialysis or renal transplants and liver transplants or portosystemic shunts for liver failure. Systemic hypertension is the most common comorbidity associated with ARPKD, but the pathogenesis of ARPKD-related hypertension remains unclear.

Notes

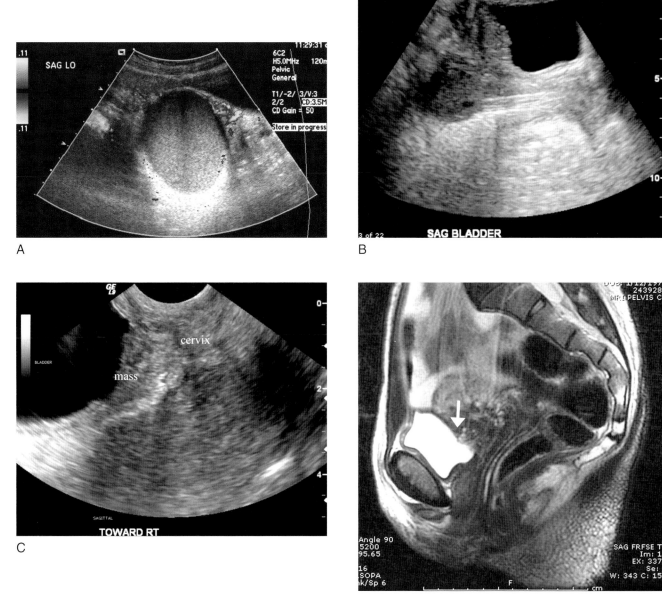

A

B

C

D

1. In this 30-year-old woman with pelvic "fullness" on the left side on bimanual pelvic examination, what are the ultrasound findings and the most likely diagnosis? (Fig. A)?

2. Is there a characteristic or common appearance of an endometrioma on an ultrasound examination? What is it? A second patient shown in Figures B, C, and D is an unusual case and had pelvic pain and hematuria monthly. Figure B is a transabdominal sagittal ultrasound image through the full bladder; Figure C is a sagittal coned-down transvaginal view of the same patient at the level of the bladder; Figure D is the sagittal MRI T_2-weighted image of this second patient, showing effacement of the posterosuperior bladder wall by a mass (see arrow) originating from the surface of the uterus.

3. Is ultrasound sensitive in the detection of abnormalities in this entity?

4. Does endometriosis adversely affect fertility?

5. Does endometriosis occur outside of the female pelvis?

Endometriosis

1. Complex adnexal cystic lesion, likely ovarian with homogeneous low internal echoes. Endometrioma.

2. Yes. Homogeneous, low level echoes.

3. No; ultrasound identifies only 11%.

4. Yes.

5. Yes.

References

Bazot M, Darai E, Hourani R, et al: Deep pelvic endometriosis: MR imaging for diagnosis and prediction of extension of disease. *Radiology* 232:379–389, 2004.

Kuligowska E, Deeds L, Lu K III: Pelvic pain: Overlooked and underdiagnosed gynecologic conditions. *Radio-Graphics* 25:3–20, 2005.

Kupfer MC, Schwimer SR, Lebovic J: Transvaginal sonographic appearance of endometriomata: Spectrum of findings. *J Ultrasound Med* 11:129–133, 1992.

Woodward PF, Sohaey R, Mezzetti Jr TP: Endometriosis: Radiologic-pathologic correlation. *RadioGraphics* 21:193–216, 2001.

Cross-Reference

Ultrasound: THE REQUISITES, 2nd ed, pp 570–571, 573–574.

Comment

Endometriosis is a disorder in which benign endometrial glands and stroma are located outside of the uterus. The diagnosis is made definitively with laparoscopy. Implants of endometrial tissue are commonly seen on the ovary, uterus, and ligament in the cul-de-sac and can be found less commonly on the rectosigmoid colon, bladder (Figures B, C, and D), cervix, and vagina. If small, these implants are not seen with ultrasound, accounting for the low sensitivity of ultrasound to detect endometriosis. Magnetic resonance imaging (MRI) has been shown to be more sensitive because of the ability to detect small endometriomas (<1 cm) and to accurately characterize blood based on signal intensity. In addition, MRI can reveal implants or evidence of hemosiderin along the peritoneum and adhesions that are the sequelae of endometriosis. Endometriosis can seed abdominal scars.

The endometrioma is a cyst that contains altered blood, usually arises from an ovary, and is often bilateral. On ultrasound, endometriomas usually have internal echoes and often demonstrate homogeneous low-level echoes (see Fig. A). The internal material can be hyperechoic. Internal septations or fluid-fluid levels may be present. Blood flow on Doppler is not seen in fine septations but can be seen in thick septations. An endometrioma is the only form of endometriosis that can be readily diagnosed with transvaginal ultrasound.

Using MRI, endometriomas are often hyperintense on T_1-weighted images. On T_2-weighted sequences, they may demonstrate a relative decrease in signal intensity ("shading") or they can be hyperintense (see Fig. D). The presence of shading is the most accurate criterion to distinguish an endometrioma from other hemorrhagic or nonhemorrhagic adnexal masses. MRI has been found to aid in the detection of deep pelvic endometriosis also referred to as deep infiltrating endometriosis, under the surface of the peritoneum.

Notes

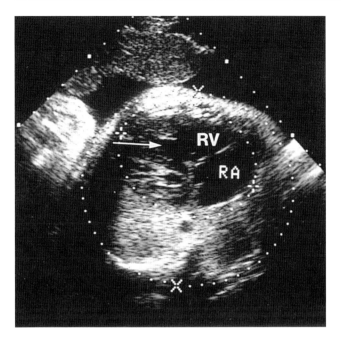

1. In this axial view of the fetal chest, the four-chamber view of the heart is shown. What is the most likely cause of the ventricular discordance? RA = right atrium; RV = right ventricle; arrow = left ventricle.

2. Which ventricle is enlarged with coarctation of the aorta?

3. Which ventricle is enlarged with a ductus occlusion?

4. Which ventricle is enlarged with intrauterine growth restriction?

Ventricular Discordance

1. Hypoplastic left heart.

2. Right ventricle.

3. Right ventricle.

4. Right ventricle.

References

Brown DL, DiSalvo DN, Frates MC, et al: Sonography of the fetal heart: Normal variants and pitfalls. *AJR* 160: 1251–1255, 1993.

Weil SR, Huhta JC: Sonographic differential diagnosis of fetal cardiac abnormalities. *Semin Ultrasound CT MR* 14:298–317, 1993.

Cross-Reference

Ultrasound: THE REQUISITES, 2nd ed, pp 240–243.

Comment

The four-chamber heart view is standard in any obstetric ultrasound screening examination. Although anomalies can be missed using this view only, the sizes of the ventricles are very important and can indicate various cardiac malformations. An important normal variant is a prominent moderator band. This hypoechoic to iso-echoic (relative to myocardium) band of tissue in the apex of the right ventricle makes the ventricular cavity appear smaller than that of the left ventricle in the normal heart. The apices of both ventricles should extend to the cardiac apex in a normal four-chamber view. The ventricles typically measure 1:1, and the measurement is obtained just behind the atrioventricular valves.

In the normal fetus, the right ventricular width mildly increases compared with the left with advancing gestational age, which is an important anatomic relationship to recognize. However, enlargement or diminution of the left ventricle can indicate various cardiac malformations. If the left ventricle is small and the right ventricle is enlarged, left-sided obstructing lesions should be considered. Coarctation of the aorta or the more severe hypoplastic left side of the heart (shown in this case) and interrupted aortic arch cause diminution of the left ventricle. Additional causes of small left ventricle with right ventricular enlargement include a double-outlet right ventricle.

A small left ventricle has also been reported with intrauterine growth restriction in fetuses that also develop right ventricular dilatation; this results from redistribution of blood flow to the fetal head with increased venous return to the right side of the heart.

Enlargement of the left ventricle with a normal right ventricle usually indicates left ventricular myocardial dysfunction. Specifically, critical aortic stenosis and primary endocardial fibroelastosis should be considered.

Notes

Challenge

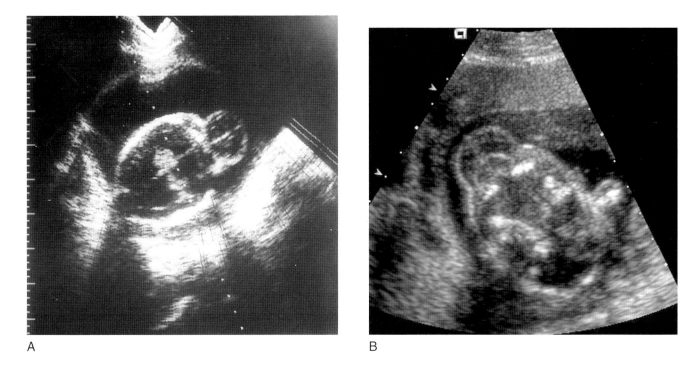

A   B

1. What entity is shown in these two coronal images of second-trimester fetal heads?

2. Would the α-fetoprotein (AFP) level usually be elevated in these cases?

3. What is Meckel-Gruber syndrome?

4. What is the prognosis in this case?

Encephalocele

1. Encephalocele.

2. No.

3. Microcephaly with an occipital meningoencephalocele, enlarged kidneys with cystic renal dysplasia, hepatic fibrosis, and polydactyly.

4. Poor.

Reference

Goldstein RB, LaPidus AS, Filly RA: Fetal cephaloceles: Diagnosis with US. *Radiology* 180:803–808, 1991.

Cross-Reference

Ultrasound: THE REQUISITES, 2nd ed, pp 390-391, 409–410, 462–463.

Comment

Encephaloceles are midline cranial defects that occur in approximately 1 in 10,000 pregnancies. A cephalocele describes a herniation of central nervous system (CNS) meninges through the midline defect in the cranium. It may contain only cerebrospinal fluid (CSF) (cranial meningocele) or brain and CSF fluid (encephalocele). Both have a poor prognosis. For an encephalocele, the mortality rate is estimated at 50%, and 75% of the survivors are mentally retarded. Both types have associated anomalies: CNS (up to 75%), systemic (70%), and karyotype (44%).

All encephaloceles, except those secondary to amniotic band syndrome, are midline. In the Western hemisphere, most encephaloceles (80%) occur in the occipital region, and the frontal and parietal locations constitute the remaining 20%. Frontal cephaloceles, more common in the Eastern hemisphere, have a better prognosis.

The ultrasound appearance of an encephalocele may be entirely cystic or solid, a cyst-within-a-cyst, or cystic and solid. The cranial defect is present but is not always apparent. Secondary findings include microcephaly, lemon-head deformity (30%), beaked tectum (70%), and ventriculomegaly (50%). Associated CNS anomalies include migrational abnormalities, agenesis of the corpus callosum, and cerebellar abnormalities.

Associated non-neurologic malformations include intrauterine growth restriction and abnormalities of amniotic fluid volume. Cardiac anomalies, facial clefts, and renal cystic disease have been reported.

In contrast to the findings with myelomeningoceles, the AFP level is usually not elevated in encephalocele because skin covers the anomaly.

Notes

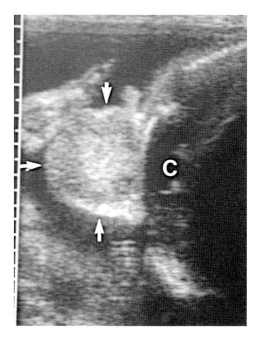

1. In a third-trimester fetus, what is the differential diagnosis of this facial abnormality (arrows) arising from the cheek (c) on this oblique image? Which diagnosis is favored considering its echogenicity and compressibility by fetal limbs on real-time observation?

2. Which tumor may arise in the brain and extend into the face?

3. What is the significance of associated polyhydramnios?

4. What is the differential diagnosis of a mass arising from the inside of the mouth?

Facial Mass

1. Hemangioma, lymphangioma, teratoma, neurofibroma, granular cell tumor (epulis), retinoblastoma, dacryocystocele, mucocele, cyst, and malignant melanoma. The most likely diagnosis is hemangioma.

2. Teratoma.

3. Worsened outcome.

4. Gingival granular cell tumor (oropharyngeal epulis), teratoma, or simple cyst.

References

Merhi, ZO, Haberman S, Robert JL, Sobol-Benin G: Prenatal diagnosis of palatal teratoma by 3-dimensional sonography and color Doppler imaging. *J Ultrasound Med* 24:1317–1320, 2005.

Shipp TD, Bromley B, Benacerraf B: The ultrasound appearance and outcome for fetuses with masses distorting the fetal face. *J Ultrasound Med* 14:673–678, 1995.

Woodward PJ, Sohaey R, Kennedy A, Koeller KK: A comprehensive review of fetal tumors with pathological correlation. *RadioGraphics* 24:215–242, 2005.

Cross-Reference

Ultrasound: THE REQUISITES, 2nd ed, pp 389–390.

Comment

Facial masses are rare fetal anomalies. They can arise from any region of the face (e.g., nose, orbit, oropharynx) or from the neck or brain and extend to involve the face. The differential diagnosis includes benign (e.g., hemangioma, lymphangioma, gingival granular cell tumor [epulis], teratoma, neurofibroma, dacryocystocele, mucocele, cyst) and malignant (e.g., teratoma, retinoblastoma, melanoma) lesions. Hemangiomas and lymphangiomas are vascular lesions considered by many to represent developmental malformations rather than true neoplasms. Accurate diagnosis is essential because proper airway management may be crucial for neonatal survival.

The location may aid in determining the etiology. With large masses, it can be difficult to accurately determine the site of origin. Hemangiomas usually arise from the scalp or skin. They are often soft, easily compressible, and often of uniform echogenicity (see figure).

Masses that arise from the mouth include the gingival granular cell tumor (congenital epulis), teratoma, or simple cyst. The teratoma is the most common mass in neonates. It can arise from many regions of the head and neck (e.g., nose, palate, thyroid, neck, brain). A dacryocystocele is a dilatation of the lacrimal duct. Retinoblastoma arises from the globe of the eye.

Two-dimensional sonography has been used to evaluate these masses. Color Doppler imaging may be useful in tumors that may have high flow (e.g., teratomas) and also in malignancies. Three-dimensional sonography has helped more clearly characterize some facial masses.

The outcomes depend on the histopathology of the mass and the extent of head and neck involvement. Hemangiomas and granular cell tumors may be completely excised. Teratomas that arise in the brain and extend into the face have a uniformly poor prognosis; they generally destroy the intracranial structures. A dacryocystocele can resolve without treatment.

Detection of polyhydramnios in association with one of the masses carries a poor prognosis because it often suggests an obstruction to swallowing.

Notes

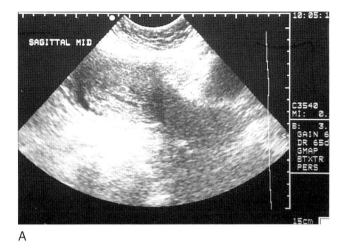

A

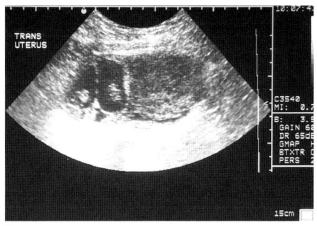

B

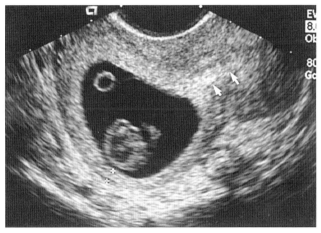

C

1. Early first-trimester fetus. Figure A shows the transabdominal sagittal image of the uterus. Figure B shows the transabdominal transverse image of the uterus at the level of the fundus. What is the diagnosis?

2. What entities can cause a gestational sac to appear eccentric?

3. What is the interstitial line sign?

4. What is Ruge-Simon syndrome?

CASE 99

Cornual (Interstitial) Ectopic Pregnancy

1. Cornual ectopic twin pregnancy.

2. Cornual ectopic, myoma, myometrial contraction, bicornuate uterus, and septate uterus.

3. A thin hyperechoic line extending from the central endometrial stripe to the periphery of the ectopic cornual gestational sac.

4. A cornual ectopic that rotates the uterus, making the sac appear to be centrally located.

References

Ackerman TE, Levi CS, Dashefsky SM, et al: Interstitial line: Sonographic finding in interstitial (cornual) ectopic pregnancy. *Radiology* 189:83–87, 1993.

Frates MC, Laing FC: Sonographic evaluation of ectopic pregnancy: An update. *AJR* 165:251–259, 1995.

Cross-Reference

Ultrasound: THE REQUISITES, 2nd ed, pp 358, 359, 362.

Comment

An interstitial or cornual ectopic pregnancy is an unusual form of ectopic implantation, occurring in less than 5% of all ectopic pregancies. Because of the proximity of the interstitial portion of the tube to the uterine cavity, the diagnosis can be challenging. Patients present later than those with the typical ectopic pregnancy, as late as the beginning of the second trimester. The cornua is partially protected by the myometrium and is capable of expanding more than the remainder of the tube to accommodate an enlarging gestational sac. As a result of this late presentation, a rupture can be catastrophic and can occasionally lead to life-threatening hemorrhage.

The ectopic gestational sac is usually eccentrically located (see Fig. B showing a twin gestation) in a cornual ectopic pregnancy. (See also images from Case 81.) Ruge-Simon syndrome refers to the rare occurrence of a cornual ectopic pregnancy that does not appear eccentric because the uterus has rotated. Uterine anomalies such as septate or bicornuate uterus can also result in an eccentric sac location. Focal myometrial contractions, leiomyomata, and a retroverted uterus result in a similar appearance. Although some literature suggests that a myometrium less than 5 mm surrounding the sac indicates a cornual ectopic, this was found to be an unreliable indicator in one important study. The absence of surrounding myometrium would suggest an interstitial pregnancy; however, the apparent presence of myometrium around the sac does not exclude it. This is shown in a cornual ectopic pregnancy in a third patient in a transvaginal coronal image (Fig. C showing the apparent myometrium). The ectopic pregnancy may be a live fetus, or a mass of solid, vascularized tissue.

The interstitial line sign (see Fig. C) has been reported as an important finding in a cornual ectopic pregnancy; a straight, thin hyperechoic line extends from the endometrium to the ectopically placed gestational sac. It is thought to represent either the interstitial portion of the fallopian tube or the endometrial canal. This sign has been shown to be more sensitive than either the eccentric sac location or myometrial thinning in confirming the presence of a cornual ectopic pregnancy.

Notes

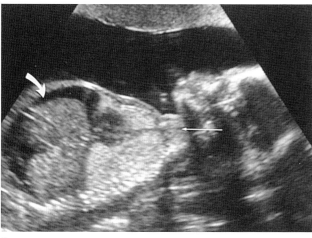

A

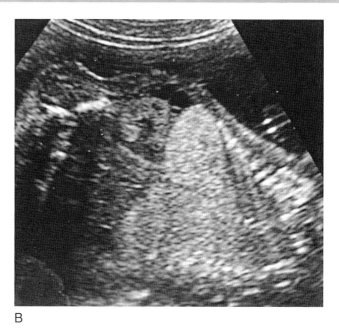

B

1. In this late second-trimester fetus, what is the differential diagnosis of bilateral lung abnormality shown in Figures A (sagittal view) and B (coronal view) of the fetal chest? In Figure A, what do the straight and curved arrows denote?

2. What causes the increased echogenicity of the lungs in laryngotracheal obstruction?

3. Are the lungs pathologically immature, developmentally normal, or of advanced maturity?

4. What is Fraser's syndrome?

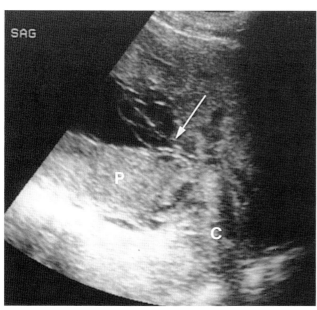

A

1. What is the pathology, and what are risk factors for the abnormality shown on this prenatal sonogram of the lower uterine segment of a pregnancy near term? (Fig. A; arrow = cord insertion; P = placenta; C = cervix.)

2. What are the clinical indicators?

3. What fetal monitoring is conducted once this condition is diagnosed?

4. What is the treatment?

CASE 100

Laryngotracheal Obstruction

1. Laryngotracheal obstruction, bilateral cystic adenomatoid malformation type III, and sequestration (rare). Straight arrow = fluid-filled trachea; curved arrow = ascites.

2. Alveolar distention with fluid.

3. Advanced maturity.

4. Tracheal or bronchial stenosis, renal agenesis, microphthalmia, cryptophthalmos, and polydactyly or syndactyly.

References

De Hullu JA, Kornman LH, Beekhuis JR, Nikkels PGJ: The hyperechogenic lungs of laryngotracheal obstruction. *Ultrasound Obstet Gynecol* 6:271–274, 1995.

Kassanos D, Christodoulou CN, Agapitos E, et al: Prenatal ultrasonographic detection of the tracheal atresia sequence. *Ultrasound Obstet Gynecol* 10: 133–136, 1997.

Cross-Reference

Ultrasound: THE REQUISITES, 2nd ed, pp 424–426.

Comment

Fetal laryngotracheal obstruction is a severe, uncommon anomaly with a grave prognosis. Associated syndromes include Fraser's syndrome (described above), vertebral defects, imperforate anus, tracheoesophageal fistula, radial and renal dysplasia, and limb anomalies (VATER), DiGeorge developmental field defect, and rhizomelic chondrodysplasia punctata.

On prenatal ultrasound, the lungs appear uniformly enlarged and hyperechoic (see Figs. A and B). This is because of expansion of the alveoli with fluid. A secondary mass effect may be present, with compression of the diaphragm, heart, and mediastinal structures. Fetal ascites and polyhydramnios can develop, probably because of obstruction of the esophagus and venous return to the heart (see Fig. A). Oligohydramnios has been described in one case. In addition, a dilated, fluid-filled tracheobronchial tree below the level of obstruction has been described in at least one case and definitively proves the diagnosis if this finding is detected (see Fig. A).

Pathologically, the lungs show advanced maturity. The expansion of air spaces with fluid induces alveolar proliferation, which accounts for the advanced maturity.

Most fetuses die at birth as a result of respiratory distress. Monitoring with ultrasound throughout the pregnancy has been advised, as well as delivery at a medical center where emergency tracheostomy or laryngotracheoplasty can be performed.

Notes

CASE 101

Obligate Cord

1. Obligate presentation of the umbilical cord. Breech positioning and small fetuses, particularly if premature.

2. Fetal heart decelerations during uterine contractions.

3. Nonstress tests and follow-up ultrasound imaging.

4. Surgery: cesarean section delivery.

References

Pelosi MA: Antepartum ultrasonic diagnosis of cord presentation. *Am J Obstet Gynecol* 162:599–601, 1990.

Sakamoto H, Takagi K, Masaoka N, et al: Clinical application of the perineal scan: Prepartum screening for cord presentation. *Am J Obstet Gynecol* 155:1041–1043, 1986.

Cross-Reference

Ultrasound: THE REQUISITES, 2nd ed, pp 489–490.

Comment

Obligate presentation of the cord refers to presentation of the umbilical cord before the fetus at the time of birth. The condition is more common in the setting of a fetal breech position (particularly a footling breech) as well as with small fetuses, including those delivered prematurely. Other risk factors include multiple gestations, polyhydramnios, multiparity, disproportion, incompetent cervix, and "hourglass membranes." Diagnosis of this condition is essential, because prolapse of the cord into the cervix during delivery can be catastrophic for the fetus. In addition, the obligate positioning of the cord results in cord compression and variable fetal cardiac decelerations or bradycardia during uterine contractions.

Diagnosis can be made at the time of delivery by palpation; in some cases the umbilical cord can be palpated in the lower uterine segment on pelvic digital examination. An antenatal diagnosis has also been made with ultrasound. As this case demonstrates, the umbilical cord can be identified overlying the internal os (see Fig. A). Transperineal scanning is helpful in imaging the lower uterine segment and determining the presenting part.

If obligate cord is diagnosed prenatally, a management scheme has been outlined. Nonstress fetal cardiac monitoring is performed at weekly intervals or more frequently if clinically warranted. Application of fundal and suprapubic pressure may provoke fetal bradycardia, indicating cord entrapment. If the cord remains in a primary presenting position, prompt delivery by cesarean section is required at term.

Notes

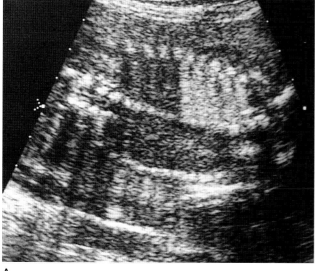

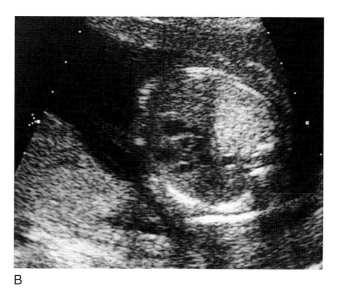

A   B

1. What is the differential diagnosis of the isolated left-sided hyperechoic (echogenic) abnormality shown in the chest of this middle second-trimester fetus? Figure A is a sagittal image, and Figure B is a coronal image of the fetal chest.

2. What lesion may have a systemic arterial supply?

3. Which type of congenital diaphragmatic hernia (CDH) appears as a solid mass?

4. What accounts for the echogenicity of the lung in bronchial obstruction or atresia?

Mucous Plug

1. Sequestration, cystic adenomatoid malformation type III, or mucous plug/bronchial atresia.

2. Extralobar or intralobar sequestration.

3. Right-sided hernias containing liver.

4. Alveolar distention with fluid.

Reference

Meizner I, Rosenak D: The vanishing fetal intrathoracic mass: Consider an obstructing mucous plug. *Ultrasound Obstet Gynecol* 6:275–277, 1995.

Cross-Reference

Ultrasound: THE REQUISITES, 2nd ed, pp 422–426.

Comment

A laryngotracheal obstruction appears on an antenatal ultrasound with enlarged, bilaterally hyperechoic lungs. The only differential considerations would be bilateral cystic adenomatoid malformation (CAM) type III or sequestrations. Bronchial atresia or an obstruction with a mucous plug can cause an isolated region of obstructed lung to enlarge and increase in echogenicity, which is demonstrated in this case. On prenatal ultrasound, a hyperechoic pulmonary mass is seen, raising the possibility of several diagnoses: CAM, sequestration, and CDH containing liver or another solid organ (if right-sided).

A focal hyperechoic lung "mass" due to bronchial obstruction is caused by distended alveoli that contain fluid. Pathologically, the lung tissue shows advanced maturity, with alveolar proliferation induced by fluid distension of the air space. The enlarged region of lung may cause a mass effect and a mediastinal shift. Detection of branching bronchi within this region would assist in making an accurate diagnosis.

An improvement or a relative decrease in the size of a hyperechoic lung mass, and even resolution, has been described on prenatal ultrasound with several entities: CAM, sequestration, and CDH (except for those containing intestine or stomach). These have been reported to improve in case reports or small series. In addition, obstruction of a bronchus with a mucous plug can cause a hyperechoic mass that improves or resolves in utero.

Notes

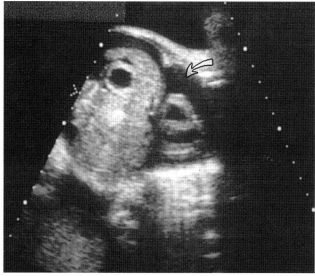

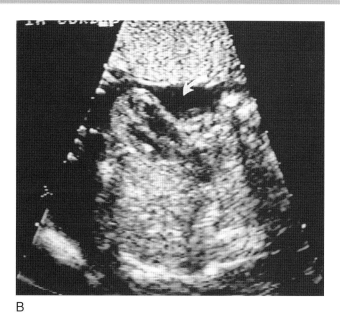

A   B

1. What rare anomaly is demonstrated in the axial images of the fetal chest in these two cases? The curved arrows point to amniotic fluid.

2. What is the most common location?

3. Are chromosomal defects associated?

4. What are the most common associated intracardiac anomalies?

Ectopia Cordis

1. Ectopia cordis (the heart outside the thorax).

2. Thoracic.

3. Yes.

4. Conotruncal anomalies.

Acknowledgment
Figure B for Case 103 courtesy of Dennis Woods.

References
Hornberger LK, Colan SD, Lock JE, et al: Outcome of patients with ectopia cordis and significant intracardiac defects. *Circulation* 94:32–37, 1996.

Liang RI, Huang SE, Chang FM: Prenatal diagnosis of ectopia cordis at 10 weeks of gestation using two-dimensional and three-dimensional ultrasonography. *Ultrasound Obstet Gynecol* 10:137–139, 1997.

Tongsong T, Wanapirak C, Sirivatanapa P, Wongtrangan S: Prenatal sonographic diagnosis of ectopia cordis. *J Clin Ultrasound* 27:440–445, 1999.

Cross-Reference
Ultrasound: THE REQUISITES, 2nd ed, pp 446–447.

Comment
Ectopia cordis is defined as partial or complete displacement of the heart outside the thorax. The heart is most commonly located adjacent to the thorax (60%). However, the heart can exist outside the body cavity in other locations: abdominal (30%), thoracoabdominal (7%), or even cervical (3%). Ectopia cordis is one of the malformations that constitute the pentalogy of Cantrell, which also includes congenital cardiac defects, a supraumbilical omphalocele, a distal sternal cleft, and ventral diaphragmatic hernia.

The ultrasound diagnosis can be made as early as the first trimester and is always made by the second trimester. The fetal heart is seen outside the thorax, as shown by these two cases. The key features in one series were thoracic or thoracolumbar wall defect with an extrathoracic pulsating mass containing Doppler waveforms appearing as intracardiac flow. Because of the associated malformations in the pentalogy of Cantrell, a careful evaluation must be made for other anomalies. In addition to these midline malformations, cranial anomalies, cleft lip and palate, gastrointestinal and genitourinary abnormalities, and pulmonary hypoplasia have been associated.

The prognosis is serious for infants with ectopia cordis, particularly the thoracic type. The associated cardiac malformations, which are most commonly conotruncal anomalies, account for the poor outcome. One series of infants with ectopia cordis has been reported; two thirds of the infants survived beyond the newborn period following surgical correction of the cardiac defects, which included tetralogy of Fallot and a double-outlet right ventricle with a ventriculoseptal defect.

Notes

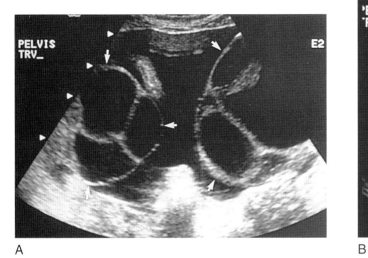

A

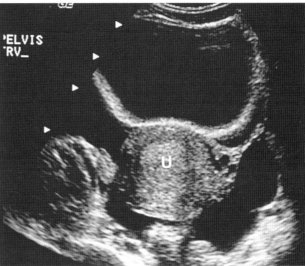

B

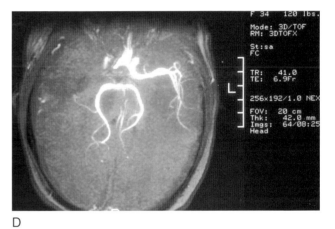

C

D

1. Which patients develop the syndrome shown in these transabdominal axial images of the pelvis (Figs. A and B; U = uterus) and sagittal image of the right upper quadrant (Fig. C; L = liver)? What do the arrows denote in Figure A?

2. Who is at increased risk?

3. What are the signs and symptoms of this syndrome?

4. What is the pathophysiology of this disorder?

5. What complication of this entity is seen in the MRA and CT images of the head in Figures D and E, respectively, in a second infertility patient?

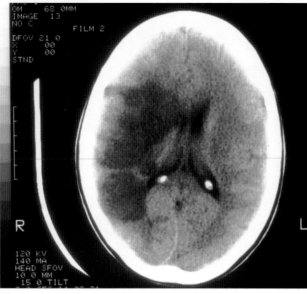

E

Ovarian Hyperstimulation Syndrome

1. Ovarian hyperstimulation caused by ovulation induction or assisted reproduction. Enlarged cystic ovaries.

2. Young, lean women with either a "necklace sign" of peripheral ovarian follicles or polycystic ovarian syndrome.

3. Ovarian enlargement and development of ascites.

4. Increased capillary permeability due to large ovarian cysts.

5. Lack of vascular flow in the right middle cerebral artery and a resultant infarct of the right cerebral hemisphere.

Reference

Berendonk CCM, Van Dop PA, Braat DDM, Merkus JMWM: Ovarian hyperstimulation syndrome: Facts and fallacies. *Obstet Gynecol Surv* 53:439–449, 1998.

Cross-Reference

Ultrasound: THE REQUISITES, 2nd ed, pp 561–563.

Comment

Ovarian hyperstimulation syndrome (OHSS) occurs in women undergoing ovulation induction or hyperstimulation for assisted reproduction. Increased capillary permeability due to the large ovarian cysts leads to third spacing, which can result in hypovolemic shock and stroke and electrolyte abnormalities. Diagnosis is made by measuring serum estradiol (E_2) levels in a patient with enlargement of the ovaries on ultrasound. Risk factors include a previous history of OHSS as well as the risk of being a young, thin woman. Women with the "necklace sign" of multiple peripheral follicles in the ovary prior to assisted reproduction or polycystic ovary disease are also at an increased risk.

Luteinization is an integral contributor to the development of OHSS. In particular, the administration of human chorionic gonadotropin increases the risk. Therefore, women who become pregnant are at higher risk for the more severe forms of OHSS.

The ultrasound findings include enlarged ovaries (see Fig. A) and ascites (see Figs. A to C). Unilateral pleural effusion has been described but is rarely as an isolated finding.

Complications in addition to hypovolemic shock (and rarely death) include thromboembolic disease, including stroke (Figs. D and E), liver and kidney dysfunction, and acute respiratory distress syndrome. The enlarged ovaries are susceptible to torsion. Treatment is supportive to maintain hemodynamic stability. Transabdominal or transvaginal ultrasound-guided paracentesis has been shown to be an effective treatment. Whereas mild forms can be managed on an outpatient basis, severe OHSS requires hospitalization and even monitoring in an intensive care unit.

Notes

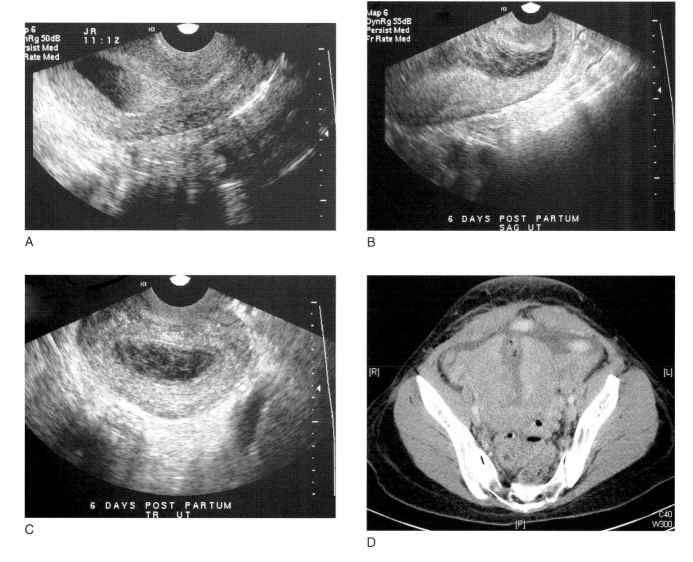

A

B

6 DAYS POST PARTUM
SAG UT

C

6 DAYS POST PARTUM
TR UT

D

1. A 16-year-old patient presents with fever, a history of a tender painful uterus on physical examination, and pelvic pain (Fig. A = transvaginal ultrasound image). Her pregnancy test is negative. Figures B and C are from a second patient with the same symptoms. What is the most likely diagnosis?

2. What are the causes of endometritis?

3. Figure D is a pelvic computed tomography image from another patient who is postpartum following premature rupture of the membranes with ensuing chorioamnionitis and one week status post emergency cesarean section. Her blood cultures grew *Escherichia coli*. What are the salient findings?

4. Which mode of delivery carries a higher risk of postpartum uterine infection?

5. Does the detection of small foci of gas within the endometrial canal in a postpartum woman confirm the diagnosis of infection? Does mucopurulent discharge indicate an infection postpartum?

6. What percentage of ultrasound studies are normal in the setting of acute infection?

Endometritis and Endomyometritis

1. Endometritis.

2. Pelvic inflammatory disease (causing an ascending infection from the vagina), postpartum period, post-instrumentation status, and intrauterine devices.

3. Uterine dehiscence with gas foci within the endometrial cavity. There is also a small amount of hemoperitoneum.

4. Cesarean section.

5. No. No. Mucopurulent discharge can last for 6 weeks postpartum.

6. Up to 50%.

Acknowledgment

CT image contributed by Cheryl Sadow, M.D.

References

Brown DL: Pelvic ultrasound in the postabortion and postpartum patient. *Ultrasound Q* 21:27–37, 2005.

Di Salvo DN: Sonographic imaging of maternal complications of pregnancy. *J Ultrasound Med* 22:69–89, 2003.

Lev-Toaff AS, Baka JJ, Toaff ME, et al: Diagnostic imaging in puerperal febrile morbidity. *Obstet Gynecol* 78:50–55, 1991.

Leyendecker JR, Gorengaut V, Brown JJ: MR imaging of maternal diseases of the abdomen and pelvis during pregnancy and the immediate postpartum period. *RadioGraphics* 24:1301–1316, 2004.

Wachsberg RH, Kurtz AB: Gas within the endometrial cavity at postpartum US: A normal finding after spontaneous vaginal delivery. *Radiology* 183:425–429, 1992.

Cross-Reference

Ultrasound: THE REQUISITES, 2nd ed, pp 539, 573.

Comment

Endometritis, an infection of the endometrial canal, is seen in pelvic inflammatory disease (whether microbacterial or venereal), in the puerperium (postpartum) period (Figs. B and C), and post-instrumentation (e.g., after dilatation and curettage). An intrauterine device can predispose a woman to endometritis. Pelvic inflammatory disease causes an ascending infection through the vagina, which if left untreated will infect the uterus and then the fallopian tubes and adnexa. These infections, which may spread into the pelvis, can cause peritoneal signs and very infrequently present with right flank pain and even periheptic pain caused by an ascending infection.

The incidence of endometritis or more severe endomyometritis, with inflammation extending into the myometrium, is much higher following a cesarean section compared with a vaginal delivery: 13% to 39% versus less than 2.7%, respectively. Ultrasound detects a normal postpartum uterus in up to 50% of women with endometritis or endomyometritis. Endometritis is usually a clinical diagnosis.

When abnormalities are detected, endometrial fluid, debris, or a fluid level (Fig. A) and gas may be identified. However, endometrial gas is more commonly a *normal* postpartum finding, even increasing in quantity or appearing over time. A focal abnormality that may contain gas in the anterior uterine wall, however, is suggestive of myometritis. This should not be confused with the normal cesarean scar that is seen as a well-defined oval hyperechoic area or a small (<1.5 cm) subclinical hematoma visualized in or adjacent to the incision in many normal women.

Complications of endomyometritis include wound or pelvic abscess, phlegmon, ovarian vein thrombosis, uterine dehiscence, bacteremia, and death from sepsis. Computed tomography and magnetic resonance imaging (MRI) are better than ultrasound in detecting parametrial inflammation. MRI is particularly useful because of its ability to display in the sagittal plane and is better suited than computed tomography for evaluating the endometrium and anterior myometrium. Retained products of conception and uterine dehiscence (see Fig. D) can be diagnosed with MRI.

Notes

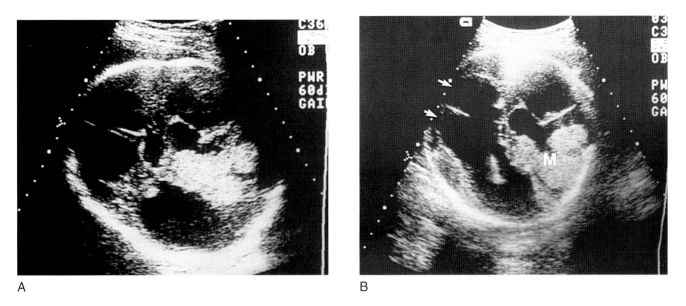

A   B

1. In this late second-trimester fetus, the fetal head is markedly enlarged and the parenchyma is greatly distorted (Fig. A). What is the differential diagnosis of this supratentorial parenchymal fetal central nervous system (CNS) abnormality?

2. Where do most fetal CNS tumors arise: supratentorially or infratentorially?

3. What is the most common fetal intracranial neoplasm?

4. How do these patients usually present?

Intracranial Teratoma

1. Teratoma, glioblastoma, astrocytoma, lipoma of the corpus callosum, and hemorrhage.

2. Supratentorially.

3. Teratoma.

4. Polyhydramnios and craniomegaly.

References

DiGiovanni LM, Sheikh Z: Prenatal diagnosis, clinical significance and management of fetal intracranial teratoma: A case report and literature review. *Am J Perinatol* 11:420–422, 1994.

Sherer DM, Onyeije CI: Prenatal ultrasonographic diagnosis of fetal intracranial tumors: A review. *Am J Perinatol* 15:319–328, 1998.

Cross-Reference

Ultrasound: THE REQUISITES, 2nd ed, p 225.

Comment

The most common fetal intracranial mass is a supratentorial teratoma. Although it is usually histologically benign, the potential complications from mass effect and high-output cardiac failure yield a very poor prognosis; most of the neonates die soon after birth. These patients often present with polyhydramnios, and the diagnosis is usually made after 20 weeks' gestation. Once detected, the goal is to minimize maternal morbidity at delivery, because the neonatal prognosis is poor. Decompression of any cystic portions by cephalocentesis may aid in delivery; cesarean section is often required owing to the large circumference of the fetal head.

On ultrasound, an intracranial solid hyperechoic and cystic mass is seen with secondary hydrocephalus (Fig. B, a slightly different projection from Fig. A; M = mass; arrows = dilated lateral ventricles). The head is often enlarged. Such findings are characteristic of a teratoma. Calcification may be present. Polyhydramnios develops, and hydrops with high-output heart failure may also occur.

Other solid CNS tumors are much less common but include glioblastoma and astrocytoma, choroid plexus papilloma (intraventricular with increased cerebrospinal fluid), and medulloblastoma (infratentorial). A parenchymal hemorrhage can appear as a solid, hyperechoic mass. Non-neoplastic causes of a CNS solid mass include heterotopia and hemimegalencephaly. A corpus callosum lipoma is usually midline with variable degrees of agenesis of the corpus callosum as well as additional associated malformations (e.g., encephalocele or meningomyelocele, hypertelorism, median clefting).

Conditions that mimic a cystic mass include porencephaly, hydranencephaly, and holoprosencephaly, all of which can be distinguished by findings specific to these entities.

Notes

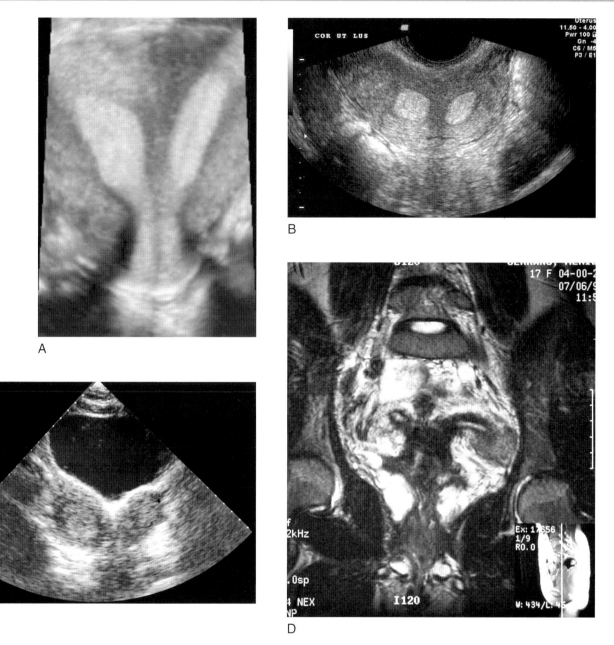

A

B

C

D

1. What is shown on this coronal transvaginal three-dimensional reconstructed image of the uterus (Fig. A)?

2. What is the most common congenital uterine anomaly?

3. What is the embryologic precursor of the uterus? Is this the precursor of the vagina as well?

4. What organ system anomaly is associated?

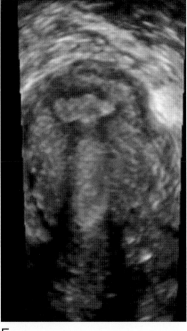

E

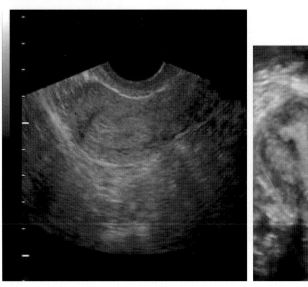

F   G

Congenital Uterine Anomalies

1. Septate uterus.

2. Septate uterus.

3. Müllerian or paramesonephric ducts. No; only the upper two thirds of the vagina.

4. Genitourinary anomaly.

References

Bega G, Lev-Toaff AS, O'Kane P, et al: Three-dimensional ultrasonography in gynecology. *J Ultrasound Med* 22:1249–1269, 2003.

Benacerraf B: Three-dimensional ultrasound in gynecology: Where is it applicable? Personal communication, 2003.

Dunitz M: Uterine factors in infertility. In Goldstein SR, Benson CB (eds): *Imaging of the Infertile Couple.* Blackwell Science, Inc, 2001, pp 41–53.

Imaoka I, Wada A, Matrsuo M, et al: MR imaging of disorders associated with female infertility: Use in diagnosis, treatment, and management. *RadioGraphics* 23:1401–1421, 2003.

Ratani RS, Cohen HL, Fiore E: Pediatric gynecologic ultrasound. *Ultrasound Q* 20:127–139, 2004.

Troiano RN, McCarthy SM: Mullerian duct anomalies: Imaging and clinical issues. *Radiology* 233:19–34, 2004.

Cross-Reference

Ultrasound: THE REQUISITES, 2nd ed, pp 536–538.

Comment

The uterus and proximal two thirds of the vagina arise embryologically from the müllerian or paramesonephric ducts. Uterine anomalies are classified into seven classes. Class I includes hypoplasia or segmental agenesis. The unicornuate uterus is class II. Class III is the uterus didelphys (see Fig. D which is a coronal T$_2$-weighted MRI). A bicornuate uterus (Fig. C) is class IV, and the septate uterus (Figs. A and B) is class V. The arcuate uterus is class VI. The congenital anomalies that result from maternal exposure to diethylstilbestrol (DES) (Figs. E and F) during pregnancy constitute class VII.

Since the uterine anomalies involve the embryologic precursor of the genitourinary system, renal anomalies are present in 25% of the above uterine cases and include renal agenesis, ectopia, malrotation, fusion, and duplication.

Comparative studies have shown that magnetic resonance imaging (MRI) is a more sensitive and accurate modality than transvaginal ultrasound (US) or a hysterosalpingogram for the detection and classification of uterine anomalies. Currently MRI is the study of choice to diagnose uterine anomalies because of its high accuracy and detailed uterovaginal anatomy. However, for distinguishing a septate uterus, MRI and transvaginal US are very accurate and noninvasive. Recently, three-dimensional US has been shown to improve the accuracy of detection and differentiation of uterine anomalies, especially with the coronal reconstructed view, compared with two-dimensional transvaginal imaging. One study showed that the accuracy was comparable with a hysterosalpingography; in addition, three-dimensional US can distinguish a bicornuate uterus from a septate uterus, which is one limitation of hysterosalpingography.

A septate uterus (Fig. B) is distinguished from a bicornuate uterus (Fig. C) on transvaginal US and MRI by demonstrating that the fundus is convex, flat, or indented no more than 1 cm. In addition, the superior portion of the septum is similar in echogenicity (US) or signal intensity (MRI) to myometrial muscle. The inferior portion is fibrous and hypoechoic on US or shows decreased signal intensity on MRI. A bicornuate uterus has divergent uterine horns and a fundal cleft greater than 1 cm (see Fig. C).

Notes

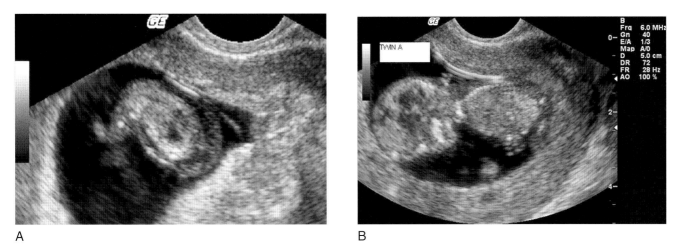

A   B

1. In this second-trimester twin pregnancy, one of the twins appears normal. What is the diagnosis?

2. What type of twin pregnancy is this?

3. What pathologic abnormality leads to this condition?

4. What is the prognosis for the normal twin?

Acardiac Twin

1. Acardiac twin (acardiac monster).

2. Monochorionic.

3. Abnormal intraplacental arterial-to-arterial and intraplacental venous-to-venous anastomoses.

4. Variable.

References

Fouron J-C, Leduc L, Grigon A, et al: Importance of meticulous ultrasonographic investigation of the acardiac twin. *J Ultrasound Med* 13:1001–1004, 1994.

Hecher K, Ville Y, Nicolaides KH: Color Doppler ultrasonography in the identification of communicating vessels in twin-twin transfusion syndrome and acardiac twins. *J Ultrasound Med* 14:37–40, 1995.

Sepulveda W, Hasbun J, Dezerega V, Devoto JC: Successful sonographically guided laser ablation of a large acardic twin at 26 weeks' gestation. *J Ultrasound Med* 23:1663–1666, 2004.

Cross-Reference

Ultrasound: THE REQUISITES, 2nd ed, p 516.

Comment

Acardiac twinning, or reversed arterial perfusion sequence, is a rare anomaly that arises in twin gestations that share a placenta (monochorionic). It occurs in 1% of monozygotic twins. Similar to the twin-twin transfusion syndrome, intraplacental vascular anastomoses result in shunting of blood between the normal or pump twin and the acardiac fetus. Unlike the twin-twin transfusion with arteriovenous anastomoses, the connections in this syndrome are different—arterial-arterial and venous-venous. The acardiac fetus is a large dependent mass, which places a large cardiovascular burden on the normal twin. The cardiovascular overload can be fatal.

Ultrasound demonstrates a partially imaged normal fetus (twin A, Fig. B) and a large perfused tissue mass lacking the upper body (see Fig. A). Limbs may be present but truncated and the mass is usually acephalic, as in Figure A. With time, the acardiac twin grows larger than the normal twin, thus creating a large cardiovascular burden in the third trimester. The normal twin develops heart failure and polyhydramnios. Reversal of umbilical artery blood flow is usually present. Reports in the literature have described identification of the communicating intraplacental vessels with color Doppler imaging.

Treatment begins with systemic administration of digitalis. Interrupting blood flow to the acardiac twin may be the only way to prevent perinatal death of the pump twin. More aggressive treatment options include induction of intravascular thrombosis by injection of substances, selective cesarean delivery, uterotomy, and ligation of the umbilical cord.

Notes

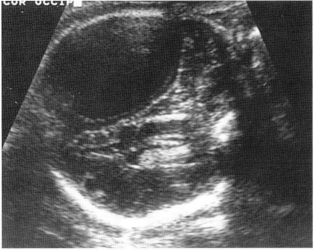

A

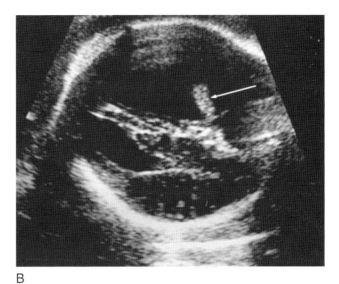

B

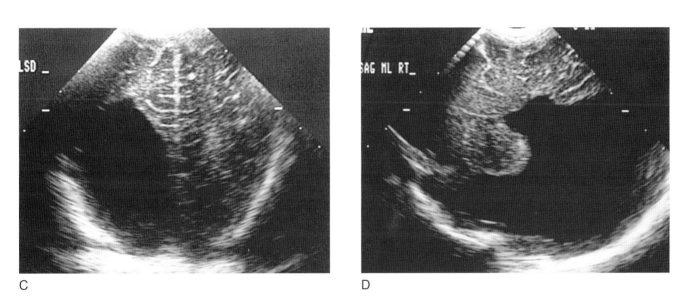

C

D

1. What abnormality is seen in these axial images of a third-trimester fetal brain (Figs. A and B)?

2. What is the antenatal differential diagnosis of a nonhydrocephalic cystic central nervous system (CNS) lesion?

3. Which of these communicate with the ventricle?

4. What are three causes of porencephaly?

Porencephaly

1. A cystic lesion replacing a normal brain with associated ventricular dilatation.

2. Arachnoid cyst, porencephalic cyst, hydranencephaly, holoprosencephaly (dorsal cyst), schizencephaly, absent corpus callosum with an interhemispheric cyst, Dandy-Walker malformation, vein of Galen malformation, and teratoma.

3. Porencephaly, dorsal cyst of holoprosencephaly, Dandy-Walker malformation, and schizencephaly.

4. Periventricular leukomalacia, hemorrhage, and infarct.

References

McGahan JP, Ellis W, Lindfors KK, et al: Congenital cerebrospinal fluid-containing intracranial abnormalities: A sonographic classification. *J Clin Ultrasound* 16: 531–544, 1988.

Meizner I, Elchalal U: Prenatal sonographic diagnosis of anterior fossa porencephaly. *J Clin Ultrasound* 24:96–99, 1996.

Cross-Reference

Ultrasound: THE REQUISITES, 2nd ed, pp 399-400.

Comment

Various congenital disorders can cause cystic brain lesions in the fetus. Determining the cause requires a careful ultrasound examination of the cystic abnormality and the remainder of the brain. In some cases, when the definitive diagnosis cannot be made by ultrasound, magnetic resonance imaging is often helpful.

This case of a large cystic lesion in the brain parenchyma (see Fig. A) with a dilated lateral ventricle (see Fig. B) is an example of porencephaly. The postnatal images (Fig. C, coronal view and Fig. D, sagittal view) show a large cyst replacing much of the right side of the neonatal brain. Porencephaly is defined as a cystic parenchymal lesion that communicates with the ventricular system. Potential causes include brain ischemia, hemorrhage, cortical venous thrombosis or vein of Galen thrombosis, infection (e.g., varicella), and periventricular leukomalacia. A pertinent example of an ischemic etiology is the porencephaly detected in early hydranencephaly, or "hydranencephaly in evolution." In these cases, the infarcted parenchyma is replaced by cystic lesions. The porencephalic cyst enlarges with time and can even bulge through the fontanelles as a result of cerebrospinal fluid (CSF) excretion by the choroid plexus. With time, the entire cerebral cortex may become replaced by fluid, with only the brainstem and some occipital lobe remaining.

The differential diagnosis of congenital cystic lesions includes an arachnoid cyst and the interhemispheric cyst seen with agenesis of the corpus callosum. Open lip schizencephaly may present as a fluid-filled structure representing the connection between the ventricle and CSF surrounding the cerebral cortex. Holoprosencephaly can present with a dorsal cyst that connects to the ventricle, and the Dandy-Walker malformation consists of a large cyst connected to the fourth ventricle. A congenital teratoma can have cystic components but with vascularized solid tissue.

Notes

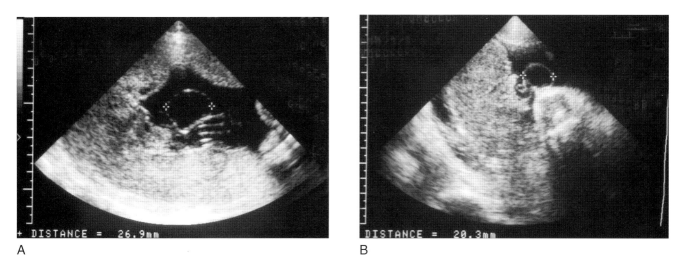

DISTANCE = 26.9mm

A

DISTANCE = 20.3mm

B

1. What is the differential diagnosis of the cystic abnormality (depicted by + signs) arising from the umbilical cord in this third-trimester fetus?

2. Which specific genitourinary anomaly is associated with an allantoic cyst?

3. On which end of the cord are allantoic duct remnants or omphalomesenteric duct remnants usually found?

4. What embryologic arrangement could potentially aid in distinguishing an allantoic duct cyst from an omphalomesenteric duct cyst?

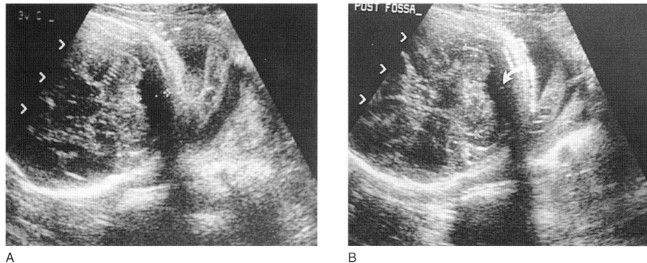

A

B

1. What is the normal size range of this anechoic structure (+ signs) within the fetal head (Fig. A)?

2. In this case, this structure measures 15 mm. What is the significance if this structure is enlarged but is an isolated finding on a prenatal sonogram?

3. With which anomalies is enlargement associated?

4. What does the presence of linear echoes (curved arrow) within this structure suggest in the setting of enlargement (Fig. B)?

Umbilical Cord Cyst

1. True umbilical cord cysts (including allantoic or omphalomesenteric cysts), Wharton's jelly cyst, umbilical cord hematoma or hemangioma, and umbilical vessel dilatation.

2. A patent urachus.

3. The fetal end.

4. Allantoic duct remnants are surrounded by umbilical vessels and are located in the center of the cord. Omphalomesenteric duct cysts arise eccentrically.

References

Dudiak CM, Salomon CG, Posniak HV, et al: Sonography of the umbilical cord. *Radiographics* 15:1035–1050, 1995.

Kalter CS, Williams MC, Vaughn V, Spellacy WN: Sonographic diagnosis of a large umbilical cord pseudocyst. *J Ultrasound Med* 13:487–489, 1994.

Cross-Reference

Ultrasound: THE REQUISITES, 2nd ed, pp 491–493.

Comment

Cystic masses of the umbilical cord may be true cysts (allantoic duct or omphalomesenteric duct remnants), dilated vasculature, or pseudocysts (e.g., Wharton's jelly cysts). Once a cystic mass is detected, it is difficult to determine the exact etiology with antenatal ultrasound. Color Doppler imaging should be used to determine if the vessels of the cord are compressed or thrombosed and to exclude a vascular anomaly as the cause of the cyst. Follow-up scans should be performed throughout the gestation period.

Cysts that arise from either allantoic or omphalomesenteric ducts can be associated with genitourinary (GU) and gastrointestinal (GI) anomalies. Specific associations include a bowel or GU obstruction, hernia, omphalocele, and patent urachus. The association with patent urachus is essential to recognize to avoid the complication of transection of the urachus when cutting the umbilical cord, particularly if the cyst arises close to the anterior abdominal wall of the fetus.

Omphalomesenteric duct cysts are lined with epithelium that can differentiate into gastric epithelia and possibly secrete acid. Ulceration can occur, resulting in a fetal hemorrhage.

Pseudocysts are collections of liquefied Wharton's jelly that may resolve but have also been reported in association with trisomy 18 and trisomy 13 syndromes.

Notes

Large Cisterna Magna

1. Two to 10 mm.

2. Probably a normal variant.

3. Dandy-Walker malformation, trisomy 18 syndrome.

4. A normal variant.

References

Haimovici JA, Doubilet PM, Benson CB, Frates MC: Clinical significance of isolated enlargement of the cisterna magna (>10 mm) on prenatal sonography. *J Ultrasound Med* 16:731–734, 1997.

Pretorius DH, Kallman CE, Grafe MR, et al: Linear echoes in the fetal cisterna magna. *J Ultrasound Med* 11:125–128, 1992.

Cross-Reference

Ultrasound: THE REQUISITES, 2nd ed, pp 327, 374, 390–394.

Comment

The routine obstetric ultrasound study of the fetal head includes an evaluation of the posterior fossa: the cerebellum and cisterna magna (the latter is the fluid-filled structure directly posterior to the cerebellum). The posterior fossa should be imaged in an axial plane through the thalami, with 10 to 15 degrees of angulation. Proper technique is essential, because more coronal imaging can create a false enlargement of the cisterna magna, which should range in anteroposterior diameter from 2 to 10 mm. The normal cisterna magna usually has linear echoes that run perpendicular to the occipital bone, particularly if it measures more than 3 mm. These echoes are believed to represent dural folds, the falx cerebelli, or subarachnoid septa.

Effacement or enlargement of the cisterna magna raises concern for associated anomalies, particularly if the cerebellum is abnormal. Effacement suggests a Chiari II malformation; the hindbrain defect includes a malformed (banana-shaped) cerebellum. Enlargement of the cisterna magna with cerebellar vermian agenesis indicates a Dandy-Walker malformation. Cisterna magna enlargement has also been associated with trisomy 18, but these fetuses usually have either cerebellar or additional structural anomalies.

This case demonstrates a normal variant enlargement of the cisterna magna. The cerebellum and brain must be normal to classify this finding as a normal variant, and there can be no other structural anomalies. One series reported that 15 cases of isolated enlargement of the cisterna magna (from 11 to 19 mm) were associated with a normal neonatal outcome. The enlargement associated with a Dandy Walker malformation is more commonly anechoic, although this is not an absolute rule.

Notes

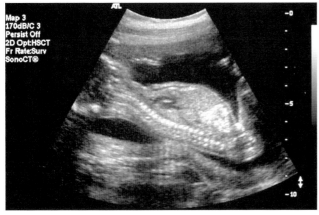

A

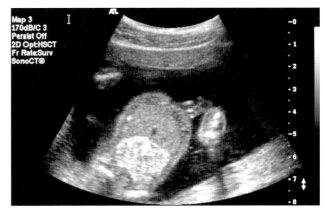

B

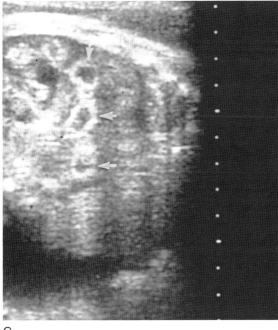

C

1. In this second trimester fetus, there is increased echogenicity of the lower abdominal area. What is the diagnosis? Figure A shows the sagittal image of the fetus. Figure B is the axial image of the fetal lower abdomen.

2. What degree of bowel echogenicity is considered abnormal?

3. Are there associated abnormalities?

4. True or false: echogenic bowel that resolves in the third trimester has no clinical significance?

Echogenic Bowel

1. Echogenic bowel.

2. If equal to or more echogenic (hyperechoic) than bone such as the spine or iliac crests.

3. Yes.

4. False.

References

Grignon A, Dubois J, Ouellet MC, et al: Echogenic dilated bowel loops before 21 weeks' gestation: A new entity. *AJR* 168:833–837, 1997.

Nyberg DA, Dubinsky T, Resta RG, et al: Echogenic fetal bowel during the second trimester: Clinical importance. *Radiology* 188:527–531, 1993.

Paulson EK, Hertzberg BS: Hyperechoic meconium in the third trimester fetus: An uncommon normal variant. *J Ultrasound Med* 10:677–680, 1991.

McNamara A, Levine D: Intraabdominal fetal echogenic masses: A practical guide to diagnosis and management. *RadioGraphics* 2005; 25:633–645.

Cross-Reference

Ultrasound: THE REQUISITES, 2nd ed, pp 441-443.

Comment

Echogenic fetal bowel, the most common echogenic mass in the fetal abdomen, is probably a combination of mesentery and small bowel. It is seen in 1% of second-trimester fetuses. The cause of the increased echogenicity has been hypothesized to be decreased fluid content of the meconium. Fifty percent of the time this echogenic mass resolves with no clinical sequelae. It is important, however, to recognize that meconium can be echogenic in the third trimester, particularly late in the gestation, as a normal variant.

Echogenic bowel can occur in any part of the abdomen but is most common in the right lower quadrant. The prognosis depends on the other concomitant abnormalities: in utero infection, cystic fibrosis, meconium ileus, intra-amniotic bleeding, and chromosomal anomalies, most commonly Down syndrome but also trisomy 18, trisomy 13, and triploidy. Because of the associated anomalies, the prognosis must remain guarded, even if the echogenic bowel resolves.

All echogenic bowel is not abnormal. To be considered abnormal, the area is expected to have an echogenicity (brightness) that does not shadow and is greater than bone such as the spine or iliac crests. The echogenic bowel is expected to be larger than 4 cm and to often exhibit a mass effect on adjacent structures. The findings in Figures A and B are abnormal and meet the aforementioned criteria.

Echogenic dilated bowel loops (EDBL) (Fig. C; arrows) are a distinct abnormality—either an isolated (one quadrant) or diffuse (more than one quadrant) gastrointestinal abnormality. They are detected in the second trimester as bowel 2 to 10 mm in diameter with an echogenic wall. In almost all cases, the finding resolves by the third trimester. As an isolated finding, it is benign. However, the complex form has a worse outcome because of associated anomalies. Such abnormalities include gastroschisis, meconium peritonitis, VATER (imperforate anus), malrotation, and bowel atresia. The etiology is believed to be bowel obstruction and is confirmed by decreased amniotic fluid disaccharidase activity.

Detection of either of these findings in the second trimester warrants prenatal and postnatal follow-up. A careful search for associated anomalies is imperative.

Notes

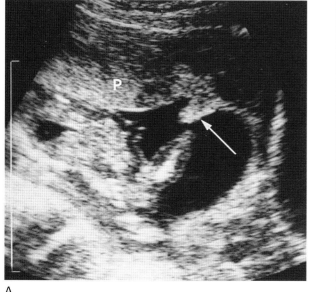
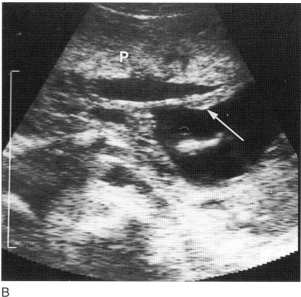

A   B

1. In this third-trimester pregnancy, what is the name of this outpouching (arrow) at the edge of the placenta (P) into the amniotic fluid (Fig. A)?

2. What complications have been associated?

3. Is ultrasound a sensitive screening tool to detect this placental abnormality?

4. What are the diagnosis and differential diagnosis of this large soft tissue band (arrow) in another third-trimester pregnancy (Fig. B; P = placenta)?

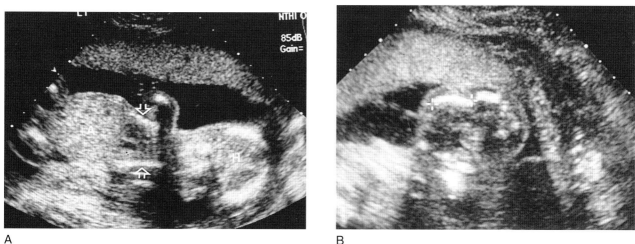

A   B

1. In this 20-week-old fetus, what abnormality is shown in the coronal image (Fig. A; H = head, A = abdomen; open arrows = chest) and the long axis image of one of its femurs (Fig. B; + signs = femoral shaft)? What is the likely diagnosis?

2. Which calvarial anomaly is frequently described as associated with this disorder?

3. What is the outcome?

4. How many spine ossification centers are typically present at each vertebral level in this disorder, and what is their significance?

Circumvallate Placenta
(Placenta Extrachorialis)

1. Circumvallate placenta.

2. Low birth weight, premature labor, placental abruption, intrauterine growth retardation, fetal anomalies, and perinatal death.

3. No.

4. Amniotic shelf (or amniotic sheet). The differential diagnosis is a circumvallate placenta and an amniotic band.

References

Harris RD, Wells WA, Black WC, et al: Accuracy of prenatal sonography for detecting circumvallate placenta. *AJR* 168:1602–1608, 1997.

McCarthy J, Thurmond AS, Jones MK, et al: Circumvallate placenta: Sonographic diagnosis. *J Ultrasound Med* 14:21–26, 1995.

Cross-Reference

Ultrasound: THE REQUISITES, 2nd ed, p 520.

Comment

Circumvallate placenta or placenta extrachorialis is not an uncommon disorder. Complete circumvallate placenta occurs in 1% of pregnancies; partial circumvallate placenta is estimated to occur 10 to 20 times more commonly. It results from a mismatch in growth at the placental margin. In typical placentation, there is a smooth transition from the parenchymal villous chorion to the membranous chorion. In circumvallate placenta, either partial or complete, the parenchymal villous chorion overgrows and bulges into the amniotic fluid. This leaves villous tissue of the chorionic frondosum that is not completely covered by the amniochorionic membrane: hence the term placenta extrachorialis. As a result, the parenchymal villous chorionic tissue bulges out peripherally, and the edge of the placenta develops a rolled appearance (see Fig. A).

Amniotic shelves or sheets (see Fig. B), thought to be due to synechiae covered by amniochorionic membrane, are usually larger but otherwise similar in appearance to a circumvallate placenta.

The clinical significance of a circumvallate placenta is uncertain. It has been associated with low birth weight, prematurity, intrauterine growth retardation, placental abruption, and perinatal death. In addition, congenital anomalies may be present, although the exact etiology of this finding is uncertain. Unfortunately, ultrasonography is neither sensitive nor specific for diagnosis, as shown by one study done by experienced sonologists.

Notes

Thanatophoric Dysplasia
(Thanatophoric Dwarfism)

1. Narrow thorax (see Fig. A) and shortened bowed long bone (see Fig. B). Thanatophoric dysplasia or dwarfism.

2. Cloverleaf skull.

3. Lethal.

4. Three ossification centers; this finding distinguishes this abnormality from achondrogenesis, which often has fewer centers.

Acknowledgment

Figures for Case 114 courtesy of Beryl Benacerraf, MD.

References

Bowerman RA: Anomalies of the fetal skeleton: Sonographic findings. *AJR* 164:973–979, 1995.

Pretorius DH, Rumack CM, Manc-Johnson ML, et al: Specific skeletal dysplasias in utero: Sonographic diagnosis. *Radiology* 159:237–242, 1986.

Cross-Reference

Ultrasound: THE REQUISITES, 2nd ed, pp 476–477, 479–480.

Comment

Thanatophoric dysplasia or dwarfism is a lethal dwarfism with many characteristic findings. The differential diagnosis of short-limbed dwarfism includes achondrogenesis, campomelic dwarfism, homozygous achondroplasia, severe hypophosphatasia, and severe osteogenesis imperfecta.

The features of thanatophoric dysplasia common to the other lethal dysplasias include a narrow thorax caused by too-short ribs (see Fig. A) and shortened bowed long bones (see Fig. B). Characteristic findings that aid in distinguishing thanatophoric dysplasia include macrocephaly with frontal bossing and hydrocephalus. A cloverleaf skull, also known as *kleeblattschädel*, is a classic finding but is present in only 14% of cases. The "telephone receiver" configuration of the shortened, bowed long bones is also characteristic of this disorder (see Fig. B). The skin may be thickened, and vertebral bodies flattened (platyspondyly). However, the spine ossification is normal.

The narrowed chest results in pulmonary hypoplasia, contributing to the high mortality rate. Polyhydramnios and hydrops often develop in utero. The presence of *kleeblattschädel* is important, because this may represent a subtype of thanatophoric dysplasia that is transmitted as an autosomal recessive trait with a risk of recurrence of 25%.

Notes

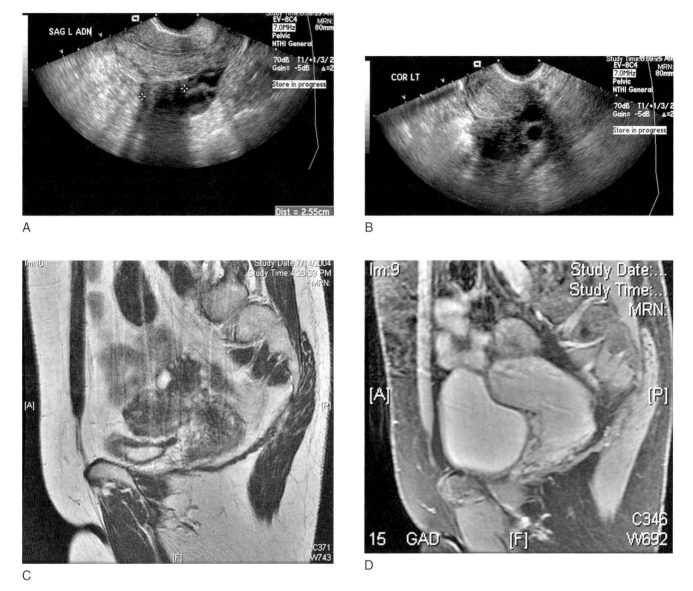

A

B

C

D

1. This 35-year-old woman was presenting for baseline assessment for infertility. Figure A is sagittal image of the left ovary and Figure B is a coronal image through the same ovary. Figures C and D are sagittal MRI images, the latter with gadolinium enhancement. What are the findings, and what is the most likely diagnosis?

2. Which subtype of this tumor is more likely to be malignant?

3. What is a Call-Exner body?

4. Which subtype is more likely to have an associated endometrial cancer?

CASE 115

Sex Cord Stromal (Thecoma-Fibroma) Tumor

1. Hypoechoic solid ovarian mass with shadowing. Diagnosis: a sex cord stromal tumor.

2. Granulosa stromal cell type.

3. Call-Exner bodies are the microfollicular and macrofollicular patterns (rosette-like) that are seen with granulosa cells when viewed cytologically.

4. Thecoma.

References

Cronje HS, Niemand I, Bam RH, Woodruff JD: Review of the granulosa-theca cell tumors from the Emil Novak Ovarian Tumor Registry. *Am J Obstet Gynecol* 180:323–327, 1999.

Green EG, Schwartz PE, McCarthy SM: Sclerosing stromal tumor of the ovary. *J Women's Imaging* 7:50–53, 2005.

Jung SE, Rha SE, Lee JM, et al: CT and MRI findings of sex cord-stromal tumor of the ovary. *AJR* 185:207–218, 2005.

Lee MS, Cha Cho H, Lee Y-H, Hong SR: Ovarian sclerosing stromal tumors. *J Ultrasound Med* 20:413–417, 2001.

Morikawa K, Hatabu H, Togashi K, et al: Granulosa cell tumor of the ovary: MR findings. *J Comput Assist Tomogr* 21:1001–1004, 1997.

Cross-Reference

Ultrasound: THE REQUISITES, 2nd ed, pp 579–580.

Comment

The sex cord stromal tumors represent an uncommon subset of ovarian neoplasms, representing about 8% of all ovarian neoplasms. They are benign. These stromal tumors usually occur in patients in the second or third decades of life. Most common symptoms are menstrual irregularities and pelvic pain. Sex cord–stromal tumors of the ovary include most of the hormonally active ovarian tumors. The subtypes include the granulosa-stromal cell, thecoma-fibroma, and Sertoli-Leydig cell tumors. The first two types can secrete estrogens, whereas the latter may secrete androgenic hormones and cause virilization.

Granulosa stromal cell tumors and thecomas, which produce estrogen, can result in endometrial hyperplasia or endometrial cancer. This case demonstrates an ovarian thecoma-fibroma tumor. Thecomas are more commonly estrogenic and have a higher incidence of associated endometrial abnormality than do granulosa cell stromal tumors. However, the granulosa cell tumor is prone to rupture and is more likely to be malignant, with a propensity for late recurrences.

Histologically, Call-Exner bodies may be seen; these are macrofollicles or microfollicles. Gross pathologic studies have shown that these tumors are often large and that they have a mean size of 10 cm. Theca cell tumors are more commonly solid. Granulosa cell tumors are usually large multiloculated cystic masses with solid portions. Both of these types of sex cord–stromal tumors can cause ovarian torsion. In many cases, hemorrhage is detected within the mass, which may be seen on ultrasound or magnetic resonance imaging (MRI). The masses usually have cystic and solid components and are vascular, especially in the periphery and around cysts. Ultrasound and MRI may also reveal any associated uterine enlargement and endometrial thickening that result from the hormonal secretion.

The detection of a multicystic or solid ovarian mass associated with endometrial thickening via ultrasound should prompt consideration of one of these sex cord stromal tumors. Most of these tumors have a good prognosis.

Notes

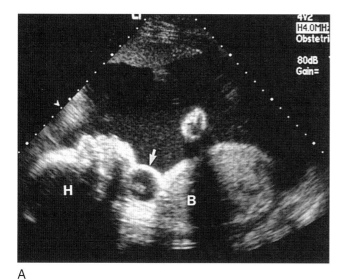

A

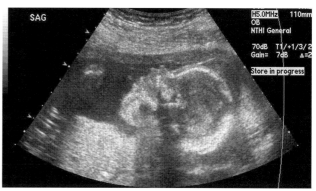

B

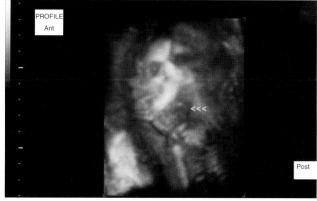

C

1. What is the differential diagnosis for the neck abnormality (arrows) noted in these third-trimester fetuses? (Fig. A = sagittal image of fetus 1; Figs. B and C = sagittal and three-dimensional sagittal images of fetus 2, respectively; H = head; B = body.)

2. How does the location aid in narrowing the differential?

3. What abnormality of amniotic fluid can be seen with a cervical teratoma (see Fig. A)?

4. What ultrasound finding would aid in distinguishing a teratoma from a cystic hygroma?

Cervical Teratoma

1. Cervical teratoma is the most likely diagnosis, but the differential diagnoses are cystic hygroma, fetal goiter, thyroglossal duct cyst or branchial cleft cyst, and congenital neuroblastoma.

2. Teratomas, thyroglossal duct cyst, and goiter are more commonly anterior; branchial cleft cysts are lateral; cystic hygromas are more commonly posterior/lateral (but may occur anteriorly).

3. Polyhydramnios in 20% of cervical teratomas.

4. Calcifications can be seen with teratoma, which can have solid and cystic components; a cystic hygroma is cystic with septations.

References

Kerner B, Flaum E, Mathews H, et al: Cervical teratoma: Prenatal diagnosis and long-term follow-up. *Prenat Diagn* 18:51–59, 1998.

Morof D, Levine D, Grable I, et al: Oropharyngeal teratoma: Prenatal diagnosis and assessment using sonography, MRI, and CT with management by ex utero intrapartum treatment procedure. *AJR* 183: 493–496, 2004.

Tsuda H, Matsumoto M, Yamamoto K, et al: Usefulness of ultrasonography and magnetic resonance imaging for prenatal diagnosis of fetal teratoma of the neck. *J Clin Ultrasound* 24:217–219, 1996.

Cross-Reference

Ultrasound: THE REQUISITES, 2nd ed, p 389.

Comment

A fetal neck mass can arise from various locations, which may aid in narrowing the differential diagnosis; however, these rules are not always valid. A cystic hygroma classically arises from the posterior and lateral parts of the neck, but a subtype can arise anteriorly and even extend into the superior mediastinum. Because of their thyroid origin, fetal goiter and thyroglossal duct cysts arise anteriorly. Branchial cleft cysts are generally found in the lateral neck. The cervical teratoma can present in any part of the neck but more commonly is seen anteriorly.

This case demonstrates a large cystic and solid teratoma in the anterior cervical region (see Figs. A to C). Fetal teratomas can arise anywhere in the body; the cervical region is rare (10%). These masses are composed of all three germ layers and represent 25% to 35% of all neonatal tumors. On ultrasound, a cystic and solid mass is seen; calcifications are present in 50% of cases. Teratomas are believed to result from a migration and entrapment of mesoderm and endoderm with ectoderm during embryogenesis. Because of the solid nature of the mass, the head is often forced into a fixed extended position. Polyhydramnios is also present in this case and develops in 20% of cases because of the inability of the fetus to swallow amniotic fluid. Pathologically, these teratomas are usually benign and encapsulated. The α-fetoprotein (AFP) level can be elevated. No associated anomalies are present.

Malignant degeneration of a cervical teratoma in utero is rare. Morbidity and mortality are related to respiratory distress at birth. Prenatal detection is essential for proper delivery and immediate stabilization of the airway. Surgical resection improves mortality from 100% to 23%. Factors associated with a poor prognosis include a large size (>8 cm diameter), rapid growth, invasion of vital structures (e.g., carotid artery, trachea, larynx), or, rarely, a malignancy.

Notes

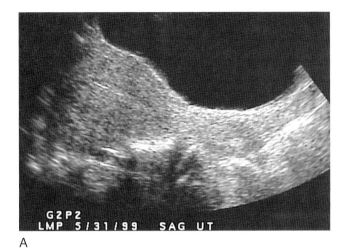

A

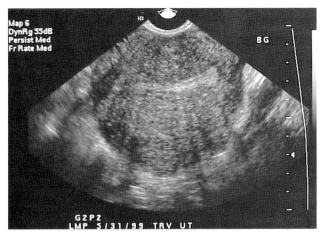

B

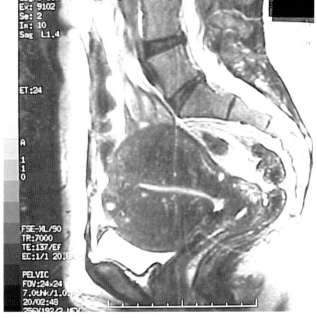

C

1. What findings are shown in this transabdominal sagittal ultrasound image (Fig. A) and the transvaginal coronal ultrasound image (Fig. B) of the uterus in a 50-year-old postmenopausal woman with history of vaginal bleeding? What are the differential possibilities?

2. What are the magnetic resonance imaging (MRI) findings of the uterus in the same patient (Fig. C)? Figure C is a T$_2$-weighted sagittal image.

3. What signs and symptoms do women with adenomyosis have?

4. Can this entity present as a mass that mimics a myoma?

Adenomyosis

1. An indistinct junctional zone (between the endometrium and the myometrium), inhomogeneity of the myometrium, thick posterior myometrium, and perhaps some myometrial cysts. The differential diagnosis is adenomyosis versus multiple small fibroids.

2. A prominent globular uterus with thickening of the junctional zone with high signal foci in the myometrium.

3. Menorrhagia, dysmenorrhagia, and uterine enlargement.

4. Yes.

References

Andreotti RF, Fleischer AC: The sonographic diagnosis of adenomyosis. *Ultrasound Q* 21:167–170, 2005.

Imaoka I, Wada A, Matsuo M, et al: MR imaging of disorders associated with female infertility: Use in diagnosis, treatment, and management. *RadioGraphics*; 23:1401–1421, 2003.

Kido A, Togashi K, Koyama T, et al: Diffusely enlarged uterus: Evaluation with MR imaging. *RadioGraphics* 23:1423–1439, 2003.

Reinhold C, McCarthy S, Bret PM, et al: Diffuse adenomyosis: Comparison of endovaginal US and MR imaging with histopathologic correlation. *Radiology* 199:151–158, 1996.

Tamai K, Togashi K, Tsuyoshi I, et al. MR imaging findings of adenomyosis: Correlation with histopathologic features and diagnostic pitfalls. *RadioGraphics* 25:21–40, 2005.

Cross-Reference

Ultrasound: THE REQUISITES, 2nd ed, pp 534, 541, 549, 553, 571.

Comment

Adenomyosis is defined as a non-neoplastic condition of migration of ectopic endometrial glands and stroma in the myometrium, with associated hyperplastic smooth muscle. Unlike endometriosis, only 13% of these glandular implants respond to endogenous estrogen and progesterone stimulation. Women present with menorrhagia or dysmenorrhagia and enlargement of the uterus.

This case of adenomyosis demonstrates loss of the discrete junctional zone, which appears heterogeneous with a thick posterior myometrium (see Fig. A). In most cases, the uterus is enlarged and globular. Detection of irregular, cystic spaces in the myometrium is the finding most specific for adenomyosis on ultrasound. However, several studies have shown findings that can be much more subtle on ultrasound, including loss of the junctional zone, a slight decrease in the echogenicity of the uterus, posterior uterine wall thickening, and displacement of the endometrial lining. A focal region of adenomyosis, called an adenomyoma, can be seen in some cases. This may have a more irregular shape than the characteristic rounded appearance of a leiomyoma. Adenomyomas are often more subtle than leiomyomas when compared to the background normal uterine tissue. Limited spatial resolution makes ultrasonography not as accurate a modality as magnetic resonance imaging (MRI) to diagnose adenomyosis.

MRI is highly accurate for making the diagnosis of adenomyosis. On MRI, many of the findings reflect smooth muscle proliferation in reaction to the heterotopic endometrial tissue. The junctional zone is thickened, and a cutoff measurement of 12 mm is used to suggest the diagnosis. Small foci with high-signal intensity are seen within the myometrium on T_2-weighted sequences (see Fig. C, the same patient as in Figs. A and B) and sometimes on a T_1-weighted image.

It is important to distinguish focal adenomyosis from a leiomyoma because the treatment differs for each. MRI is helpful in this role, particularly when subtle ultrasound findings are present and additionally because the appearance of an adenomyoma as a calcified uterine mass, mimicking a myoma on ultrasound, has been reported in the literature. On MRI, the borders of an adenomyoma are irregular, and the presence of the high signal foci in the myometrium on T_2-weighted sequences should aid in the distinction of these two entities. Adenomyosis can now be diagnosed and differentiated with a high degree of accuracy by both ultrasonography and MRI.

Notes

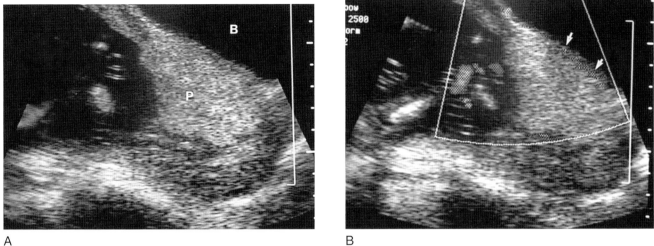

A   B

1. In this third-trimester pregnancy, Figure A is a sagittal transabdominal scan of the lower uterine segment (P = placenta; B = urinary bladder). Figure B, a Doppler image of Figure A, shows flow denoted by arrows. What is the diagnosis, and which three entities constitute its spectrum of abnormality?

2. Name three risk factors for this diagnosis.

3. List three potential complications of this diagnosis.

4. What are three characteristic ultrasound findings of this diagnosis?

Placental Invasion (Accreta, Increta, and Percreta)

1. Placenta percreta. Placental invasion of the uterine wall is categorized as placenta accreta (up to), increta (into), and percreta (through), depending on the depth of myometrial invasion.

2. Risk factors include previous uterine surgery (particularly a cesarean section), a placenta previa, or a history of a retained placenta.

3. Bladder invasion and rupture, uterine infection or wall rupture, and uterine inversion.

4. An anterior placenta, ranging from a low-lying previa to a total previa; absence of the normal subplacental anechoic/hypoechoic zone composed of the myometrium and junctional zones; subplacental vascular spaces.

Reference

Comstock CH, Lee W, Vettraino IM, Bronsteen RA: The early sonographic appearance of placenta accreta. *J Ultrasound Med* 22:19–23, 2003.

Hoffman-Tretin JC, Koenigsberg M, Rabin A, et al: Placenta accreta: Additional sonographic observations. *J Ultrasound Med* 1:29–34, 1992.

Kim H, Hill MC, Winick AB, et al: Residents' teaching files; prenatal diagnosis of placenta accreta with pathologic correlation. *RadioGraphics* 18:237–242, 1998.

Levine D, Hulka CA, Ludmir J, et al: Placenta accreta: evaluation with color Doppler US, power Doppler US, and MR imaging. *Radiology* 205: 773–776, 1997.

Nagi JN, Ofili-Yebovi D, Marsh M, Jurkovic D: First-trimester cesarean scar pregnancy evolving into placenta previa/accreta at term. *J Ultrasound Med* 24:1569–1573, 2005.

Cross-Reference

Ultrasound: THE REQUISITES, 2nd ed, pp 495–496.

Comment

Placental invasion of the uterine wall is categorized as placenta accreta, percreta, or increta, depending on the depth of the myometrial invasion. Myometrial contact by villi without invasion is called accreta. Invasion into the myometrium or through the myometrium with serosal penetration is labeled increta or percreta. The case shown here demonstrates invasion through the myometrium to the bladder. Villi penetrate into the myometrium as a result of a deficiency of the decidua basalis, typically caused by prior disruption of the endometrium. At delivery, hemorrhage results because the placenta cannot detach.

The most common predisposing risk factors are placenta previa, previous uterine surgery (cesarean section, myomectomy, or curettage), a history of a retained placenta, advanced maternal age, or multiparity. If the placenta implants over a site of disrupted endometrium, such as the anterior lower uterine segment of a post–cesarean uterus, the risk of invasion is quite high. The presence of a low-lying gestational sac near the cervix should suggest the possibility of placenta accreta in the patient who has had prior uterine surgery. Attachment to the old scar may be seen. The diagnosis can be made during the first trimester. The decidua is derived from the endometrium of the maternal uterus and when normally formed, it prevents the trophoblastic villi from invading the myometrium.

If an invasion is not detected antenatally, patients can present with massive hemorrhage at delivery because the placenta fails to detach normally. The diagnosis can be suggested by recognizing several important ultrasound findings. The placenta is anterior, ranging from low-lying to complete previa. Invasion may be reflected by the absence of the normal subplacental anechoic/hypoechoic zone, composed of a junctional zone. This can be focally or entirely absent. In percreta, extension may involve the bladder wall. Other associated findings include a heterogeneous echotexture of the placenta, the presence of a few or numerous subplacental vascular spaces, and enlargement of parauterine veins. If the subplacental myometrium is only thinned, this could represent a normal finding; however, accreta cannot then be excluded, particularly if risk factors are present. Gray scale ultrasound is adequate for evaluating most placentas.

In this case, Figures A and B show an anterior placenta previa (P), which is invading the bladder wall (B). The abnormal blood vessels are detected by color Doppler imaging. The diagnosis of a placenta percreta was made prior to delivery.

Complications include bladder invasion and rupture, uterine infection, uterine wall rupture, and uterine inversion. Despite attempts to control blood loss with a hysterectomy, patients may still lose substantial quantities of blood. Control of the bleeding with interventional embolization techniques has been attempted to facilitate a hysterectomy with less blood loss.

Notes

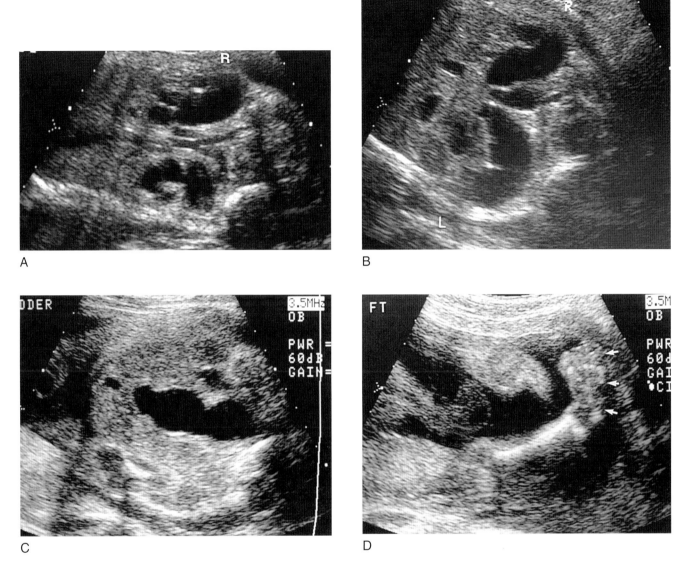

A

B

C

D

1. What is the differential diagnosis of this third-trimester fetus (Figs. A to C)? Figure A is a coronal image of the kidneys; Figure B is a coronal image of the lower abdomen below the kidneys; and Figure C is an axial image of the pelvis. R = fetal right side; L = fetal left side in Figures A and B.

2. Which condition occurs more commonly in males?

3. For which condition is vesicoamniotic shunting more appropriate?

4. Which condition has associated musculoskeletal anomalies (Fig. D; arrows point to a fetal foot)?

Prune-Belly Syndrome

1. Prune-belly syndrome, urethral stenosis or agenesis, and posterior urethral valves.

2. Both posterior urethral valves and prune-belly syndrome; posterior urethral valves occur exclusively in males.

3. Posterior urethral valves and urethral agenesis.

4. Prune-belly syndrome.

References

Brinker MR, Palutsis RS, Sarwark JF: The orthopedic manifestations of prune-belly (Eagle-Barrett) syndrome. *J Bone Joint Surg* 77-A:251–257, 1995.

Smith CA, Smith Edwin A, Parrott TS, et al: Voiding function in patients with the prune-belly syndrome after Monfort abdominoplasty. *J Urol* 159:1675–1679, 1998.

Woodard JR: Lesson learned in three decades of managing the prune-belly syndrome (Editorial). *J Urol* 159:1680, 1998.

Cross-Reference

Ultrasound: THE REQUISITES, 2nd ed, pp 463–465, 468.

Comment

Prune-belly syndrome is believed by many to be a generalized mesenchymal disorder as opposed to an obstructive uropathy. It is manifested by dilatation of the renal collecting systems, absence or hypoplasia of the abdominal musculature, and cryptorchidism. The absence of normal abdominal muscles results in a wrinkled appearance to the skin of the anterior abdominal wall, and the abdomen is protuberant. Prune-belly syndrome, also known as Eagle-Barrett syndrome, is much more common in males.

On prenatal ultrasound, various forms of dilatation of the pelvicaliceal system and ureters are seen. This case demonstrates bilateral renal pelvicaliceal dilatation (see Fig. A), bilateral ureteral dilatation (see Fig. B), and a thick-walled prominent and unusually shaped urinary bladder (see Fig. C). The anterior abdominal wall abnormality can be difficult to visualize. The differential diagnosis of a bilateral ureteral obstruction includes posterior urethral valves, which occur exclusively in males, and urethral atresia.

Several musculoskeletal anomalies are associated with prune-belly syndrome and can be sought if the diagnosis is suspected on prenatal ultrasound. The most common abnormality is subluxation or dislocation of the hip, which is often resistant to traditional treatment. Scoliosis, chest wall deformity (pectus excavatum), and renal osteodystrophy have also been described in children with prune-belly syndrome. In this case, the fetus had a clubfoot (see Fig. D).

Vesicoamniotic shunting has not necessarily been shown to improve the renal function. Postnatal treatment is directed at reconstruction of the urinary system, orchiopexy, and surgical repair of the anterior abdominal wall. The genitourinary function correlates with bladder function as well. Furthermore, repair of the anterior abdominal wall improves bowel and bladder functions.

Notes

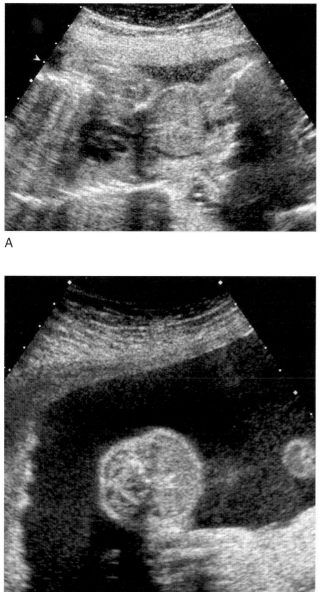

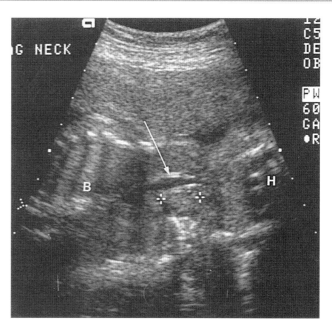

A

B

C

1. What is the mass in the neck of this third trimester fetus shown in the coronal images (Figs. A and B) and axial image (Fig. C)?

2. What is the linear anechoic area between the parts of the neck mass in Figure B?

3. What is the usual etiology of this disorder?

4. What are the potential consequences if the disorder is left untreated?

Fetal Goiter

1. Right and left lobes of an enlarged thyroid.

2. The trachea.

3. Treatment of maternal Graves' disease with propylthiouracil (PTU).

4. Obstruction of the airway or esophagus; hyperextension of the neck. Lower intelligence scores.

Reference

Van Loon AJ, Derksen JTM, Bos AF, Rouwe CW: In utero diagnosis and treatment of fetal goitrous hypothyroidism, caused by maternal use of propylthiouracil. *Prenat Diagn* 15:599–604, 1995.

Cross-Reference

Ultrasound: THE REQUISITES, 2nd ed, pp 244, 246–247.

Comment

Enlargement of the fetal thyroid gland may be associated with a hypothyroid or hyperthyroid state. Fetal goiter, demonstrated by these coronal images of the fetal neck, can be detected and followed after treatment with prenatal ultrasound. The differential diagnosis of an anterior neck mass in utero includes teratoma, thyroglossal duct cyst (midline), and branchial cleft cyst (usually lateral). Rarely, a cystic hygroma may present anteriorly.

In patients with Graves' disease, the thyroid-stimulating immunoglobulins cross the placenta and cause fetal hyperthyroidism. Despite early neonatal treatment, developmental disorders can result.

Alternatively, fetal hypothyroidism is caused by the transplacental transfer of medications (e.g., PTU) used to treat maternal hyperthyroidism. Agenesis or hypoplasia of the fetal thyroid is an additional cause. Polyhydramnios may be present. The neonate may develop cardiovascular or respiratory abnormalities as well as mental retardation.

Cordocentesis is the only accurate method to determine fetal thyroid hormone levels. Treatment of hyperthyroidism is possible with maternally administered PTU; however, hypothyroidism requires fetal intramuscular, intravascular, or intra-amniotic infusion of thyroxine.

Notes

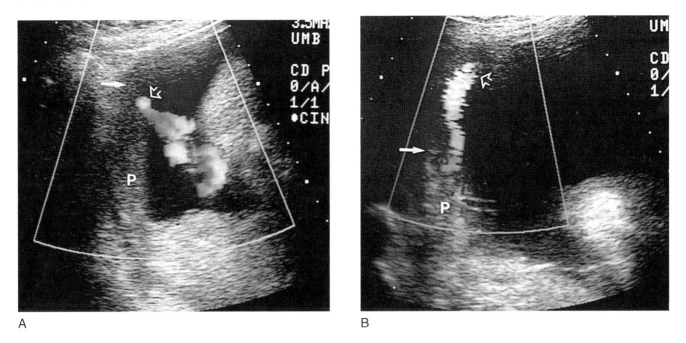

A   B

1. What is the difference between the cord insertion in the color Doppler images of the placenta (P) in Figures A and B? Closed arrow = margin of the placenta; open arrow = insertion of the umbilical cord.

2. Are there problems associated with a marginal cord insertion?

3. Is a velamentous cord insertion more common in multiple pregnancies?

4. What are the complications or anomalies associated with velamentous cord insertion?

Velamentous Insertion of the Umbilical Cord

1. Figure A shows a marginal cord insertion. Figure B shows a velamentous cord insertion, an insertion of the umbilical cord into the amniochorionic membranes beyond the placental margin.

2. No.

3. Yes, ten times more common.

4. Rupture during labor causing fetal exsanguination, preterm delivery, intrauterine growth restriction (IUGR), single umbilical artery anomalies, and other congenital anomalies.

References

Pretorius DH, Chau C, Poelter DM, et al: Placental cord insertion visualization with prenatal ultrasonography. *J Ultrasound Med* 15:585–593, 1996.

Raga F, Ballester MJ, Osborne NG, Bonilla-Musoles F: Role of color flow Doppler ultrasonography in diagnosing velamentous insertion of the umbilical cord and vasa previa. *J Reprod Med* 40:804–808, 1995.

Cross-Reference

Ultrasound: THE REQUISITES, 2nd ed, pp 489–490.

Comment

Marginal cord insertion is defined as peripheral insertion of the cord in the placenta, within 2 cm of the edge. Velamentous insertion is distinguished by aberrant vessels traversing between the amnion and chorion before placental insertion. Velamentous cord insertion occurs in 1.1% of single intrauterine gestations, with a ten times higher incidence in multiple pregnancies. It is also associated with uterine anomalies and indwelling intrauterine devices (IUDs).

A velamentous insertion carries the risk of several complications. During active labor, a velamentous insertion is not anchored and can tear, resulting in exsanguination. Preterm delivery occurs in 17% of cases. IUGR, single umbilical artery, congenital anomalies, and low Apgar scores have also been reported. A vasa previa caused by a velamentous insertion in front of the presenting part of the fetus also may occur.

Ultrasound studies have reported a 42% sensitivity for detection of an abnormal placental cord insertion, particularly later in the gestation period. Nonetheless, this is an important portion of the prenatal sonogram evaluation. The use of color Doppler imaging facilitates visualization of the insertion site.

Notes

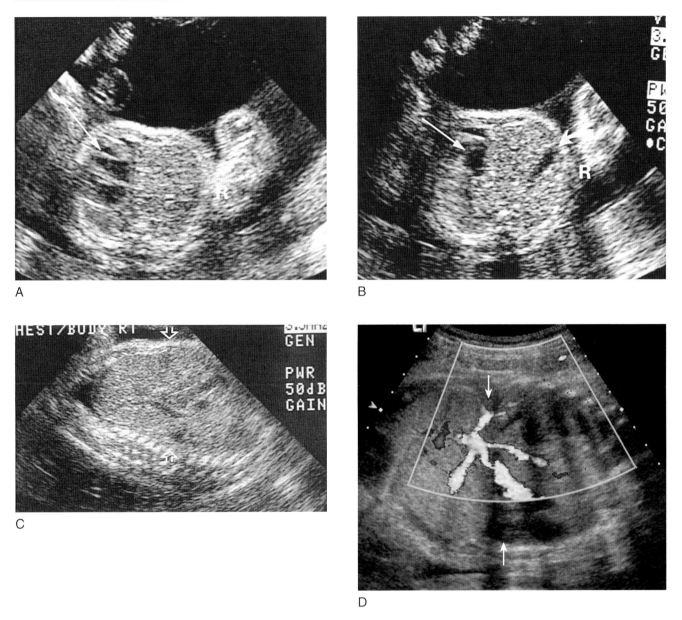

A

B

C

D

1. In this second-trimester fetus, what is the differential diagnosis of this axial image of the chest (Fig. A: R = right side of the fetus; arrow = the heart)? What is the diagnosis once Figure B is also taken into account? What does the curved arrow denote?

2. In the same case, what does the sagittal image of the right side of the fetal chest show (Fig. C)? Open arrows show the bottom of the chest.

3. Can the liver herniate into a left-sided diaphragmatic hernia?

4. How can color Doppler imaging be used, as in Figure D?

Congenital Diaphragmatic Hernia, Right-Sided Bochdalek

1. Cystic adenomatoid malformation (CAM) type III, sequestration, herniation of the liver into a diaphragmatic hernia in a right-sided Bochdalek hernia. Right-sided Bochdalek hernia. The curved arrow denotes the gallbladder.

2. Herniation of the liver above the right hemidiaphragm.

3. Yes, the left lobe.

4. Doppler imaging can be used to show the hepatic vessels. Figure D demonstrates hepatic vessels above the level of the diaphragm (arrows), confirming that part of the liver has herniated into the chest.

References

Guibaud L, Filiatrault D, Garel L, et al: Fetal congenital diaphragmatic hernia: Accuracy of sonography in the diagnosis and prediction of the outcome after birth. *AJR* 166:1195–1202, 1996.

Hubbard AM, Adzick NS, Crombleholme TM, Haselgrove JC: Left-sided congenital diaphragmatic hernia: Value of prenatal MR imaging in preparation for fetal surgery. *Radiology* 203:636–640, 1997.

Cross-Reference

Ultrasound: THE REQUISITES, 2nd ed, pp 422–424.

Comment

A left-sided congenital diaphragmatic hernia (CDH) is much more common than a right-sided hernia (~7:1), and a right-sided CDH carries a worse prognosis. Bochdalek hernias are located laterally and more commonly on the left. Morgagni hernias are positioned medially, and when these hernias occur the abdominal contents can herniate into the pericardium. The lateral and left-sided hernias are easier to detect with prenatal ultrasound than are the medial and right-sided ones.

It is important to try to determine the side of herniation. The fetal gallbladder (right-sided hernia) may be confused with the fetal stomach (left-sided hernia) (see Fig. B). In most right-sided CDHs, the stomach lies in its normal position. This case demonstrates a large right-sided hernia with the liver in the right hemithorax (see Figs. A to D). The left lobe of the liver can herniate into the left hemithorax with a left-sided diaphragmatic hernia. Magnetic resonance imaging (MRI) has been shown to be more accurate than ultrasound in confirming herniation of the liver.

Prenatal diagnosis is essential for counseling and surgical planning. The differential diagnosis includes other pulmonary masses, such as sequestration, bronchogenic cyst, and CAM. Because of the large cysts that can be seen with CAM type I, it can be more difficult to distinguish from the herniated bowel of a CDH. The paucity of abdominal structures on imaging aids in diagnosing CDH.

Notes

A

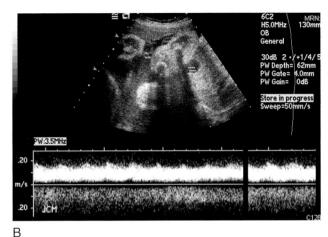

B

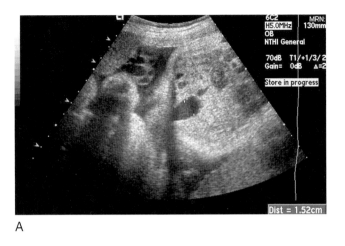

C

1. What finding (Fig. A fetal abdomen without color Doppler imaging) is detected anteriorly at the cord insertion (CI) site in the fetal abdomen of this second-trimester fetus? Figure B is a spectral waveform through this structure and Figure C shows the bladder flanked by the iliac arteries.

2. What is the normal caliber of the intra-abdominal portion of the umbilical vein?

3. Is this finding associated with other abnormalities?

4. Can Doppler imaging be valuable on follow-up examinations?

Umbilical Vein Varix

1. Umbilical vein varix.

2. The normal intra-abdominal umbilical vein measures 3 mm at 15 menstrual weeks and increases linearly to 8 mm at term.

3. Yes; there has been a reported association with third-trimester hydrops fetalis and fetal outcome.

4. Yes; it can evaluate the complication of varix thrombosis.

References

Dudiak CM, Salomon CG, Posniak HV, et al: Sonography of the umbilical cord. *RadioGraphics* 15:1035–1050, 1995.

Mahony BS, McGahan JP, Nyberg DA, Reisner DP: Varix of the fetal intra-abdominal umbilical vein: Comparison with normal. *J Ultrasound Med* 11:73–76, 1992.

Rahemtullah A, Lieberman E, Benson C, Norton ME: Outcome of pregnancy after prenatal diagnosis of umbilical vein varix: *J Ultrasound Med* 20:135–139, 2001.

White SP, Kofinas A: Prenatal diagnosis and management of umbilical vein varix of the intra-amniotic portion of the umbilical vein. *J Ultrasound Med* 13:992–994, 1994.

Cross-Reference

Ultrasound: THE REQUISITES, 2nd ed, p 434.

Comment

The normal umbilical cord has two arteries and one vein. The single left umbilical vein, coursing with both umbilical arteries in the umbilical cord, joins the fetal left portal vein. It carries oxygenated blood to the fetus from the placenta. The umbilical arteries arise from the internal iliac arteries.

On ultrasound, the umbilical vein can be seen from its insertion at the anterior abdominal wall and can be followed into the liver on sagittal and oblique/transverse images. The normal size for the intra-abdominal extrahepatic portion of the umbilical vein is 3 mm at 15 weeks. The vein grows throughout the gestation period to measure 8 mm at term. An umbilical vein varix is defined as a focal dilatation of the umbilical vein just inside the anterior abdominal wall (see Fig. A).

A varix more commonly involves the intra-amniotic portion (within the umbilical cord). The intra-amniotic varix can cause fetal demise as a result of thrombosis, and some recommend delivery as soon as lung maturity permits. An autopsy series has shown thrombosis of the varix to be a cause of stillbirth. An isolated intra-abdominal extrahepatic umbilical vein varix, which is demonstrated here, is rare. The literature is controversial with regard to its significance, and some report an increased risk of third-trimester fetal hydrops and adverse fetal outcomes. The varicosity can thrombose and compromise delivery of oxygenated blood to the fetus. Color Doppler imaging should be performed on all umbilical vein varicosities to document their patency, and close follow-up with serial ultrasound studies is advised. Detection of an umbilical vein varix should initiate a thorough examination of the fetus, including a fetal survey and echocardiogram. Isoimmunization should be ruled out and the consideration of karyotyping should be discussed.

The differential diagnosis of an intra-abdominal umbilical vein varix includes other cystic abdominal structures, such as the fetal gallbladder; a choledochal cyst; a mesenteric, ovarian, or urachal cyst; and a dilated bowel or genitourinary structure. Color Doppler imaging will document that the structure represents the umbilical vein varix, unless the varicosity has become thrombosed. Because of the risk of complications, some advocate delivery as soon as the fetal lungs mature.

Notes

1 Tamoxifen, 3–4

2 Pleural Effusions, 5–6

3 Cystic Abdominal Mass, 7–8

4 Ureteropelvic Junction Obstruction, 9–10

5 Choroid Plexus Cysts, 11–12

6 Turner's Syndrome, 13–14

7 Oligohydramnios (Secondary to Spontaneous Rupture of the Membranes), 15–16

8 Ovarian Cancer (Cystadenocarcinoma), 17–18

9 Appendicitis, 19–20

10 Sacrococcygeal Teratoma, 21–22

11 Dandy-Walker Malformation, 23–24

12 Central Nervous System Arteriovenous Malformation, 25–26

13 Placenta Previa, 27–28

14 Anencephaly, 29–30

15 Duodenal Atresia, 31–32

16 Nuchal Skin Measurement: Second Trimester, 33–34

17 Myelomeningocele, 35–36

18 Aqueductal Stenosis, 37–38

19 Omphalocele, 39–40

20 Congenital Uterine Anomalies and Pregnancy, 41–42

21 Normal First-Trimester Intrauterine Pregnancy with Extrauterine Mass, a Cystic Teratoma (Dermoid), 43–44

22 Conjoined (Siamese) Twins in the First Trimester, 45–47

23 Cystic Adenomatoid Malformation, 49–50

24 Holoprosencephaly, 51–52

25 Polycystic Ovarian Disease, 53–54

26 Hydrocephalus, 55–56

27 Sequestration, 57–58

28 Intrauterine Contraceptive Device, 59–61

29 Enlarged Fetal Stomach, 63–64

30 Clubfoot, 65–66

31 Renal Agenesis, 67–68

32 Ectopic Pregnancy, 69–70

33 Pericardial Effusion, 71–72

34 Multicystic Dysplastic Kidney, 73–74

35 Trisomy 21 (Down Syndrome)—Basic, 75–76

36 Polyhydramnios, 77–78

37 Placental Infarct, 79–80

38 Papillary Muscle Calcification (Intraventricular Hyperechoic Focus), 81–82

39 Tetralogy of Fallot, 83–84

40 Ventriculoseptal Defect, 85–86

41 Endometrial Cancer, 87–88

42 In Utero Infection, 89–90

43 Cystic Hygroma, 91–92

44 Oligohydramnios (Secondary to Renal Agenesis), 93–94

45 Endocardial Cushion Defect, 95–96

46 Gastroschisis, 97–98

47 Dermoid, 99–101

48 Congenital Diaphragmatic Hernia, Left-Sided Bochdalek, 103–104

49 Subchorionic Hemorrhage, 105–106

50 Single Umbilical Artery (Two-Vessel Umbilical Cord), 107–108

51 Myelomeningocele, 109–110

52 Hydronephrosis, 111–112

53 Ruptured Ectopic Pregnancy, 113–114

54 Ebstein's Anomaly, 115–116

55 Ovarian Cyst, 119–121

56 Trisomy 18, 123–124

57 Myelomeningocele Versus Sacrococcygeal Teratoma, 125–126

58 Ovarian Torsion, 127–128

59 Umbilical Artery Doppler, 129–130

60 Posterior Urethral Valves, 131–132

61 Early Intrauterine Gestational Sac, 133–135

62 Hydranencephaly, 137–138

63 Retained Products of Conception, 139–140

64 Nonimmune Fetal Hydrops, 141–142

65 Uterine Masses, 143–144

66 Incompetent Cervix, 145–146

67 Intracranial Hemorrhage, 147–148

68 Calvarial Abnormalities, 149–150

69 Small Bowel (Jejunoileal) Obstruction, 151–152

70 Cystic Fibrosis, 153–154

71 Fetal Liver Calcifications, 155–156

72 Placental Abruption, 157–158

73 Cleft Lip and Palate, 159–160

74 Esophageal Atresia, 161–162

75 Nuchal Skin Measurement: First Trimester, 163–164

76 Ovarian Vein Thrombosis, 165–166

77 Large Bowel (Anorectal) Atresia, 167–168

78 Second-Trimester Twin Gestation and Fetal Demise, 169–170

79 Osteogenesis Imperfecta, 171–173

80 Fetal Ovarian Cyst, 175–176

81 Heterotopic Pregnancy, 177–178

82 Fetal Gallbladder, 179–180

83 Transposition of the Great Vessels, 181–182

84 Cardiac Rhabdomyoma, 183–184

85 Endometrial Polyp, 185–186

86 Posterior Neck Mass, 187–188

87 Pelvic Inflammatory Disease (Hydrosalpinx), 189–190

88 Trisomy 13, 191–192

89 Gestational Trophoblastic Disease, 193–194

90 Cervical Ectopic Pregnancy, 195–196

91 Succenturiate Lobe, 197–198

92 Twin-Twin Transfusion, 199–200

93 Trisomy 21 (Down Syndrome)—Advanced, 201–202

94 Autosomal Recessive Polycystic Kidney Disease, 203–204

95 Endometriosis, 205–206

96 Ventricular Discordance, 207–208

97 Encephalocele, 211–212

98 Facial Mass, 213–214

99 Cornual (Interstitial) Ectopic Pregnancy, 215–216

100 Laryngotracheal Obstruction, 217–218

101 Obligate Cord, 217–218

102 Mucous Plug, 219–220

103 Ectopia Cordis, 221–222

104 Ovarian Hyperstimulation Syndrome, 223–224

105 Endometritis and Endomyometritis, 225–226

106 Intracranial Teratoma, 227–228

107 Congenital Uterine Anomalies, 229–231

108 Acardiac Twin, 233–234

109 Porencephaly, 235–236

110 Umbilical Cord Cyst, 237–238

111 Large Cisterna Magna, 237–238

112 Echogenic Bowel, 239–240

113 Circumvallate Placenta (Placenta Extrachorialis), 241–242

114 Thanatophoric Dysplasia (Thanatophoric Dwarfism), 241–242

INDEX OF CASES

115 Sex Cord Stromal (Thecoma-Fibroma) Tumor, 243–244

116 Cervical Teratoma, 245–246

117 Adenomyosis, 247–248

118 Placental Invasion (Accreta, Increta, and Percreta), 249–250

119 Prune-Belly Syndrome, 251–252

120 Fetal Goiter, 253–254

121 Velamentous Insertion of the Umbilical Cord, 255–256

122 Congenital Diaphragmatic Hernia, Right-Sided Bochdalek, 257–258

123 Umbilical Vein Varix, 259–260

A

Abdominal mass in fetus, cystic, 7–8
Abdominal wall defect
    in gastroschisis, 97–98
    in omphalocele, 39–40
Abortion, spontaneous
    in progress, compared to cervical ectopic pregnancy, 195–196
    retained products of conception in, 139–140
    in subchorionic hemorrhage, 105–106
    in twin pregnancy, 170
Abruption, placental, 157–158
Acardiac twin, 233–234
Adenomatoid malformation, cystic, 49–50, 218, 220
    differentiated from congenital diaphragmatic hernia,
        103–104, 258
    polyhydramnios in, 50, 78
Adenomyosis, 247–248
Agenesis
    of cerebellar vermis in Dandy-Walker malformation, 23–24
    renal, 10, 67–68
        oligohydramnios in, 68, 93–94
    urethral, 132, 252
    of uterus, 42, 231
Allantoic cyst, 237–238
Amniocentesis for choroid plexus cysts, 11–12
Amniotic band syndrome, 66, 242
Amniotic fluid
    in oligohydramnios. *See* Oligohydramnios
    in polyhydramnios. *See* Polyhydramnios
Amniotic shelf or sheet, 242
Anencephaly, 29–30
    polyhydramnios in, 30, 78
Anorectal atresia, 167–168
Aorta
    coarctation of
        in intracranial arteriovenous malformations, 26
        in Turner's syndrome, 13–14
        ventricular discordance in, 207–208
    overriding, in tetralogy of Fallot, 83–84
    in transposition of great vessels, 181–182
Appendicitis in pregnancy, 19–20
Aqueductal stenosis, 37–38
    hydrocephalus in, 37–38, 56
Arcuate uterus, 42, 231
Arteriovenous malformation, intracranial fetal,
        25–26
Ascites
    in meconium peritonitis, 8
    in ovarian cancer, 18
    in ovarian hyperstimulation syndrome, 224
Assisted reproduction techniques
    heterotopic pregnancy in, 177–178
    ovarian hyperstimulation syndrome in, 223–224
Atresia
    anorectal, 167–168
    duodenal, 31–32
        polyhydramnios in, 32, 78
        stomach enlargement in, 32, 64
    esophageal, 161–162
Atrioventricular canal
    in endocardial cushion defect, 95–96

Atrioventricular canal *(Continued)*
    in trisomy 21, 76, 86, 201–202
    unbalanced, 96
Autosomal dominant polycystic kidney disease, 204
Autosomal recessive polycystic kidney disease, 203–204

B

Bicornuate uterus, 41–42, 231
Bladder
    displacement in sacrococcygeal teratoma, 22
    keyhole appearance in posterior urethral valves, 131–132
Bleeding. *See* Hemorrhage
Bochdalek hernia
    left-sided, 103–104, 258
    right-sided, 257–258
Bowel
    atresia of, 31–32, 64, 78, 167–168
    echogenicity of, 239–240
    obstruction of, 151–152, 154, 167–168
Branchial cleft cyst, 246, 254
Bronchial obstruction with mucous plug, 219–220
Bronchogenic cyst, fetal, 50
Butterfly sign of choroid plexus, 52

C

Calcification
    in liver, 155–156
    in papillary muscle, 81–82
        in trisomy 21, 82, 202
    in sacrococcygeal teratoma, 22
Call-Exner bodies, 243–244
Calvarial abnormalities, 149–150. *See also* Skull, fetal
Cancer
    of breast, tamoxifen therapy in, 3–4
    of endometrium, 4, 87–88, 186
    of ovary, 17–18, 44
Cardiomegaly in fetal arteriovenous malformations, 26
Carotid artery infarction, hydranencephaly in, 138
Central nervous system anomalies
    arteriovenous malformations, 25–26
    and calvarial abnormalities, 149–150
    cisterna magna enlargement, 237–238
    encephalocele, 211–212
    hydranencephaly, 137–138
    in utero infections, 89–90
    intracranial teratoma, 227–228
    porencephaly, 235–236
    with posterior neck mass, 187–188
    in single umbilical artery, 107–108
    in trisomy 13, 192
    in trisomy 21, 202
Cephalocele, 188, 212
Cerebellar vermis agenesis in Dandy-Walker malformation,
        23–24
Cerebral artery
    Doppler imaging of, 129–130
    hemorrhage in fetus, 147–148
Cervical teratoma of neck, 245–246
Cervix
    ectopic pregnancy in, 195–196
    incompetence of, 145–146

Cesarean section
endometritis after, 226
scar and ectopic pregnancy, 69–70
Chiari malformations
hydrocephalus in, 56
myelomeningocele in, 36, 56, 126, 150
Cholelithiasis, fetal, 180
Chorioamnionitis, 16
Chorioangioma, placental, 80
Choriocarcinoma in gestational trophoblastic disease, 194
Chorionic gonadotropin levels. *See* Gonadotropin levels, human chorionic
Choroid plexus
butterfly sign of, 52
cyst of, 11–12
in trisomy 18, 12, 123–124
Circumvallate placenta, 241–242
Cisterna magna enlargement, 237–238
Cleft lip and palate, 159–160
in trisomy 13, 192
Cloverleaf skull, 149–150
in thanatophoric dysplasia, 150, 242
Clubfoot, 65–66
in oligohydramnios, 16, 66
in trisomy 13, 66, 192
in trisomy 18, 66, 124
Coarctation of aorta
in intracranial arteriovenous malformations, 26
in Turner's syndrome, 13–14
ventricular discordance in, 207–208
Colonic obstruction, 167–168
differentiated from small bowel obstruction, 151–152
Conjoined twins, 45–47
Contraceptive device, intrauterine, 59–61
Cornual ectopic pregnancy, 215–216
Corpus luteum cyst, 18, 44, 114
hemorrhagic, 119, 121
Cyst
abdominal fetal, 7–8
choroid plexus, 11–12, 123–124
corpus luteum, 18, 44, 114
hemorrhagic, 119, 121
decidual, 70
enteric duplication, 7–8
of kidney
in autosomal recessive polycystic disease, 203–204
in multicystic dysplastic kidney, 8, 10, 73–74
ovarian. *See* Ovary, cysts of
pulmonary fetal, 49–50
umbilical cord, 237–238
Cystadenocarcinoma, ovarian, 17–18, 44
Cystic fibrosis, 153–154
small bowel obstruction in, 152, 154
Cystic hygroma. *See* Hygroma, cystic
Cytomegalovirus infections, 72, 89–90

D

Dandy-Walker malformation, 23–24
cisterna magna enlargement in, 238
polyhydramnios in, 78
Decidual casts, 70
Decidual cysts, 70
Decidual reaction in ectopic pregnancy, 70, 113–114
Delivery
endometritis after, 225–226
obligate presentation of umbilical cord in, 217–218

Delivery (*Continued*)
ovarian vein thrombosis after, 165–166
in velamentous insertion of umbilical cord, 256
Dermoid cyst of ovary, 8, 18, 43–44, 99–101
DES-related uterine anomalies, 42
Diaphragmatic hernia, fetal, 50, 219–220
differentiated from cystic adenomatoid malformation, 103–104, 258
left-sided Bochdalek, 103–104, 258
right-sided Bochdalek, 257–258
Dichorionic pregnancy
conjoined twins in, 45–47
fetal demise in, 169–170
Didelphic uterus, 42, 231
Diethylstilbestrol-related uterine anomalies, 42
Double bubble sign in duodenal atresia, 32
Double decidual reaction, 70
Down syndrome. *See* Trisomy 21
Duodenal atresia, 31–32
polyhydramnios in, 32, 78
stomach enlargement in, 32, 64
Duplication cyst, enteric, 7–8
Dwarfism, thanatophoric, 241–242
Cloverleaf skull in, 150, 242
Dysplasia
renal multicystic, 8, 10, 73–74
thanatophoric, 241–242
Cloverleaf skull in, 150, 242

E

Eagle-Barrett syndrome, 252
Ebstein's anomaly, 115–116
Ectopia cordis, 221–222
Ectopic pregnancy, 69–70
cervical, 195–196
cornual, 215–216
decidual reaction in, 70, 113–114
interstitial, 114, 215–216
methotrexate therapy in, 113–114, 196
in pelvic inflammatory disease, 189–190
rupture of, 113–114
with simultaneous intrauterine pregnancy, 177–178
Edward's syndrome. *See* Trisomy 18
Effusions
pericardial, 71–72
pleural, 5–6
Emphysema, lobar, 50
Encephalocele, 211–212
neck mass in, 92, 187–188
Endocardial cushion defect, 95–96
Endometrioma, 18, 44, 205–206
Endometriosis, 205–206
Endometritis, 225–226
Endometrium
cancer of, 4, 87–88, 186
hyperplasia of, 4, 87–88, 186
polyps of, 4, 185–186
tamoxifen-associated abnormalities of, 3–4, 88
thickness of, 3–4, 87–88, 186
Endomyometritis, 225–226
Enteric duplication cysts, 7–8
Esophageal atresia, 161–162
Estriol levels in triple screen test, 164. *See also* Triple screen test

F

Facial mass, fetal, 213–214
Fallopian tubes in hydrosalpinx, 189–190

Fallot, Tetralogy of, 83–84
    endocardial cushion defect in, 95–96
    ventricular septal defect in, 84, 86
Femur
    in osteogenesis imperfecta, 171–173
    in thanatophoric dysplasia, 150, 242
α-Fetoprotein levels
    in anencephaly, 30
    in encephalocele, 211–212
    in myelomeningocele, 109–110, 212
    in placental infarction, 80
    in posterior neck mass, 187–188
    in triple screen test, 164. *See also* Triple screen test
Fetus. *See also specific disorders*
    abdominal mass in, cystic, 7–8
    adenomatoid malformation in, cystic, 49–50
    anencephaly in, 29–30, 78
    anorectal atresia in, 167–168
    aqueductal stenosis in, 37–38, 56
    bowel echogenicity in, 239–240
    calvarial abnormalities in, 149–150, 242
    cardiac rhabdomyoma in, 183–184
    choroid plexus cyst in, 11–12, 123–124
    cisterna magna enlargement in, 237–238
    cleft lip and palate in, 159–160, 192
    clubfoot in, 65–66, 124, 192
    cystic hygroma in, 91–92
    Dandy-Walker malformation in, 23–24, 78, 238
    diaphragmatic hernia in, 50, 103–104, 219–220, 257–258
    duodenal atresia in, 31–32, 64, 78
    Ebstein's anomaly in, 115–116
    ectopia cordis in, 221–222
    encephalocele in, 92, 187–188, 211–212
    endocardial cushion defect in, 95–96
    esophageal atresia in, 161–162
    facial mass in, 213–214
    gallbladder visualization in, 179–180, 258
    gastroschisis in, 40, 97–98
    goiter in, 246, 253–254
    holoprosencephaly in, 51–52, 192
    hydranencephaly in, 137–138, 236
    hydrocephalus in, 37–38, 55–56
    hydronephrosis in, 9–10, 22, 111–112, 126
    hydrops in, 92, 141–142
    infections in, 89–90
    intracranial arteriovenous malformation in, 25–26
    intracranial hemorrhage in, 147–148
    intracranial teratoma in, 227–228
    laryngotracheal obstruction in, 217–218, 220
    liver calcifications in, 155–156
    multicystic dysplastic kidneys in, 8, 10, 73–74
    myelomeningocele in, 35–36, 56, 109–110, 125–126, 149–150
    neck mass in, 187–188, 245–246
    nuchal skin measurements in, 33–34, 75–76, 163–164
    in oligohydramnios and spontaneous rupture of membranes, 15–16
    omphalocele in, 39–40
    osteogenesis imperfecta in, 171–173
    ovarian cyst in, 8, 175–176
    papillary muscle calcification in, 81–82, 202
    papyraceous, 170
    pericardial effusion in, 71–72
    pleural effusions in, 5–6
    polycystic kidney disease in, autosomal recessive, 203–204
    porencephaly in, 235–236
    pulmonary hypoplasia in, 16
    pulmonary sequestration in, 50, 57–58, 220
    renal agenesis in, 10, 67–68

Fetus. *See also specific disorders (Continued)*
    sacrococcygeal teratoma in, 21–22, 125–126
    small bowel obstruction in, 151–152, 154
    stomach absence in, 161–162
    stomach enlargement in, 32, 63–64
    tetralogy of Fallot in, 83–84, 86, 95–96
    thanatophoric dysplasia in, 150, 241–242
    transposition of great vessels in, 26, 181–182
    trisomy 13 in, 191–192
    trisomy 18 in, 123–124
    trisomy 21 in, 75–76, 201–202
    Turner's syndrome in, 13–14, 91–92
    in twin pregnancy, 45–47, 169–170, 199–200, 215–216, 233–234
    ureteropelvic junction obstruction in, 9–10
    urethral valves in, posterior, 131–132, 252
    ventricular discordance in, cardiac, 207–208
Fibroids, uterine, 143–144
    intrauterine contraceptive device in, 60
Fibroma of ovary, 244
Fibrosis, cystic, 153–154
    small bowel obstruction in, 152, 154
Folic acid deficiency, neural tube defects in, 30
Fossa ovalis in Ebstein's anomaly, 115–116
Fraser's syndrome, 217–218

G

Gallbladder, fetal, 179–180, 258
    differentiated from umbilical vein varix, 180, 260
Gastroschisis, 97–98
    differentiated from omphalocele, 40, 97–98
Gestational sac, 133–135
    in cervical ectopic pregnancy, 195–196
    in cornual ectopic pregnancy, 215–216
    in heterotopic pregnancy, 178
    and pseudogestational sac, 69–70
Gestational trophoblastic disease, 193–194
Goiter, fetal, 246, 253–254
    neck mass in, 246, 253–254
Gonadotropin levels, human chorionic
    and diameter of intrauterine gestational sac, 134
    in gestational trophoblastic disease, 193–194
    in ruptured ectopic pregnancy, 113–114
    in triple screen test, 164. *See also* Triple screen test
Granulosa cell tumors of ovary, 243–244
Graves' disease, 254
Growth restriction, intrauterine, ventricular discordance in, 207–208

H

Hair in dermoid cyst, 100
Hamartoma, pulmonary, 50
Heart
    in acardiac twinning, 233–234
    in Ebstein's anomaly, 115–116
    in ectopia cordis, 221–222
    in endocardial cushion defect, 95–96
    in papillary muscle calcification, 81–82, 202
    in rhabdomyoma, 183–184
    in transposition of great vessels, 181–182
    in trisomy 13, 191–192
    in trisomy 21, 82, 201–202
    in ventricular discordance, 207–208
Hemangioma, facial mass in, 214
Hemorrhage
    in adenomyosis, 247–248
    in corpus luteum cyst, 119, 121
    in endometrial cancer, 88

Hemorrhage *(Continued)*
  in endometrial polyp, 185–186
  intracranial fetal, 147–148
  in placental abruption, 158
  in retained products of conception, 139–140
  subchorionic, 105–106, 158
Hernia, diaphragmatic fetal. *See* Diaphragmatic hernia, fetal
Herpes simplex virus infections, 89–90
Heterotopic pregnancy, 177–178
Hirschsprung's disease, 168
HIV infections, 72, 89–90
Holoprosencephaly, 51–52
  in trisomy 13, 52, 192
Hydatidiform mole, 193–194
Hydranencephaly, 137–138
  porencephaly in, 236
Hydrocephalus, fetal, 55–56
  in aqueductal stenosis, 37–38, 56
  in arteriovenous malformations, intracranial, 26
  in Dandy-Walker malformation, 24
  differentiated from hydranencephaly, 138
Hydronephrosis, 111–112
  in sacrococcygeal teratoma, 22, 126
  in ureteropelvic junction obstruction, 9–10
Hydrops
  immune, 142
  nonimmune, 141–142
    in cystic hygroma, 92, 142
Hydrosalpinx, 189–190
Hygroma, cystic, 91–92
  hydrops fetalis in, 92, 142
  neck mass in, 91–92, 187–188, 245–246
  spoke-wheel appearance in, 188
  in trisomy 13, 92, 192
  in trisomy 21, 92, 202
Hyperplasia, endometrial, 87–88, 186
  in tamoxifen therapy, 4
Hyperstimulation syndrome, ovarian, 223–224
  ovarian torsion in, 128, 224
Hypoplasia
  of cardiac ventricle, 207–208
  pulmonary fetal, 16
    in Bochdalek hernia, 104
    in renal agenesis, 68
  of uterus, 42, 231
Hypothyroidism, fetal
  in goiter, 254
  in ovarian cyst, 176

I

Ileal obstruction, fetal, 151–152
Ileus, meconium, 152, 154
Iliac angle in trisomy 21, 202
Iliac artery, internal, 260
  in two-vessel umbilical cord, 108
Incompetent cervix, 145–146
Infarction
  carotid artery, hydranencephaly in, 138
  placental, 79–80
Infections
  chorioamnionitis in, 16
  endometritis in, 225–226
  in utero, 89–90
  pelvic inflammatory disease in, 189–190, 225–226
  pericardial effusions in, 71–72
Interstitial ectopic pregnancy, 114, 215–216
Interstitial line sign in cornual ectopic pregnancy, 216

Intracranial arteriovenous malformations, 25–26
Intracranial hemorrhage, fetal, 147–148
Intradecidual sign, 70
Intrauterine contraceptive device, 59–61
Intrauterine growth restriction, ventricular discordance in, 207–208

J

Jejunal obstruction, 151–152

K

Keyhole appearance of bladder in posterior urethral valves, 131–132
Kidneys
  agenesis of, 10, 67–68
    oligohydramnios in, 68, 93–94
  hydronephrosis, 9–10, 22, 111–112, 126
  multicystic dysplastic, 8, 10, 73–74
  pelvic diameter of, 10
  pelvic location of, 44, 68
  polycystic disease of
    autosomal dominant, 204
    autosomal recessive, 203–204

L

Large bowel
  atresia of, 167–168
  obstruction of, 167–168
    differentiated from small bowel obstruction, 151–152
Laryngotracheal obstruction, fetal, 217–218, 220
Leiomyoma, uterine, 143–144
  differentiated from adenomyosis, 247–248
Leiomyosarcoma, uterine, 143–144
Lemon sign in myelomeningocele, 36, 56, 110, 126, 149–150
Leukocytosis in appendicitis and pregnancy, 19–20
Levonorgestrel intrauterine contraceptive device, 61
Limb-body wall complex differentiated from omphalocele, 40
Lip, cleft, 159–160
  in trisomy 13, 192
Lipoleiomyoma, uterine, 143–144
Lithium therapy in pregnancy, and Ebstein's anomaly in fetus, 115–116
Liver calcification in fetus, 155–156
Lungs, fetal
  in Bochdalek hernia, 103–104, 257–258
  in cystic adenomatoid malformation, 49–50, 218, 220
  hypoplasia of, 16, 68, 104
  in laryngotracheal obstruction, 217–218, 220
  mucous plug in, 219–220
  sequestration in, 50, 57–58, 220
Luteoma, ovarian, 44

M

Magnetic resonance imaging
  in adenomyosis, 247–248
  in appendicitis and pregnancy, 20
  in endometritis, 226
  in myelomeningocele, 36
  in ovarian vein thrombosis, 166
  in uterine anomalies, congenital, 42, 231
Meckel-Gruber syndrome, 211–212
Meconium
  ileus, 152, 154
  peritonitis, 8, 152, 153–154
  plug syndrome, 168
  pseudocyst from, 8, 154
Megacystis-megaureter syndrome, 132
Membrane rupture, spontaneous, oligohydramnios in, 15–16
Meningomyelocele. *See* Myelomeningocele

Methotrexate therapy in ectopic pregnancy, 113–114, 196
Molar pregnancy, 193–194
Monochorionic pregnancy, 46, 169–170
  acardiac twin in, 233–234
  twin-twin transfusion syndrome in, 199–200
Morgagni hernia, 104, 258
Mucous plug, fetal pulmonary, 219–220
Multicystic dysplastic kidney, 8, 10, 73–74
Myelomeningocele, 35–36, 109–110
  encephalocele compared to, 212
  hydrocephalus in, 56
  lemon sign in, 36, 56, 110, 126, 149–150
  neck mass in, 92, 188
  sacrococcygeal teratoma compared to, 125–126
Myoma, endometrial, differentiated from endometrial polyps, 185–186

N

Nasal bones, absence in trisomy 21, 202
Neck mass, 187–188
  in cystic hygroma, 91–92, 187–188, 245–246
  in encephalocele, 92, 187–188
  in goiter, 246, 253–254
  in myelomeningocele, 92, 188
  in teratoma, 245–246, 254
Necklace sign in ovarian hyperstimulation syndrome, 224
Nephroma, mesoblastic, polyhydramnios in, 78
Neural tube defects
  anencephaly in, 29–30
  myelomeningocele in, 35–36, 109–110
  neck mass in, 188
Nuchal skin measurements
  in first trimester, 76, 163–164
  in hydrops, 142
  in second trimester, 33–34, 76
  in trisomy 21, 75–76, 164, 202
Nyberg classification of cleft lip and palate, 160

O

Obligate presentation of umbilical cord, 217–218
Oligohydramnios
  clubfoot in, 16, 66
  with intact membranes, 16
  in renal agenesis, 68, 93–94
  in spontaneous rupture of membranes, 15–16
  in twin-twin transfusion syndrome, 199–200
  umbilical artery Doppler imaging in, 16, 94, 130
Omphalocele, 39–40
  differentiated from gastroschisis, 40, 97–98
  and holoprosencephaly, 52
Omphalomesenteric cyst, 237–238
Osteogenesis imperfecta, 171–173
Ovarian vein thrombosis, 165–166
Ovary
  cancer of, 17–18, 44
  cysts of, 17–18, 119–121
    in cystadenocarcinoma, 17–18, 44
    dermoid, 8, 18, 43–44, 99–101
    fetal, 8, 175–176
    in hyperstimulation syndrome, 224
    in polycystic disease, 53–54
    postmenopausal, 119–121
  hyperstimulation syndrome of, 223–224
    ovarian torsion in, 128, 224
  sex cord stromal tumors of, 243–244
  torsion of, 44, 127–128
    in dermoid cyst, 100
    in ovarian hyperstimulation syndrome, 128, 224

P

Palate, cleft, 159–160
  in trisomy 13, 192
Paper fetus, 170
Papillary muscle calcification, 81–82
  in trisomy 21, 82, 202
Parallel great vessels, 182
Parvovirus infections, 72
Patau's syndrome. *See* Trisomy 13
Pelvic inflammatory disease, 189–190
  endometritis in, 225–226
Pelvic kidney, 44, 68
Pelvocaliectasis, 111–112
Pericardial effusions, fetal, 71–72
Peritonitis, meconium, 8, 152, 153–154
Placenta
  abruption of, 157–158
  accreta, 249–250
  circumvallate, 241–242
  extrachorialis, 241–242
  increta, 249–250
  infarction of, 79–80
  invasion of uterine wall, 249–250
  percreta, 249–250
  previa, 27–28, 249–250
  succenturiate lobe of, 197–198
Plasma protein A, pregnancy-associated, 164
Pleural effusions, fetal, 5–6
Polycystic disease
  of kidney
    autosomal dominant, 204
    autosomal recessive, 203–204
  of ovary, 53–54
Polydactyly
  and holoprosencephaly, 52
  in trisomy 13, 192
Polyhydramnios, 77–78
  in anencephaly, 30, 78
  in cervical teratoma and neck mass, 245–246
  in cystic adenomatoid malformation, 50, 78
  in duodenal atresia, 32, 78
  in esophageal atresia, 162
  in facial mass, 213–214
  in intracranial teratoma, 228
  in sacrococcygeal teratoma, 22, 78
Polyps, endometrial, 185–186
  in tamoxifen therapy, 4
Porencephaly, 235–236
Postmenopausal women
  adenomyosis in, 247–248
  endometrial cancer in, 87–88
  ovarian cyst in, 119–121
Postpartum period
  endometritis in, 225–226
  ovarian vein thrombosis in, 165–166
Potter's syndrome, 68
Pourcelot index in ovarian cancer, 18
Pregnancy
  appendicitis in, 19–20
  cervical incompetence in, 145–146
  in congenital uterine anomalies, 41–42
  cystic teratoma in, 43–44
  ectopic. *See* Ectopic pregnancy
  fetal imaging in. *See* Fetus
  gestational sac in. *See* Gestational sac
  gestational trophoblastic disease in, 193–194
  Graves' disease treatment in, 254

Pregnancy *(Continued)*
  heterotopic, 177–178
  lithium therapy in, and Ebstein's anomaly in fetus, 115–116
  oligohydramnios in. *See* Oligohydramnios
  ovarian torsion in, 127–128
  placenta in. *See* Placenta
  polyhydramnios in. *See* Polyhydramnios
  spontaneous rupture of membranes in, 15–16
  subchorionic hemorrhage in, 105–106
  trauma in, and fetal intracranial hemorrhage, 148
  umbilical cord in. *See* Umbilical cord
Products of conception, retained, 139–140
Protein A in plasma, pregnancy-associated, 164
Prune-belly syndrome, 251–252
  differentiated from posterior urethral valves, 132, 252
Pseudocyst, meconium, 8, 154
Pseudogestational sac, 70
Pulmonary artery
  in parallel great vessels, 182
  in tetralogy of Fallot, 84
  in transposition of great vessels, 181–182
Pulsatility index in ovarian cancer, 17–18
Pyelectasis, 111–112

R

Rastelli classification of endocardial cushion defects, 96
Resistive index in ovarian cancer, 17–18
Retained products of conception, 139–140
Retinoblastoma, 214
Retroplacental bleeding, 158
Rhabdomyoma, cardiac, 183–184
Rubella, 89–90
Ruge-Simon syndrome, 216

S

Sacrococcygeal teratoma, 21–22, 78, 125–126
  differentiated from myelomeningocele, 125–126
  hydronephrosis in, 22, 126
  polyhydramnios in, 22, 78
Sclerosis, tuberous, cardiac rhabdomyoma in, 183–184
Scoliosis in omphalocele, 40
Septal defects, ventricular, 85–86
  in tetralogy of Fallot, 84, 86
  in trisomy 21, 76, 86
Septate uterus, 42, 229–231
Sequestration, pulmonary, in fetus, 50, 57–58, 220
Sertoli-Leydig cell tumors, 244
Sex cord stromal tumors, 243–244
Siamese twins, 45–47
Simian crease in trisomy 21, 202
Single umbilical artery, 107–108
Skull, fetal, 149–150
  cloverleaf deformity of, 149–150, 242
  in lemon head and myelomeningocele, 36, 56, 110, 126, 149–150
  in osteogenesis imperfecta, 171–173
  strawberry-shape in trisomy 18, 12, 124, 149–150
  in thanatophoric dysplasia, 150, 242
Small bowel
  atresia of, 31–32, 64, 78
  echogenicity of, 239–240
  obstruction of, 151–152, 154
Snowstorm appearance in gestational trophoblastic disease, 193–194
Spalding's sign, 149–150
Spina bifida, 35–36, 109–110

Spoke-wheel appearance in cystic hygroma, 188
Stein-Leventhal syndrome, 54
Stomach
  absence in fetus, 161–162
  enlargement in fetus, 63–64
    in duodenal atresia, 32, 64
Strawberry-shaped calvarium in trisomy 18, 12, 124, 149–150
Struma ovarii, 100, 101
Stuck twin syndrome, 200
Subchorionic hemorrhage, 105–106, 158
Succenturiate lobe of placenta, 197–198

T

Tachyarrhythmias, hydrops fetalis in, 142
Tamoxifen therapy, endometrial abnormalities in, 3–4, 88
Teratoma
  facial mass in, 214
  intracranial, 227–228
  neck mass in, 245–246, 254
  ovarian, 8, 18, 43–44, 99–101
  sacrococcygeal, 21–22, 78, 125–126
Tetralogy of Fallot, 83–84
  endocardial cushion defect in, 95–96
  ventricular septal defect in, 84, 86
Thanatophoric dysplasia, 241–242
  cloverleaf skull in, 150, 242
Thecoma, 243–244
Thrombosis of ovarian vein, 165–166
Thyroglossal duct cyst, 246, 254
Thyroid disorders
  in dermoid cyst, 100, 101
  in goiter, 253–254
  in ovarian cyst, 176
Thyrotoxicosis in dermoid cyst, 100, 101
TORCH infections, 89–90, 142
Torsion, ovarian, 44, 127–128
  in dermoid cyst, 100
  in ovarian hyperstimulation syndrome, 128, 224
Toxoplasmosis, 89–90
Transfusion syndrome, twin-twin, 199–200
Transposition of great vessels, 26, 181–182
Trauma in pregnancy, fetal intracranial hemorrhage in, 148
Tricuspid valve
  Ebstein's anomaly of, 115–116
  regurgitation in twin-twin transfusion syndrome, 199–200
Triple screen test
  in anencephaly, 30
  in choroid plexus cyst, 12
  in trisomy 21, 76, 164
  in Turner's syndrome, 14
Trisomy 13, 191–192
  clubfoot in, 66, 192
  cystic hygroma in, 92, 192
  holoprosencephaly in, 52, 192
Trisomy 18, 123–124
  choroid plexus cysts in, 12, 123–124
  clubfoot in, 66, 124
  cystic hygroma in, 92
  single umbilical artery in, 108
  strawberry-shaped calvarium in, 12, 124, 149–150
Trisomy 21, 75–76, 201–202
  atrioventricular canal in, 76, 86, 201–202
  choroid plexus cysts in, 12
  cystic hygroma in, 92, 202
  duodenal atresia in, 32
  endocardial cushion defect in, 96
  hydronephrosis in, 111–112

Trisomy *(Continued)*
   nuchal skin thickening in, 75–76, 164, 202
   papillary muscle calcification in, 82, 202
   ventricular septal defect in, 76, 86
Trophoblastic disease, gestational, 193–194
Tuberous sclerosis, cardiac rhabdomyoma in,
        183–184
Turner's syndrome, 13–14
   cystic hygroma in, 91–92
Twin pregnancy
   acardiac twin in, 233–234
   conjoined twins in, 45–47
   cornual ectopic, 215–216
   fetal demise in, 169–170
   twin-twin transfusion syndrome in, 199–200

U

Umbilical artery, 260
   Doppler imaging of, 129–130
     in oligohydramnios, 16, 94, 130
   single, 107–108
Umbilical cord
   cysts of, 237–238
   marginal insertion of, 255–256
   obligate presentation of, 217–218
   two-vessel, 107–108
   velamentous insertion of, 255–256
Umbilical vein
   in two-vessel umbilical cord, 108
   varix of, 259–260
     differentiated from fetal gallbladder, 180, 260
Unicornuate uterus, 42, 231
Urachus, patent, 238
Ureteropelvic junction obstruction, fetal, 9–10
Urethral agenesis, 132, 252
Urethral valves, posterior, 131–132
   differentiated from prune-belly syndrome, 132, 252

Urethral valves, posterior, *(Continued)*
   vesicoamniotic shunting in, 132, 252
Uterus
   adenomyosis of, 247–248
   cervical incompetence of, 145–146
   congenital anomalies of, 41–42, 229–231
   contraceptive device in, 59–61
   Didelphic, 42, 231
   endometrial portion. *See* Endometrium
   masses in, 143–144
   placental invasion of, 249–250

V

VACTERL syndrome
   anorectal atresia in, 168
   esophageal atresia in, 162
Varix of umbilical vein, 259–260
   differentiated from fetal gallbladder, 180, 260
Vein of Galen malformation, 26
Velamentous insertion of umbilical cord, 255–256
Ventricular calcification, cardiac, 81–82
Ventricular discordance, cardiac, 207–208
Ventricular septal defect, 85–86
   in tetralogy of Fallot, 84, 86
   in trisomy 21, 76, 86
Ventriculomegaly
   in Dandy-Walker malformation, 23–24
   in myelomeningocele, 36
Vesicoamniotic shunting in posterior urethral valves, 132, 252

W

Wharton's jelly cysts, 238
Whirlpool sign in ovarian torsion, 128

Y

Yolk sac, 133–135
   in heterotopic pregnancy, 178